GUEST EDITORS

WILLIAM J. BRADY, MD, Professor and Vice Chair, Department of Emergency Medicine; Medical Director, Life Support Learning Center, University of Virginia School of Medicine, Charlottesville, Virginia

WYATT W. DECKER, MD, Associate Professor and Chair, Department of Emergency Medicine, Mayo Clinic College of Medicine, Rochester, Minnesota

AMAL MATTU, MD, Associate Professor and Program Director, Department of Emergency Medicine, University of Maryland School of Medicine, Baltimore, Maryland

CONTRIBUTORS

JENNIFER M. AVILES, MD, Department of Emergency Medicine, University of Maryland School of Medicine, Baltimore, Maryland

RONNIER J. AVILES, MD, Cardiovascular Branch, Division of Intramural Research, National Heart, Lung, and Blood Institute, National Institutes of Health, Bethesda, Maryland

KEVIN BARLOTTA, MD, Senior Resident, Department of Emergency Medicine, University of Virginia, Charlottesville, Virginia

KATRINA BARNETT, MD, Department of Emergency Medicine, Boston Medical Center/ Boston University School of Medicine, Boston, Massachusetts

ERIC T. BOIE, MD, FAAEM, Vice Chair, Clinical Practice Chair, Department of Emergency Medicine, Mayo Clinic, Rochester, Minnesota; Assistant Professor of Emergency Medicine, Mayo College of Medicine, Rochester, Minnesota

WILLIAM J. BRADY, MD, Professor and Vice Chair, Department of Emergency Medicine; Medical Director, Life Support Learning Center, University of Virginia School of Medicine, Charlottesville, Virginia

DAVID R. BURT, MD, Associate Medical Director, Emergency and Cardiovascular Medicine, Spectrum Health System, Grand Rapids, Michigan

THEODORE CHAN, MD, Department of Emergency Medicine, University of California, San Diego, San Diego, California

WYATT W. DECKER, MD, Associate Professor and Chair, Department of Emergency Medicine, Mayo Clinic College of Medicine, Rochester, Minnesota

STEPHEN DOBMEIER, BSN, CSPI, Managing Director, Blue Ridge Poison Center, Division of Medical Toxicology, Department of Emergency Medicine, University of Virginia, Charlottesville, Virginia

BRIAN EUERLE, MD, RDMS, Assistant Professor of Surgery, Division of Emergency Medicine, University of Maryland School of Medicine; Director, Emergency Ultrasound, Emergency Medicine Residency Program, University of Maryland School of Medicine, Baltimore, Maryland

JAMES A. FELDMAN, MD, Vice Chair, Research, Department of Emergency Medicine, Boston Medical Center; Associate Professor of Emergency Medicine, Boston University School of Medicine, Boston, Massachusetts

GUS M. GARMEL, MD, FACEP, FAAEM, Senior Staff Emergency Physician, The Permanente Medical Group, Kaiser Santa Clara Medical Center, Santa Clara, California; Co-Program Director, Stanford/Kaiser Emergency Medicine Residency Program, Stanford University School of Medicine, Stanford, California

CHRIS A. GHAEMMAGHAMI, MD, Associate Professor of Emergency Medicine, Director, Chest Pain Center, Department of Emergency Medicine, University of Virginia Health System, Charlottesville, Virginia

RACHEL M. GILMORE, MB, MRCPI, Department of Emergency Medicine, Mayo Clinic College of Medicine, Rochester, Minnesota

DANIEL G. HANKINS, MD, FACEP, Assistant Professor, Department of Emergency Medicine, Mayo Clinic, Rochester, Minnesota

LUIS H. HARO, MD, Consultant, Department of Emergency Medicine, Mayo Clinic Rochester, and Instructor of Emergency Medicine, Mayo Clinic College of Medicine, Rochester, Minnesota

RICHARD A. HARRIGAN, MD, Associate Professor, Department of Emergency Medicine, Temple University, Philadelphia, Pennsylvania

CHRISTOPHER P. HOLSTEGE, MD, FACMT, FAAEM, FACEP, Medical Director, Blue Ridge Poison Center; Director, Division of Medical Toxicology; Associate Professor, Department of Emergency Medicine; University of Virginia, Charlottesville, Virginia

BRIAN S. KELLY, MD, Senior Resident, Emergency Medicine Residency, University of Maryland Medical Center, Baltimore, Maryland

MICHELLE KRAJICEK, MD, Chief Resident, Department of Emergency Medicine, Mayo Clinic College of Medicine, Mayo School of Graduate Education, Rochester, Minnesota

BRIAN LENTZ, MD, Fellow in Cardiovascular Emergencies, Department of Emergency Medicine, University of Virginia, Charlottesville, Virginia

JOEL T. LEVIS, MD, PhD, Staff Emergency Physician, The Permanente Medical Group, Kaiser Santa Clara Medical Center, Santa Clara, California; Clinical Instructor, Emergency Medicine, Stanford University School of Medicine, Stanford, California

theclinics.com

EMERGENCY MEDICINE CLINICS OF NORTH AMERICA

Emergency Cardiology: Challenges, Controversies, and Advances

GUEST EDITORS
William J. Brady, MD,
Wyatt W. Decker, MD and
Amal Mattu, MD

November 2005 • Volume 23 • Number 4

SAUNDERS

An Imprint of Elsevier, Inc.
PHILADELPHIA LONDON TORONTO MONTREAL SYDNEY TOKYO

W.B. SAUNDERS COMPANY
A Division of Elsevier Inc.

1600 John F. Kennedy Boulevard, Suite 1800 • Philadelphia, Pennsylvania 19103-2899

http://www.theclinics.com

EMERGENCY MEDICINE CLINICS OF NORTH AMERICA
November 2005
Editor: Karen Sorensen

Volume 23, Number 4
ISSN 0733-8627
ISBN 1-4160-2713-0

Emergency Medicine Clinics of North America (ISSN 0733-8627) is published quarterly by W.B. Saunders Company. Corporate and Editorial Offices: 1600 John F. Kennedy Boulevard, Suite 1800, Philadelphia, PA 19103-2899. Accounting and Circulation Offices: 6277 Sea Harbor Drive, Orlando, FL 32887-4800. Periodicals postage paid at Orlando, FL 32862, and additional mailing offices. Subscription prices are $175.00 per year (US individuals), $275.00 per year (US institutions), $235.00 per year (international individuals), $325.00 per year (international institutions), $215.00 per year (Canadian individuals), and $325.00 per year (Canadian institutions). International air speed delivery is included in all *Clinics'* subscription prices. All prices are subject to change without notice. POSTMASTER: Send address changes to *Emergency Medicine Clinics of North America*, W.B. Saunders Company, Periodicals Fulfillment, Orlando, FL 32887-4800. **Customer Service: 1-800-654-2452 (US). From outside of the US, call 1-407-345-4000. E-mail: hhspcs@harcourt.com.**

Emergency Medicine Clinics of North America is covered in *Index Medicus, Current Contents/Clinical Medicine, EMBASE/Excerpta Medica, BIOSIS, SciSearch, CINAHL, ISI/BIOMED,* and *Research Alert.*

Printed in the United States of America.

JOSEPH K. LOBL, MD, Consultant, Department of Emergency Medicine, Mayo Clinic Rochester, and Assistant Professor of Emergency Medicine, Mayo Clinic College of Medicine, Rochester, Minnesota

ANURADHA LUKE, MD, Clinical Instructor, Department of Emergency Medicine, Mayo Clinic, Rochester, Minnesota

AMAL MATTU, MD, Associate Professor and Program Director, Department of Emergency Medicine, University of Maryland School of Medicine, Baltimore, Maryland

JOSEPH P. MARTINEZ, MD, Assistant Professor, Division of Emergency Medicine, and Assistant Clinical Director, Emergency Department, University of Maryland School of Medicine, Baltimore, Maryland

MICHAEL A. MCCULLOCH, MD (Fellow), Department of Pediatrics, Division of Cardiology, University of Virginia Health System, Charlottesville, Virginia

ERIN MCNUTT, MD, Assistant Professor of Medicine, University of California San Francisco School of Medicine, San Francisco, California

THOMAS D. MELOY, MD, Assistant Professor of Emergency Medicine, Department of Emergency Medicine, Mayo Clinic College of Medicine, Rochester, Minnesota

STEPHAN J. MILLER, MD, Department of Emergency Medicine, Mayo Clinic College of Medicine, Rochester, Minnesota

ANDREW D. PERRON, MD, Residency Program Director, Department of Emergency Medicine, Maine Medical Center, Portland, Maine

ARUN V. RAGHAVAN, MD, Emergency Medicine Resident, Department of Emergency Medicine, Mayo Clinic College of Medicine, Rochester, Minnesota

LATHA G. STEAD, MD, FACEP, Department of Emergency Medicine, Mayo Clinic College of Medicine, Rochester, Minnesota

TIMOTHY SWEENEY, MD, Attending Physician, Department of Emergency Medicine, Maine Medical Center, Portland, Maine

JEFFREY TABAS, MD, Associate Professor of Medicine, University of California San Francisco School of Medicine, San Francisco, California

ALICE TANG, DO, MPH, Ultrasound Fellow, Division of Emergency Medicine, University of Maryland School of Medicine, Baltimore, Maryland

WILLIAM A. WOODS, MD, FAAP, Departments of Emergency Medicine and Pediatrics, University of Virginia Health System, Charlottesville, Virginia

CONTENTS

GOAL STATEMENT

The goal of Emergency Medicine Clinics of North America is to keep practicing physicians up to date with current clinical practice in emergency medicine by providing timely articles reviewing the state of the art in patient care.

ACCREDITATION

The Emergency Medicine Clinics of North America is planned and implemented in accordance with the Essential Areas and Policies of the Accreditation Council for Continuing Medical Education (ACCME) through the joint sponsorship of the University of Virginia School of Medicine and Elsevier. The University of Virginia School of Medicine is accredited by the ACCME to provide continuing medical education for physicians.

The University of Virginia School of Medicine designates this educational activity for a maximum of 60 category 1 credits per year, 15 category 1 credits per issue, toward the AMA Physician's Recognition Award. Each physician should claim only those credits that he/she actually spent in the activity.

The American Medical Association has determined that physicians not licensed in the US who participate in this CME activity are eligible for AMA PRA category 1 credit.

Category 1 credit can be earned by reading the text material, taking the CME examination online at http://www.theclinics.com/home/cme, and completing the evaluation. After taking the test, you will be required to review any and all incorrect answers. Following completion of the test and evaluation, your credit will be awarded and you may print your certificate.

FACULTY DISCLOSURE/CONFLICT OF INTEREST

The University of Virginia School of Medicine, as an ACCME accredited provider, endorses and strives to comply with the Accreditation Council for Continuing Medical Education (ACCME) Standards of Commercial Support, Commonwealth of Virginia statutes, University of Virginia policies and procedures, and associated federal and private regulations and guidelines on the need for disclosure and monitoring of proprietary and financial interests that may affect the scientific integrity and balance of content delivered in continuing medical education activities under our auspices.

The University of Virginia School of Medicine requires that all CME activities accredited through this institution be developed independently and be scientifically rigorous, balanced and objective in the presentation/discussion of its content, theories and practices.

All authors/editors participating in an accredited CME activity are expected to disclose to the readers relevant financial relationships with commercial entities occurring within the past 12 months (such as grants or research support, employee, consultant, stock holder, member of speakers bureau, etc.). The University of Virginia School of Medicine will employ appropriate mechanisms to resolve potential conflicts of interest to maintain the standards of fair and balanced education to the reader. Questions about specific strategies can be directed to the Office of Continuing Medical Education, University of Virginia School of Medicine, Charlottesville, Virginia.

The authors/editors listed below have identified no financial or professional relationships for themselves, their spouse/partner:
Ronnier J. Aviles, MD; Jennifer M. Aviles, MD; Kevin S. Barlotta, MD; Katrina Barnett, MD; Eric T. Boie, MD; William J. Brady, MD; David R. Burt, MD; Theodore Chan, MD; Wyatt W. Decker, MD; Stephen Dobmeier, BSN, CSPI; Brian Euerle, MD, RDMS; James A. Feldman, MD; Gus M. Garmel, MD; Chris A. Ghaemmaghami, MD; Rachel M. Gilmore, MRCPI; Daniel G. Hankins, MD; Luis H. Haro, MD; Richard A. Harrigan, MD; Christopher P. Holstege, MD; Brian S. Kelly, MD; Michelle Krajicek, MD; Brian Keith Lentz, MD; Joel T. Levis, MD, PhD; Joseph K. Lobl, MD; Anuradha Luke, MD; Joseph P. Martinez, MD; Amal Mattu, MD; Michael A. McCulloch, MD; Erin McNutt, MD; Thomas D. Meloy, MD; Stephan J. Miller, MD; Andrew D. Perron, MD; Arun V. Raghavan, MD; Karen Sorensen, Acquisitions Editor; Latha G. Stead, MD; Timithy Sweeney, MD; Jeffrey Tabas, MD; Alice Tang, DO, MPH; and, William A. Woods, MD.

Disclosure of Discussion of Non-FDA Approved Uses for Pharmaceutical and/or Medical Devices.
The University of Virginia School of Medicine, as an ACCME provider, requires that all authors identify and disclose any "off label" uses for pharmaceutical and medical device products. The University of Virginia School of Medicine recommends that each physician fully review all the available data on new products or procedures prior to clinical use.

TO ENROLL

To enroll in the Emergency Medicine Clinics of North America Continuing Medical Education program, call customer service at 1-800-654-2452 or visit us online at www.theclinics.com/home/cme. The CME program is available to subscribers for an additional fee of $170.00

FORTHCOMING ISSUES

February 2006

The ECG in Emergency Medicine
Richard Harrigan, MD, William Brady, MD, and Ted C. Chan, MD, *Guest Editors*

May 2006

Emergency Medicine and the Public's Health
Jon Mark Hirshon, MD, MPH, and David M. Morris, MD, MPH, *Guest Editors*

August 2006

Geriatric Emergency Medicine
Brendan Magauran, MD, MBA, FACEP, Joseph Kahn, MD, FACEP, and Jonathan Olshaker, MD, FACEP, *Guest Editors*

RECENT ISSUES

August 2005

Endocrine and Metabolic Emergencies
Mary Jo Wagner, MD, FACEP, and Kathleen Cowling, DO, MS, FACEP, *Guest Editors*

May 2005

Pain and Sedation Management in the 21st Century Emergency Department
John G. McManus, Jr, MD, FACEP, and Benjamin Harrison, MD, FACEP, *Guest Editors*

February 2005

International Emergency Medicine
L. Kristian Arnold, MD, FACEP, and Jeffrey Smith, MD, MPH, *Guest Editors*

ELSEVIER
SAUNDERS

Emerg Med Clin N Am
23 (2005) xv–xvii

EMERGENCY
MEDICINE
CLINICS OF
NORTH AMERICA

Preface

Emergency Cardiology: Challenges, Controversies, and Advances

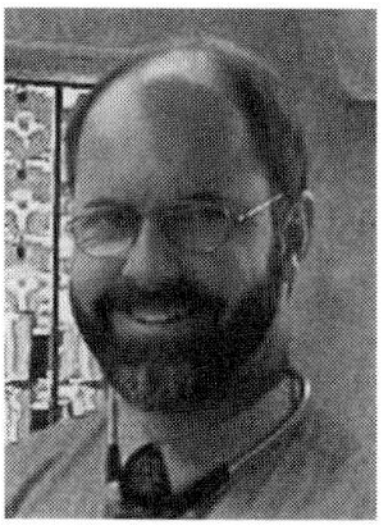
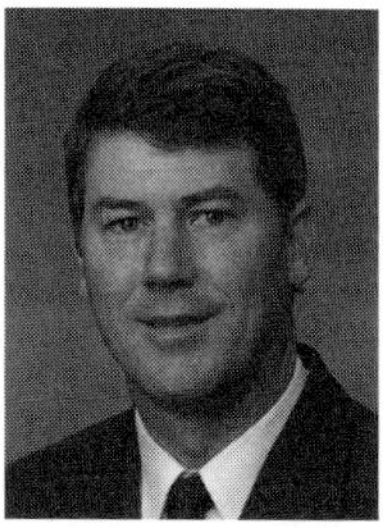
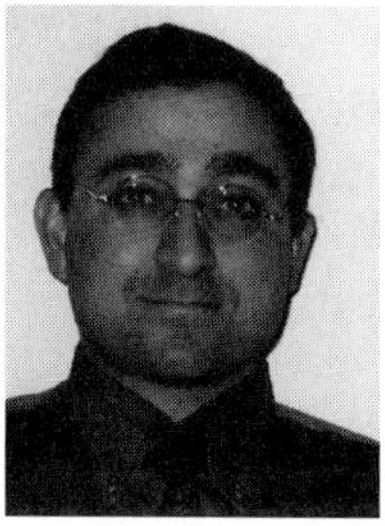

William J. Brady, MD Wyatt W. Decker, MD Amal Mattu, MD
Guest Editors

The emergency physician faces significant clinical challenges on a regular basis. One particular area of clinical challenge concerns cardiovascular emergencies, ranging from the patient with acute myocardial infarction (AMI) complicated by bradycardia to the child with respiratory failure due to a congenital heart lesion. The dyspneic patient with bradycardia and pulmonary congestion: cardiotoxic ingestion or acute coronary syndrome? The chest pain patient with the left bundle branch block electrocardiogram (ECG) pattern: AMI or noncoronary presentation? The cyanotic neonate with tachycardia: sepsis or congenital heart defect? The elderly patient with back pain presenting in shock: abdominal aortic aneurysm or pyelonephritis? The middle-aged female with headache and elevated blood pressure: a hypertensive emergency or elevated blood pressure due to cephalgia? These scenarios depict only a few diagnostic cardiovascular challenges encountered daily by the emergency physician. The most appropriate diagnostic and therapeutic approach to the patient in these and other cardiovascular presentations is constantly changing as research continues to improve emergency cardiovascular care.

The patient with acute coronary syndrome (ACS) represents numerous challenges to the emergency physician. Clearly, the diagnosis of ACS is a daily challenge; numerous obstacles are encountered by the clinician, including atypical histories, confounding ECG patterns, and equivocal

doi:10.1016/j.emc.2005.07.017

serum marker results. Advanced cardiac imaging in various forms is available in many settings, yet which investigation is most appropriate for your patient? Exercise stress testing? Stress echocardiography? Nuclear imaging? Or a combination of these methods? During the past 30 years, considerable effort has been made to improve the diagnostic evaluation of ACS. While much information is still contained within the ECG, computer-assisted and artificial intelligence algorithms have been developed to improve the diagnostic accuracy of the clinician. New, more sensitive, and more specific serum markers for myocyte injury have been developed and now play a central role in the diagnosis and risk stratification for ACS. Diagnostic tools such as echocardiography, stress testing, nuclear imaging, and the chest pain center continue to be studied for their use in effectively and safely evaluating and treating the chest pain patient with possible ACS in the emergent setting.

Once the diagnosis is established, additional questions surface. Fibrinolytic therapy and interventional, catheter-based techniques have revolutionized treatment of patients with ST segment elevation AMI (STEMI) during the 1980s. Recent work has focused on optimizing strategies, both pharmacologic and interventional, as well as expanding treatment options for Non-ST segment elevation AMI (NSTEMI) and unstable angina patients. Combination therapies with antiplatelet, antithrombotic, and fibrinolytic agents continue to be studied for STEMI patients. Interventional success has improved with the use of newer stenting devices and glycoprotein platelet inhibitors. Efforts to both establish regional cardiac centers as well as expand interventional capabilities to smaller hospitals have focused on improving timely, appropriate care for more AMI patients. This revolution in acute reperfusion therapy has made early diagnosis, as well as rapid treatment, a substantial challenge for the clinician.

Beyond the ACS presentation, numerous other cardiovascular presentations are reviewed. Toxin-mediated syndromes, such as cocaine and other cardiotoxins, are reviewed with particular emphasis on bedside diagnosis and toxin-specific therapies. Innovative therapies in pulmonary edema are suggested—treatment approaches that challenge age-old management strategies in the patient who has acute congestive heart failure. Atrial fibrillation, a common arrhythmia in the emergency department (ED), is reviewed with a focus on the most appropriate management strategies for the emergency physician: rate control versus rhythm conversion. The dilemma of hypertension in the ED (ie, When is it emergent? Urgent? Uncomplicated?) is addressed. Aortic disasters in the elderly patient and cardiovascular presentations in the child are also reviewed, rounding out the extremes of patient age in the ED population.

In this issue of the *Emergency Medicine Clinics of North America*, we have assembled a list of knowledgeable emergency physicians who have authored timely and focused reviews in these various areas of cardiovascular emergency care. These reviews address the central clinical issues with an emphasis on "what you need to know" to appropriately manage patients in the ED.

William J. Brady, MD
3020 Cove Lane
Charlottesville, VA 22911, USA

E-mail address: wb4z@hscmail.mcc.virginia.edu

Wyatt W. Decker, MD
Mayo Clinic
200 First Street SW
Rochester, MN 55905, USA

E-mail address: decker.wyatt@mayo.edu

Amal Mattu, MD
Department of Emergency Medicine
110 South Paca Street
Sixth Floor, Suite 200
Baltimore, MD 21201, USA

E-mail address: amalmattu@comcast.net

ELSEVIER
SAUNDERS

Emerg Med Clin N Am
23 (2005) 937–957

EMERGENCY
MEDICINE
CLINICS OF
NORTH AMERICA

Initial Evaluation of Chest Pain

Eric T. Boie, MD

Department of Emergency Medicine, Mayo Clinic, 200 1st Street South West, Rochester, MN 55905, USA

Chest pain is among the most frequently evaluated presenting complaints in the emergency department (ED). Diagnostic etiologies range from benign to life-threatening. Failure to diagnose the life-threatening chest emergencies—specifically acute coronary syndrome, aortic dissection, and pulmonary embolism—can lead to catastrophic medical and legal outcomes for the patient and physician respectively. This article focuses on clinical and risk management strategies to minimize misdiagnosis and produce favorable medical and medicolegal outcomes.

A 49-year-old otherwise-healthy man was lifting weights when he felt a "pop" in his chest followed by severe chest pain and shortness of breath. He presented to a California ED whereby he stated that the pain radiated into his throat and left shoulder. Vitals were stable, and ECG and cardiac enzyme testing were normal. Chest radiograph showed mild cardiomegaly. The patient was given intravenous narcotics with some pain relief and was dismissed from the ED with oral analgesics and a diagnosis of musculoskeletal chest pain. The patient was found dead the following afternoon. Survivors sued the emergency physician for failure to diagnose a life-threatening chest emergency. A settlement was reached for $530,000 [1].

This case typifies the high stakes diagnostic challenge encountered daily by emergency physicians (EPs) in the evaluation of patients who are experiencing chest pain. Visits for chest pain comprise 5% to 8% of all ED visits—roughly 5 to 6 million annual ED chest pain evaluations [2,3]. The proportion of patients presenting to the EDs and subsequently being admitted for chest pain is growing [4]. In an effort to provide best patient care, the primary goal in the evaluation of the chest pain patient is straightforward: timely and accurate diagnosis with prompt therapeutic intervention. Misdiagnosis and delayed intervention can lead to death and substantial morbidity. Given the magnitude of loss with these undesirable

E-mail address: boie.eric@mayo.edu

doi:10.1016/j.emc.2005.07.007 *emed.theclinics.com*

outcomes, medical malpractice risk is also substantial. Nearly 30% of monetary losses in emergency medicine litigation are related to missed myocardial infarction (MI) alone [5].

Achieving optimal clinical outcomes and avoiding medicolegal pitfalls requires conscientious and thorough evaluation and appropriate application of risk management strategies. As EPs, the authors first consider the five major life-threatening chest emergencies: (1) acute myocardial infarction (AMI)/unstable angina (acute coronary syndrome [ACS]), (2) pulmonary embolism, (3) aortic dissection, (4) cardiac tamponade, and (5) tension pneumothorax. This article focuses on ACS, aortic dissection (AD), and pulmonary embolism (PE) because these are the entities most commonly encountered, misdiagnosed, and litigated among ED chest pain patients. For each of these entities, epidemiology, clinical presentations, diagnostic evaluations, and initial interventions are reviewed. Risk management strategies to avoid diagnostic and therapeutic pitfalls are emphasized.

Acute coronary syndrome

A 68-year-old woman presented to a Missouri ED complaining of sharp stabbing chest pain relieved by Motrin. Before arrival, she had experienced exertional chest pain radiating down both arms and nausea. All symptoms had since abated. The patient was diagnosed with chest-wall pain. She was prescribed ibuprofen and cyclobenzaprine. Five days later she returned in cardiopulmonary arrest. ECG revealed an acute ST elevation myocardial infarction (STEMI). She was taken to the catheterization laboratory and subsequently died. A settlement for $295,000 was reached with surviving family [6].

Epidemiology and risk

Identifying patients who have ACS among the vast population of ED patients presenting with chest pain is paramount. Consequences of misdiagnosis include infarction, arrhythmia, and death. The statistics of ACS are well-known. Coronary artery disease (CAD) is the leading cause of death in the United States [3]. 1.1 million AMIs occur annually [7]. The rate of "missed" AMIs has been estimated to range from 2% to 8% [2]. Patients who experience AMI or unstable angina dismissed from the ED have short-term mortality of 25%—twice that of AMI patients admitted to the hospital [4].

Malpractice litigation targeting EDs and EPs is dominated by ACS [8]. Missed AMI remains the condition responsible for the largest dollar paid out in ED malpractice claims annually [5]. Judgments and settlements are substantial, averaging $280,000—a dollar amount exceeded only by brain and spinal cord injury claims [8]. Forty percent of claims result in some payment [9]. With the advent of aggressive and time-sensitive therapy, like thrombolytics and primary angioplasty, the nature of litigation is changing. No longer is mortality the sole endpoint and basis for suit. Now claims for "potential myocardium lost" or "reduction in ejection fraction" as a result of failed or delayed intervention are common [8].

Clinical presentation

ACS can present in various ways, including but not limited to sudden death, arrhythmia, syncope, angina, or MI. The description of "classic angina" is reflexively familiar. Substernal chest pain is characterized as crushing, aching, viselike, or pressure. The pain typically radiates to the neck, jaw, and left arm. Associated symptoms include dyspnea, nausea, vomiting, diaphoresis, and presyncope. Pain often begins abruptly lasting 5 to 15 minutes, taking several minutes to reach maximal intensity. The pain is worse with activity and improves with rest.

The challenge facing EPs is that angina often presents in atypical rather than classic fashion. Burning epigastric pain is just as suggestive of ACS as typical substernal chest pain [10]. Although sharp, stabbing, and fleeting pains are regarded as atypical for ischemic pain, such pain is seen in 5% of patients who experience AMI [11]. Some studies suggest that 20% to 60% of patients who experience AMI have symptoms that are silent or so atypical that they do not present for evaluation during the acute phase [12]. Women, diabetics, and elderly men are most at risk for such presentations. Elderly patients who develop ACS can present with a range of complaints, including generalized weakness, altered mental status, syncope, atypical chest pain, and dyspnea. Dyspnea is the single most common presenting symptom of angina in patients greater than 85 years old [13]. Women presenting with ACS tend to be older on average than their male counterparts; have more comorbid disease, such as diabetes and hypertension; and have a longer delay from symptom onset to presentation to the ED [14]. Women also present more frequently with nausea, vomiting, dyspnea, and increased radiation of pain to the neck, back, or jaw. EPs are thus compelled to consider atypical and occult presentations of ACS as common [8].

Diagnostic evaluation

General

In the evaluation of a patient experiencing chest pain suspicious for ACS, the EP has three primary objectives [15]: (1) rapid identification of patients who develop acute STEMI who need immediate intervention with thrombolytic therapy or percutaneous intervention, (2) accurate identification of patients who develop unstable angina and are in need of aggressive medical management and admission for further evaluation, and (3) clear identification of patients in need of further risk stratification through provocative testing.

History and physical

A complete and accurate history remains the cornerstone of a quality evaluation of any patient presenting with chest pain. Although history alone is insufficient to exclude CAD, it can help in risk- stratifying patients as low, medium, or high risk and allow targeting of subsequent interventions and studies [2]. The history should assess characteristics of the pain, including onset, location, severity, duration, radiation, and circumstances surrounding its appearance. Associated symptoms, such as nausea, vomiting, syncope, palpitations, and diaphoresis should also be elicited. Chest pain that awakens the patient may be an ominous predictor of underlying coronary disease [8]. Right-sided pain is as worrisome as left-sided. Cardiac risk factor assessment is traditionally considered a routine element of the patient history; however, its value has been disputed. Patient age, sex, body habitus, family history of CAD, and comorbid illness, including diabetes mellitus, hypertension, hypercholesterolemia, and tobacco abuse, are all classic coronary risk factors. Aside from age, sex, and family history of premature CAD, the actual role of risk factors in predicting ACS or AMI in ED chest pain patients seems minimal [2]. Risk factors are based on population studies and, thus, are more predictive of development of CAD over a lifetime, not on predicting whether patients experiencing chest pain in the ED are likely to have ACS [13]. Characteristics of chest pain, personal history of CAD, and ECG findings outweigh risk factors. Focusing on an absence of risk factors results in EPs underestimating the possibility of disease in a patient who experiences otherwise classical symptoms of angina [2]. The physical examination in patients who have suspected ACS is rarely helpful, but may reveal arrhythmia, evidence of heart failure, a new murmur, or cardiovascular compromise and shock.

ECG

The ECG is the most critical and valuable bedside test for a patient with suspected ACS. The ECG is most helpful when it is abnormal. Any patient with a suspected ACS should receive an ECG within five minutes of their arrival to the ED [16]. Immediate examination for ST-segment elevation consistent with AMI is necessary to identify candidates for immediate thrombolytic therapy or percutaneous intervention. The ECG, however, is insensitive for AMI because only 40% to 50% of patients who experience AMI have ST elevation present [17]. ECGs should be examined for early changes suggestive of ACS including any Q waves, ST-segment depression, inverted T waves, flat ST segments, and J-point elevations. Minor changes may be nondiagnostic but can provide support for clinical evidence of underlying coronary disease. When an ECG shows new, albeit nondiagnostic, changes, which may be a result of ischemia, further evaluation is indicated. Dismissal of these patients without further evaluation is hazardous clinically and legally [16]. Right-sided leads, posterior leads, and continuous ST-segment monitoring may be helpful in patients who a concerning history but a normal or nondiagnostic ECG [8].

Approximately 20% of ED patients who experience chest pain have a completely normal ECG. Rate of AMI in patients who present with chest pain and a totally normal ECG is 1% to 4% [17]. Although a normal ECG after 12 hours of pain has a high negative predictive value for ACS, it is not 100% reliable [17]. Failure to recognize abnormalities on ECG is one of the most frequent sources of ACS litigation.

Cardiac markers

Troponin I and Troponin T are the new gold standard markers of cardiac ischemia. They have largely supplanted creatine kinase (CKMB) because they are more sensitive, specific, useful, and prognostic [2]. Troponin I assays are heterogenous in the subforms that they measure so results are not comparable across labs or institutions. Troponin T is commonly elevated in patients who experience renal failure. Although the long-term mortality in these patients is higher, the significance of this evaluation remains unclear [2]. Serial troponins are more sensitive for detecting ischemia than isolated values. Negative serial troponins effectively rule out infarctions but do not rule out the presence of underlying coronary disease [16].

Chest pain observation units and stress testing

Chest pain observation units have been created in EDs nationwide to provide a cost-effective, yet thorough, cardiac diagnostic evaluation in patients who have suspected CAD. These specialized units were developed to rapidly evaluate lower risk patients and reduce the rate of inadvertent dismissal of higher risk patients. The safety and efficacy of chest pain observation units using strict evaluation protocols has been extensively demonstrated [18]. These units have been predicated on early cardiac stress testing. Serial cardiac biomarker testing alone has been believed to be inadequate to identify patients who have underlying coronary disease [2]. The incremental diagnostic value of cardiac stress testing is significant. When added to ECG, clinical variables, and cardiac serum markers, the sensitivity of detecting CAD increases from 60% to 90% with stress testing [2]. Observation units are not a panacea and face several challenges, including variable protocols, variable accessibility to functional testing, and use by low-risk patients who could be discharged directly without observation [15].

Recently, investigators have begun to question the necessity of advanced cardiac evaluation, particularly in low risk populations [19]. Chest pain observation units have not been widely embraced in Canada, where risk-stratification tools are used that specifically determine which patients are safe to discharge from the ED [20]. Other investigators are re-exploring the use and safety of serial marker rule-outs without cardiac stress testing [3].

Options for cardiac stress testing in ED observation units have included standard treadmill exercise testing (TMET), stress echocardiography, and nuclear perfusion studies, such as thallium and technetium 99. The clinical use of the TMET for detecting CAD in otherwise-stable patients is generally accepted, despite reports of limited sensitivity (60%–70%) and specificity (50%–70%) [21]. False-positive TMET studies are particularly common in younger women [15]. Despite this, ED-based treadmill exercise testing has been shown to provide useful prognostic information for adverse events in low- and moderate-risk patients [22,23].

Several studies have demonstrated echocardiography is greater than 80% sensitive in identifying AMI and underlying CAD in patients who demonstrate nondiagnostic ECGs [11]. Echocardiography has limitations, however. The sensitivity of echocardiography is operator-dependent. Although wall motion abnormalities appear before classic ECG changes, absence of regional wall motion abnormalities does not exclude the possibility of ischemia. Conversely, presence of regional wall abnormalities is nonspecific and not necessarily predictive of ACS or coronary event [11].

Nuclear perfusion imaging has been postulated to be the most sensitive and specific noninvasive test available for detection of underlying coronary disease in patients who exhibit normal and nondiagnostic ECGs [8].

All of these testing modalities have been used in observation unit protocols with success and safety. The specific test used depends on institution-specific protocols and resources. Stress testing acutely reduces returns to the ED for chest pain evaluation and rates of subsequent nonfatal and fatal AMI [24]. Current American Heart Association and American College of Cardiology guidelines recommend cardiac stress testing at the time of discharge from the ED, or soon thereafter [15]. Evidence and practice standards compel the EP to use observation units liberally for appropriate patients.

Risk management strategies

A 45-year-old woman presented to a Massachusetts ED the morning after a night of intermittent right-sided chest pain. The pain was associated with shortness of breath and palpitations. On arrival to the ED, the patient was clutching her throat and screaming. Examination revealed tenderness at the costochondral junction. Chest radiograph, complete blood cell count, and electrolytes were normal. Two ECGs done 90 minutes apart were read as normal, although the second differed from the first. No cardiac enzyme testing was ordered. The patient was given a discharge diagnosis of costochondritis. Later that afternoon, she returned to the hospital by ambulance, complaining of chest pain, sweating, and confusion. Shortly after arrival, she arrested and died. The jury returned a verdict for the plaintiff for $1.65 million [25].

Avoiding misdiagnosis in patients who have ACS and the subsequent litigation that follows can be successfully accomplished by several means. The first step is a conscientious and thorough diagnostic evaluation as outlined earlier.

Secondly, an appreciation of classes of patients in whom ACS is most likely to be missed is also valuable. This list includes the following patient groups [26]:

1. Young: less than 10% of AMI occur in patients under 45 years of age, but the incidence of AMI in this demographic is growing; high index of suspicion should be maintained in young patients who develop typical anginal symptoms, particularly if there is a history of tobacco abuse or a family history of premature coronary disease [8].
2. Elderly: elderly patients are more prone to atypical presentations with dyspnea as a common angina equivalent.
3. Women: women tend to present with longer delay from symptoms onset, have higher incidence of comorbid diseases, such as diabetes and hypertension, tend to be older than their male counterparts, and, more commonly, have atypical presentations [13]. Postmenopausal women assume the same risk as their male counterparts for coronary disease.
4. "Frequent flyers": with repeated visits to the ED, a tendency accumulates to minimize or dismiss this group of patients' complaints.
5. Alcoholics and drug users: negative countertransference and antipathy toward patients who drug seek or are perceived as less desirable can prevent objective evaluation for the etiology of their chest pain.
6. Diabetics: presentations are more frequently silent or atypical.

Also included are patients who have developed [26]:

1. Atypical presentations: up to 10% of new AMI and unstable angina are missed at onset because of atypical presentations. Angina equivalent symptoms are important to consider.
2. Comorbid psychiatric and somatoform disease: psychiatric disease does not preclude a patient from having coexistent CAD. Psychiatric diagnoses in patients who complain of chest pain should always be diagnoses of exclusion.
3. Pre-existing gastrointestinal (GI) disease: epigastric or chest pain in these patients may be misleading attributed to their underlying chronic diagnoses rather than ACS.

Thirdly, and in addition to having an appreciation for patient classes in whom ACS is likely to be missed, it is also valuable to have an understanding of risky practices to avoid. Five practices to avoid are [8]:

1. Discounting previous symptoms even if symptoms are resolved on presentation to the ED. The symptoms must still factor in to risk assessment and subsequent management.
2. Ignoring epigastric or upper abdominal pain as a potential sign of inferior myocardial ischemia.
3. Relying on reproducible chest wall pain to rule out ACS. In one study, 6% of patients who develop chest wall tenderness had AMI [27].

4. Using response to antacids or other treatments as definitive diagnostic aids. Patients who have ACS can become pain-free for various reasons and responsiveness to a GI cocktail does not rule out CAD [28].
5. Failing to appreciate nonspecific ECG changes. Nondiagnostic changes may be ominous signs of evolving coronary syndrome or underlying CAD.

In the case above (45-year-old woman presented to a Massachusetts ED), initial evaluation revealed chest wall pain in the face of abnormal but nondiagnostic ECGs with a catastrophic outcome.

Finally, the following practices can help reduce the medicolegal risk in the evaluation of patients who have suspected ACS [29]:

1. Adhere to risk management guidelines and chest pain protocols, which allow better, more consistent care and sharper diagnostic accuracy.
2. Document your ED record with special emphasis on history, differential diagnosis, and rationale for key decisions. Risk factors should also be documented despite their limited value in the acute setting, because it indicates an appreciation that coronary syndrome was seriously considered.
3. Use serial cardiac markers, prolonged observation, and cardiac stress testing in patients who have compelling stories but normal or nondiagnostic ECGs.
4. Maintain high index of suspicion for atypical presentations.
5. Maximize the physician-patient relationship stressing compassionate care and communication.

Aortic dissection

A 50-year-old man presented to a California ED with a sudden onset of shooting back pain, diaphoresis, and dyspnea 8 hours before arrival. The pain had resolved during the day but had returned in the back and now the upper abdomen. The patient denied any chest pain, nausea, vomiting, or presyncopal symptoms. Physical examination findings revealed only mild back and abdominal tenderness. ECG and cardiac markers were normal. Chest radiograph showed a right hilar mass. The patient was dismissed with oral narcotics and a diagnosis of musculoskeletal chest and back pain. Thirty-three hours after discharge, the patient was found dead. Autopsy revealed proximal aortic dissection (AD) with cardiac tamponade. Survivors brought suit against the EP. The jury returned the verdict for the defense [30].

Epidemiology

The described case exemplifies the formidable diagnostic challenge and catastrophic consequences of a missed diagnosis of AD, another life-threatening cause of chest pain that must be routinely considered in any patient presenting to the ED with this symptom. AD is the most common and most lethal aortic emergency [31]. Among the life-threatening causes of chest pain, AD has the highest mortality—an estimated 1% to 2% per hour for the first 48 hours [32]. Patients who experience untreated AD have a 2-week mortality rate of 66% [33]. Approximately 25,000 cases of AD are evaluated annually in EDs, making this entity two to three times more common than ruptured abdominal aortic aneurysm [34]. The absolute incidence of AD has increased two- to fourfold in the last 30 years [35]. Unfortunately, as many as 65% of ADs are missed on initial presentation [35]. A correct antimortem diagnosis is made in less than 50% of cases [36]. In fact, one study noted that in 28% of documented cases, AD was never considered as a possible diagnosis [36].

Clinical presentation

The presenting signs and symptoms of AD are dependent on the location of the dissection and the vessels effected. Chest pain is the most common presenting complaint and is present in greater than 90% of patients who experience acute AD [31]. Pain is typically abrupt and most severe at onset. Frequently, a period of latency occurs whereby pain abates, which is believed to be secondary to the dissection ceasing. A return of pain often marks further propagation of the dissection. Pain is often migratory, beginning in the chest and upper back and moving to the abdomen and low back. Migratory pain should prompt strong consideration of AD. In one study, 71% of patients who experience acute AD also experienced migratory pain [37]. Severe pain above and below the diaphragm should also heighten suspicion for AD. Pain has classically been described as ripping or tearing; however, pain is characterized differently by different patients, and some studies suggest a tearing or ripping quality to the pain is rarely reported clinically [38].

Patients may also complain of nausea, vomiting, dyspnea, syncope, and diaphoresis. Involvement of the great vessels may result in an acute stroke syndrome. Paraplegia may be observed if spinal arteries are involved. Abdominal pain may be a presenting complaint if mesenteric vasculature is involved. Lower-extremity weakness and acute neuropathies are also observed.

Diagnostic evaluation

History and physical

As for any patient presenting with chest pain, elucidation of the onset, quality, character, intensity, duration, radiation, modifying factors, and associated symptoms is necessary to obtain in a patient who is experiencing suspected AD. Risk factor assessment should be included in the history. Risk factors for AD include hypertension, male sex, nonwhite race, connective tissue disease (ie, Ehlers-Danlos Syndrome or Marfan's

Syndrome), bicuspid aortic valve, coarctation of the aorta, and drug-use including methamphetamine and cocaine [31]. Peak age of incidence is between 50 and 70 years of age. A higher incidence is also noted in women in the third trimester of their pregnancy. In any patient experiencing chest pain and one of the risk factors described earlier, AD should be considered [35].

Physical examination should assess vital signs and physical signs of vascular interruption. The physical examination is insensitive for the diagnosis of AD because it is not uncommon for the examination findings to be entirely normal. Blood pressure is elevated in more than 50% of cases, particularly in patients who are experiencing distal dissection [35]. Hypotension is much less common, suggesting the possibility of tamponade or intrathoracic rupture. Peripheral pulses should be examined to assess for blood pressure discrepancies between limbs, which may indicate interruption of blood flow. Pulse deficits are commonly transient [35]. Cardiac examination findings may reveal murmur of aortic insufficiency seen commonly in proximal dissections. Muffled heart tones and jugular venous distention may point toward cardiac tamponade secondary to a dissection. Neurologic deficits, such as hemiplegic stroke, ischemic paraparesis, peripheral myopathy, and alteration in level of consciousness can all be seen.

Imaging

Definitive imaging for AD may include computed tomography (CT), aortic angiography, transesophageal echocardiography (TEE), or MRI. Several diagnostic options for definitive evaluation exist for AD. CT is the most readily available, widely used, noninvasive technique for the diagnosis of AD. Sensitivity and specificity of CT approaches 100% for the diagnosis of AD [39]. Aortic angiography is the traditional definitive method for confirming the diagnosis of AD has a diagnostic accuracy of 95% to 99% [40]. Aortography, however, is the most highly invasive, requires the patient be out of the ED for extended period of time, and exposes the patient to a significant contrast load [31]. TEE is being used with increasing frequency and has been shown to be safe, even in critically ill patients [41]. Sensitivity of TEE for detecting proximal and distal dissections is 100% [42]. The main limitations for use of the TEE is a lack of widespread, 24-hour availability. Finally, MRI is the newest imaging method for the diagnosis of AD. It is highly sensitive and specific and does not require exposing the patient to contrast material. In ventilated or monitored patients it is not ideal and is not widely available.

Definitive imaging is indicated in any patient in whom clinical suspicion for AD exists. Given the overall low rate of antemortem diagnosis, definitive testing should occur with any patient with a compelling history for AD.

Treatment

Treatment of AD is aimed at eliminating the forces that favor progression of the dissection. Prompt production of blood pressures can be accomplished through use of sodium nitroprusside with a rate adjusted to achieve a systolic blood pressure between 100 and 120 mmHg [31]. Concomitant use of a beta-blocker to avoid reflux tachycardia secondary to the nitroprusside-use is desirable to further decrease the shear forces that promote propagation. A target heart rate of 60 to 80 beats per minute is desirable [31].

Patients who have developed acute dissection involving the ascending aorta should receive rapid surgical consultation. Conversely, distal ADs are traditionally treated medically. Surgery is indicated in distal dissections when evidence of lower extremity or visceral ischemia, renal failure, paraparesis, or paraplegia is available [31]. If surgical specialists and support resources are not readily available, rapid transport by appropriate personnel should be expeditiously pursued.

Risk management strategies

In analysis of malpractice litigation involving AD, there are several common patterns recognized. By recognizing these patients, similar pitfalls may be avoided. Common patterns include:

1. Misdiagnoses of musculoskeletal pain or radiculopathy followed by discharge from the ED. This scenario occurred in the example case. In such cases, the dismissal diagnoses only partially fit the presenting symptoms, which when taken in sum could be better explained by AD.
2. Misdiagnosis with hospitalization for rule-out MI. This pattern is particularly important to remember with the increased use of chest pain observation units for patients undergoing evaluation for ACS. The diagnostic endpoint for patients presenting with chest pain cannot simply be ruled out of underlying coronary disease. Alternative diagnoses, such as AD and pulmonary embolism (PE), always need to be strongly considered [35].
3. Failure to expedite intervention. After diagnosis of AD, admissions with delays to subspecialty evaluations are not acceptable in a disease in which mortality increases by the hour. Consultation needs to be prompt. Documentation of times of initial contact with and arrival of consultants is prudent.
4. Inappropriate management of blood pressure. Failure to do so can be postulated as causative in failing to prevent propagation of the dissection. This underscores the need for prompt intervention to lower the blood pressure and pulse in patients who develop AD.

Of the four commonly observed patterns in case law, the two involving failure to diagnose AD with the subsequent disastrous implications are by far the most commonly litigated.

Freedman [35] outlined several additional risk management strategies for evaluating patients who are experiencing chest pain and specifically for AD, which are summarized here:

1. Maintain a high index of suspicion. If AD is not routinely considered, it is not diagnosed with acceptable sensitivity. Tolerance of a high number of negative CT scans or other definitive studies for the purpose of ruling out AD must exist. A high positive work-up rate likely means many ADs are going undiagnosed.
2. Pursue a definitive workup for AD in patients presenting with chest pain with one or more risk factors or one of the identifiable clinical syndromes that include the following:

   Chest pain with neurologic symptoms
   Chest pain radiating to the back
   Chest pain with signs of vascular compromise
   Chest pain that is migratory
   Chest pain with severe abdominal or back pain
   Chest pain with a widened mediastinum on chest radiography
   Chest pain with a murmur of aortic insufficiency

3. Understand that definitive ECG evidence of AMI does not rule out concurrent presence of AD. Although a normal screening chest radiograph in the setting of AMI makes AD less likely, a rapid definitive imaging test is indicated when the clinical suspicion of AD is high. Ten to twenty percent of patients who develop AD have a normal chest radiograph [37].
4. Obtain definitive diagnostic imaging immediately in cases of suspected AD, using the test that is most readily available. Protocols should exist to avoid confusion as to the availability of tests during various circumstances and times of day.
5. Initiate treatment aimed at preventing propagation on immediate diagnosis of AD. A combination of a vasodilator and beta-blocker effectively lower blood pressure and heart rate.
6. Initiate specialty consultation on a stat basis, when AD is diagnosed or even highly suspected. If definitive care is not immediately available, expeditious transfer should be arranged according to transfer protocols.

Pulmonary embolism

A 52-year-old man presented to a New York ED 12 hours after the onset of left-sided chest pain. The pain radiated under his left arm and into his back. The pain had dissipated over the day, but he developed shortness of breath in the afternoon. On presentation, vitals were normal. Oxygen saturation was 93% on room air. Physical examination findings revealed some mild chest wall tenderness. Chest radiograph, ECG, and cardiac markers were normal. Motrin and nitroglycerin provided no relief. He was ultimately discharged with an antibiotic with the diagnosis of bronchitis, chest wall pain, and dyspnea. One week later the patient collapsed and died at home. Autopsy revealed multiple acute and PE. The patient's wife brought suit against the EP and hospital. The jury awarded $1.6 million to the plaintiff [43].

Missed PE is a major source of malpractice litigation in emergency medicine [44]. It is estimated that the diagnosis of PE is missed 400,000 times annually leading to 100,000 preventable deaths [45]. Other studies have estimated that only 30% of PE is diagnosed antemortem [46]. The mortality rate for untreated PE is 18.4%—seven times greater than that of appropriately treated PE [47]. Certainly, failure to be diagnosed is the greatest threat to the patient with PE [48]. The challenges faced in the diagnosis of PE are similar to those discussed for ACS and AD. Clinical presentation can be widely variable, presenting signs and symptoms are nonspecific, and there is no single highly sensitive, noninvasive test to make the diagnosis. Finally, and more specific to PE, difficulty exists in accurately assessing pretest probability of disease.

Clinical presentation

In general, the presentation of PE is nonspecific. Young patients who present with excellent cardiac reserve tend to have mild, transient, or no symptoms at all [48]. Patients may complain of chest pain, which is typically sudden in onset and pleuritic in nature. Dyspnea, palpitations, presyncope, or syncope may also be presenting complaints. Accurate diagnosis is clouded when clinical presentations are coexistent with underlying obstructive lung disease, pneumonia, or underlying congestive heart failure. In such cases, PE can present with the symptomatology of any of these entities [49].

Diagnostic evaluation

The diagnostic evaluation for patients who experience suspected PE continues to present considerable challenges to an ongoing controversy among EPs. A combination of an estimation of clinical pretest probability of disease combined with D-dimer or CT imaging are the most common tools used to evaluate a patient who has developed a suspected PE. Specific algorithms in the various risk populations are included in the following discussion.

Clinical scoring

The clinical likelihood of a patient having PE has long been estimated by implicit means (ie, physician judgment). Physician judgment is based on the patient's clinical presentation, history and physical evaluation, and risk factor assessment; however, studies have shown poor agreement among EPs in estimating pretest probability of disease [50]. Experience level affects pretest probability assessment with less experienced clinicians demonstrating less ability to accurately assign pretest probability [51]. Implicit assessment results in a large group of patients being placed in moderate risk category. Thus, clinical judgment has yielded disappointing results in its ability to accurately determine pretest probability of disease.

In light of this, clinical scoring systems have been developed. Wells and others have created a seven-feature bedside assessment tool to categorize patients as having low, moderate, or high pretest probability of PE [52,53]. Even with Wells criteria, studies have shown poor agreement among physicians on the assignment of pretest probability and poor accuracy for the same [54]. Until a reliable validated clinical scoring system can be developed, the assignment of pretest probability of PE remains a challenge.

History and physical

As in the entities previously described, history in a patient presenting with chest pain suspicious for PE focuses on features of the pain and associated symptoms. Particularly important in patients who have developed suspected PE is risk factor assessment. Box 1 details many risk factors that need to be considered in a patient who has developed possible PE [48]. Physical examination in a patient who has developed suspected PE should focus on vital signs and pulmonary findings. Tachycardia and tachypnea are classically described, but the former is often absent in younger patients and the later absent in up to 13% of patients who have documented PE [48]. Physical examination findings may show pleural rub or rales, or findings consistent with pulmonary consolidation. In summary, however, no physical finding exists, sensitive or specific, for the diagnosis of PE. Physical examination offers no clues to the diagnosis in 28% to 58% of cases [48].

D-dimer assays

D-dimer is a cross-linked fiber degradation product form by plasmin, which serves as a marker of clot lysis. Tremendous improvement in the sensitivity of D-dimer assays has been made through the advent of quantitative enzyme-linked amino-sorbed assay (ELISA) [55]. D-dimer is most helpful as an exclusionary test with a negative result indicating a low likelihood of PE. D-dimer assays as a whole have poor specificity with numerous conditions resulting in false-positive results.

The greatest use of the D-dimer assays is when combined with other noninvasive imaging or clinical probability assessment scoring systems. In this way, a negative D-dimer can be incorporated into diagnostic algorithms to safely withhold anticoagulation among patients who exhibit a low pretest probability for PE [55]. Negative results on quantitative rapid ELISA D-dimer assays have likelihood ratios that can create significant changes between pretest and posttest probability of disease. Recent studies reporting the negative likelihood ratios for a negative result on a quantitative rapid ELISA D-dimer make them as predictive as a normal ventilation-perfusion (V/Q) scan or negative duplex ultrasound [56].

Eleven prospective clinical studies have evaluated the role of D-dimer in excluding venous thromboembolic disease. In patients who demonstrate

Box 1. Risk factors for pulmonary embolism

Inherited disorders (thrombophilias)

- Elevated individual clotting factor levels (VIII, IX, XI)
- Factor V Leiden Mutation
- Hyperhomocystinemia
- Protein C, protein S, or antithrombin III deficiency
- Prothrombin G20210A mutation

Acquired—persistent

- Age
- Antiphospholipid antibodies (lupus anticoagulant, anticardiolipin antibody)
- History of pulmonary embolism/deep venous thrombosis
- History of superficial thrombophlebitis
- Hyperviscosity syndrome (polycythemia vera, malignant melanoma)
- Immobilization (bedridden, paresis, or paralysis)
- Malignancy
- Medical conditions:
  congestive heart failure
  obesity
  nephrotic syndrome
  tobacco abuse
  AMI
  varicose veins

Acquired—transient

- Central venous catheter/pacemaker placement
- Hormone replacement therapy
- Immobilization—isolated extremity
- Long-distance travel/air travel
- Oral contraceptive pills
- Pregnancy and puerperium
- Surgery
- Trauma

Adapted from Sadosty AT, Boie TE, Stead LG. Pulmonary Embolism. Emerg Med Clin North Am 2003;21(2):363–84; with permission.

high clinical pretest probability of PE but a negative D-dimer, not enough evidence exists to safely support stopping an investigation for PE in such a patient [49]. By contrast, for patients who exhibit low clinical pretest probability of disease and a negative quantitative rapid ELISA D-dimer, it is increasingly accepted that the diagnosis of PE is effectively ruled out [56]. Controversy still exists over the extent of work-up necessary in patients who demonstrate moderate pretest clinical probability and a negative D-dimer assay.

One significant limitation affecting widespread use of D-dimer is the numerous commercially available assays, which are not interchangable, differing significantly in sensitivity and negative likelihood ratios [55]. Latex glutination assays and whole blood qualitative assays do not demonstrate the same negative predictive value that quantitative ELISA assays do and should not be incorporated in diagnostic algorithms similarly.

Ventilation-perfusion scanning

The PIOPED investigators used V/Q scanning as the primary advanced imaging diagnostic modality for patients who develop suspected PE [57]. V/Q scans are most helpful when they are read as normal or high probability; however, results of V/Q scans fail to provide definitive indication to withhold or give anticoagulation in up to 70% of patients on whom the test is performed [48].

CT

CT is fast becoming the advanced imaging modality of choice for patients who present with suspected PE. CT is widely available, noninvasive, increasingly sensitive, and has the advantage of revealing alternative diagnoses when PE is not found. The biggest concern with conventional CT imaging is failure to detect subsegmental PE [58]. Great controversy over the clinical significance of subsegmental clot exists. Therapy in PE is aimed at preventing subsequent emboli rather than treating existing clot. In debating the significance of subsegmental PE, some investigators have argued that outcome studies of rate of subsequent or recurrent PE and death are more appropriate as a gold standard than comparisons with the gold standard of angiographic subsegmental PE detection rates [59]. Eleven such studies exist, prospective and retrospective, which demonstrate patient outcome is not adversely affected when anticoagulation is held based on a negative spiral CT [60]. The frequency of subsequent clinical diagnosis of PE after a negative spiral CT is low and in fact lower than a normal or low probability V/Q scan [60]. These studies were all based on conventional spiral CT. The advent of advanced generation, multirow scanners with increased resolution and ability to detect subsegmental PEs may further enhance the diagnostic ability of CT, but few studies using this technology are presently available. Despite its diagnostic accuracy, CT should not be the sole test on which the diagnosis of PE is ruled out. Specifically in patients who demonstrate high pretest clinical probability of disease, a CT alone does not rule out the presence of PE. CT should be combined with D-dimer assays and assessments of clinical pretest probability to determine the presence or absence of PE.

Diagnostic evaluation summary

A review by Fedullo and Tapson [61] provides rational guidance to the approach that the patient who presents with suspected PE should be addressed using a combination of pretest probability assessment, D-dimer assays, and advanced imaging modalities to effectively rule in or out the diagnosis of PE [61].

Patients who exhibit low pretest probability of PE account for 25% to 65% of all patients evaluated for PE with subsequent diagnosis of PE in 5% to 10% of cases [52,62–64]. For these patients at low clinical probability, a negative quantitative ELISA D-dimer effectively rules out the diagnosis of PE.

Patients who have a high pretest probability for PE comprise 10% to 30% of all patients evaluated for PE with subsequent diagnosis of PE in 70% to 90% [52,62–64]. D-dimer has no significant role in this patient population because a negative result does not rule out the presence of PE. Spiral CT should be performed in these patients. If CT is negative, duplex ultrasound or CT venography of the lower extremities may be indicated. If lower-extremity studies are also negative in this high-risk patient population, pulmonary angiogram is indicated to rule out the presence of PE.

Intermediate risk patients comprise 25% to 65% of all patients examined for PE, with subsequent diagnosis of PE in 25% to 45% [52,62–64]. The algorithm proposed by Fedullo and Tapson is identical to that for the high-probability group such that a negative CT and lower-extremity studies are not adequate alone to rule out PE. Some investigators would argue that a negative D-dimer in this intermediate-risk population obviates the need for any imaging [56]. This intermediate group remains the most challenging group of patients to determine a diagnostic endpoint that effectively rules out disease.

Risk management strategies

Understanding the challenges of diagnosis of PE and the poor outcomes that follow misdiagnosis, several risk management strategies can be applied to optimize medical and legal outcomes:

1. Maintain a high index of suspicion for PE. Clinical presentation can be highly variable and subtle to extreme. Risk factor assessment is a critical part of the patient history. Patients presenting with chest pain with clinical risk factors for PE should be strongly considered for work-up.
2. Consistently determine and document pretest probability for PE. Whether based on implicit means (ie, clinical judgment) or available clinical scoring tools, documentation of pretest probability of disease allows rational work-up of PE using the diagnostic tools and algorithms available. This documentation also allows justification of the clinical rationale and decision process should the diagnosis of PE be missed.
3. Establish a literature-supported algorithm of diagnostic evaluation based on pretest probability of disease to routinely apply it in patients

who present with suspected PE. Consistent evaluation is then provided, leading to rational rather than random and changing processes.
4. Do not rely solely on any single diagnostic test to rule out the presence of PE. No single test is currently available that can always effectively rule out the presence of PE. A negative quantitative ELISA D-dimer does not exclude the diagnosis in high-risk patients. CT imaging alone does not exclude the diagnosis in moderate or high-risk patients.
5. Understand that pulmonary angiography, although seldom used, continues to be recommended and has a role, particularly in high-risk patients who demonstrate negative CT imaging and negative lower extremity studies.

Summary

EPs evaluate patients presenting with chest pain in their practice daily. Although most patients have benign causes of their chest pain, accurate and timely diagnosis of the major life-threatening chest emergencies is critical. ACS, AD, and PE have the shared characteristics of being diagnostically formidable with catastrophic consequences when the diagnosis is missed. These entities comprise the highest risk encounters for the EP. By combining conscientious, thorough, evidence-based evaluation with appropriate application of risk management strategies, the likelihood of an adverse clinical and medicolegal outcome is substantially reduced.

Acknowledgments

The author thanks Ms. Cyndra Franke for her diligent and patient assistance with the preparation of this manuscript.

References

[1] Doe v Roe, California. Medical malpractice: verdicts, settlements & experts. 2004;20(9):13.
[2] Kontos MC. Evaluation of the emergency department chest pain patient. Cardiol Rev 2001; 9(5):266–75.
[3] Lai C, Noeller TP, Schmidt K, et al. Short-term risk after initial observation for chest pain. J Emerg Med 2003;25(4):357–62.
[4] Lee TH, Rouan GW, Weisberg MC, et al. Clinical characteristics and natural history of patients with acute myocardial infarction sent home from the emergency room. Am J Cardiol 1987;60(4):219–24.
[5] Hubler JR, Zimmerly JG. Don't shrug off the painful shoulder: high-risk presentations associated with a common chief complaint. ED Legal Letter 1999;10(7):53–62.
[6] Stonner v Ash, Ray County (MO) Circuit Court. Case no. 02CV103710. Medical malpractice: verdicts, settlements & experts. 2004;20(8):11–2.
[7] Pope JH, Aufderheide TP, Ruthazer R, et al. Missed diagnosis of acute cardiac ischemia in the emergency department. N Engl J Med 2000;342(16):1163–70.
[8] Dunn JD. Missed MI: costly, deadly, and sometimes unpreventable. ED Legal Letter 2002; 13(7):73–84.
[9] Acute myocardial infarction study. Rockville (MD): Physician Insurers Association of America; 1996.

[10] Lee TH, Cook EF, Weisberg M, et al. Acute chest pain in the emergency room: identification and examination of low risk patients. Arch Intern Med 1985;145(1):65–9.
[11] Lim SH, Sayre MR, Gibler WB. 2-D echocardiography prediction of adverse events in ED patients with chest pain. Am J Emerg Med 2003;21(2):106–10.
[12] Sigurdsson E, Thorgeirsson G, Sigvaldason H, et al. Unrecognized myocardial infarction: epidemiology, clinical characteristics, and the prognostic role of angina pectoris. The Reykjavik Study. Ann Intern Med 1995;122(2):96–102.
[13] Jones ID, Slovis CM. Emergency department evaluation of the chest pain patient. Emerg Med Clin North Am 2001;19(2):269–82.
[14] Boccardi L, Verde M. Gender differences in the clinical presentation to the emergency department for chest pain. Ital Heart J 2003;4(6):371–3.
[15] Diercks DB, Panacek EA. Risk and chest pain evaluation: inseparable? J Emerg Med 2003; 25(4):455–7.
[16] Lee TH, Goldman L. Evaluation of the patient with acute chest pain. N Engl J Med 2000; 342(16):1187–95.
[17] Brady WJ, Roberts D, Morris F. The nondiagnostic ECG in the chest pain patient: normal and nonspecific initial ECG presentations of acute MI. Am J Emerg Med 1999;17(4):394–7.
[18] Domanovits H, Schillinger M, Paulis M, et al. Acute chest pain—a stepwise approach, the challenge of the correct clinical diagnosis. Resuscitation 2002;55(1):9–16.
[19] Hollander JE. Evaluation of patient with chest pain: are the bells and whistles evidence based? Ann Emerg Med 2003;41(3):352–4.
[20] Christenson J, Innes G, McKnight D, et al. Safety and efficiency of emergency department assessment of chest discomfort. CMAJ 2004;170(12):1803–7.
[21] Bartel AG, Behar VS, Peter RH, et al. Graded exercise stress tests in angiographically documented coronary artery disease. Circulation 1974;49:348–56.
[22] Gibler WB, Runyon JP, Levy RC, et al. A rapid diagnostic and treatment center for patients with chest pain in the emergency department. Ann Emerg Med 1995;25(1):1–8.
[23] Diercks DB, Gibler WB, Liu T, et al. Identification of patients at risk by graded exercise testing in an emergency department chest pain center. Am J Cardiol 2000;86:289–92.
[24] Shoyeb A, Bokhari S, Sullivan J, et al. Value of definitive diagnostic testing in the evaluation of patients presenting to the emergency department with chest pain. Am J Cardiol 2003; 91(12):1410–4.
[25] Anonymous v Anonymous, Massachusetts. Medical malpractice: verdicts, settlements & experts. 2004;20(10):14.
[26] Croskerry P. Achilles heels of the ED: delayed or missed diagnoses. ED Legal Letter 2003; 14(10):109–20.
[27] Disla E, Rhim HR, Reddy A, et al. A prospective analysis in an emergency department setting. Arch Intern Med 1994;154(21):2466–9.
[28] Wrenn K, Slovis CM, Gongaware J. Using the "GI cocktail": a descriptive study. Ann Emerg Med 1996;28:104–5.
[29] Bonner S. Chest pain: reducing the legal risks. ED Legal Letter 1998;9(11):105–12.
[30] Purgason v Dunning, Sacramento County (CA) Superior Court. Case no. 00AS06766. Medical malpractice: verdicts, settlements, & experts. 2004;20(3):22–3.
[31] Salkin MS. Thoracic aortic dissection: avoiding failure to diagnose. ED Legal Letter 1997; 8(11):107–18.
[32] Hals G. Acute thoracic aortic dissection: current evaluation and management. Emerg Med Rep 2000;21:1.
[33] Miller DC. Surgical management of aortic dissections: indications, perioperative management, and long-term results. In: Doroghazi RM, Slatter EE, editors. Aortic dissection. New York: McGraw Hill; 1983. p. 193–243.
[34] Feldman JA. Thoracic and abdominal aortic aneurysms. In: Tintinalli JE, Krome RL, et al, editors. Emergency medicine: a comprehensive study guide. 3rd edition. New York: McGraw Hill; 1992. p. 1384.

[35] Freedman DL. Aortic dissection: be suspicious or the autopsy will make diagnosis. ED Legal Letter 2000;11(10):105–16.
[36] Spittell PC, Spittell JA Jr, Joyce JW, et al. Clinical features and differential diagnosis of aortic dissection: experience with 236 cases (1980–1990). Mayo Clin Proc 1993;68(7): 642–51.
[37] Slater EE, DeSanctis RW. The clinical recognition of dissecting aortic aneurysm. Am J Med 1976;60:625–33.
[38] Armstrong WF, Bach DS, Carey LM, et al. Clinical and echocardiographic findings in patients with suspected acute aortic dissection. Am Heart J 1998;136(6):1051–60.
[39] Yoshida S, Akiba H, Tamakawa M, et al. Thoracic involvement of type A aortic dissection and intramural hematoma: diagnostic accuracy—comparison of emergency helical CT and surgical findings. Radiology 2003;228(2):430–5.
[40] Eagle KA, Quertermous T, Kritzer GA, et al. Spectrum of conditions initially suggesting acute aortic dissection but with negative aortograms. Am J Cardiol 1986;57(4):322–6.
[41] Kouchoukos NT, Dougenis DD. Surgery of the thoracic aorta. N Engl J Med 1997;336: 1876–86.
[42] Nienaber CA, Spielmann RP, von Kodolitsch Y, et al. Diagnosis of thoracic aortic dissection: magnetic resonance imaging versus transesophageal echocardiography. Circulation 1992;85(2):434–47.
[43] Shepherd v State of New York Court of Claims, Syracuse. Case no. 102377. Medical malpractice: verdicts, settlements & experts. 2004;20(6):18–9.
[44] Laack TA, Goyal DG. Pulmonary embolism: an unsuspected killer. Emerg Med Clin North Am 2004;22(4):961–83.
[45] Feied C. Pulmonary embolism. In: Rosen P, Barkin R, Daniel DF, editors. Emergency medicine: concepts and clinical practice. St. Louis (MO): Mosby-Year Book, Inc.; 1998. p. 1770–2.
[46] Morgenthaler TI, Ryu JH. Clinical characteristics of fatal pulmonary embolism in a referral hospital. Mayo Clin Proc 1995;70:417–24.
[47] Carson JL, Kelley MA, Duff A, et al. The clinical course of pulmonary embolism. N Engl J Med 1992;326(19):1240–5.
[48] Sadosty AT, Boie ET, Stead LG. Pulmonary embolism. Emerg Med Clin North Am 2003; 21(2):363–84.
[49] Goldhaber SZ. Pulmonary embolism. Lancet 2004;363(7417):1295–305.
[50] Jackson RE, Rudoni RR, Pascual R. Emergency physician (EP) assessment of the pre-test probability of pulmonary embolism (PE). Acad Emerg Med 1999;6:437.
[51] Kline JA, Wells PS. Methodology for a rapid protocol to rule out pulmonary embolism in the emergency department. Ann Emerg Med 2003;42(2):266–75.
[52] Wells PS, Ginsberg JS, Anderson DR, et al. Use of a clinical model for safe management of patients with suspected pulmonary embolism. Ann Intern Med 1998;129(12): 997–1005.
[53] Anderson DR, Wells PS, Stiell I, et al. Thrombosis in the emergency department: use of a clinical diagnosis model to safely avoid the need for urgent radiological investigation. Arch Intern Med 1999;159(5):477–82.
[54] Sanson BJ, Lijmer JG, MacGillavry MR, et al. Comparison of a clinical probability estimate and two clinical models in patients with suspected pulmonary embolism. ANTELOPE-Study Group. Thromb Haemost 2000;83(2):199–203.
[55] Frost SD, Brotman DJ, Michota FA. Rational use of D-dimer measurement to exclude acute venous thromboembolic disease. Mayo Clin Proc 2003;78(11):1385–91.
[56] Stein PD, Hull RD, Patel KC, et al. D-dimer for the exclusion of acute venous thrombosis and pulmonary embolism: a systematic review. Ann Intern Med 2004;140(8):589–602.
[57] PIOPED Investigators. Value of the ventilation/perfusion scan in acute pulmonary embolism: results of the prospective investigation of pulmonary embolism diagnosis (PIOPED). JAMA 1990;263(20):2753–9.

[58] Perrier A, Howarth N, Didier D, et al. Performance of helical computed tomography in unselected outpatients with suspected pulmonary embolism. Ann Intern Med 2001;135(2): 88–97.
[59] Wolfe TR, Hartsell SC. Pulmonary embolism: making sense of the diagnostic evaluation. Ann Emerg Med 2001;37(5):504–14.
[60] Schoepf UJ, Goldhaber SZ, Costello P. Spiral computed tomography for acute pulmonary embolism. Circulation 2004;109(18):2160–7.
[61] Fedullo PF, Tapson VF. Clinical practice: the evaluation of suspected pulmonary embolism. N Engl J Med 2003;349(13):1247–56.
[62] Khorasani R, Gudas TF, Nikpoor N, et al. Treatment of patients with suspected pulmonary embolism and intermediate probability lung scans: is diagnostic imaging underused? Am J Roentgenol 1997;169(5):1355–7.
[63] Miniati M, Pistolesi M, Marini C, et al. Value of perfusion lung scan in the diagnosis of pulmonary embolism: results of the Prospective Investigative Study of Acute Pulmonary Embolism Diagnosis (PISA-PED). Am J Respir Crit Care Med 1996;154(5):1387–93.
[64] Miniati M, Monti S, Bottai M. A structed clinical model for predicting the probability of pulmonary embolism. Am J Med 2003;114(3):173–9.

ELSEVIER
SAUNDERS

Emerg Med Clin N Am
23 (2005) 959–975

EMERGENCY
MEDICINE
CLINICS OF
NORTH AMERICA

Advances in Cardiac Biomarkers

Jennifer M. Aviles, MD[a,*], Ronnier J. Aviles, MD[b]

[a]*Department of Emergency Medicine, Boston University School of Medicine, Quincy Medical Center, Quincy, MA 02169, USA*

[b]*Cardiovascular Branch, Division of Intramural Research, National Heart, Lung, and Blood Institute, National Institutes of Health, 10 Center Drive, Building 10, Room 2c713, MSC 1538, Bethesda, MD 20892-1538, USA*

The use of cardiac biomarkers for the diagnosis and risk stratification of patients in the emergency department (ED) is evolving rapidly. Previously, the role of cardiac enzymes was restricted to the diagnosis of acute myocardial infarction (AMI). The identification of new biomarkers and more sensitive assays has extended the use of biomarkers beyond the diagnosis of cardiac necrosis. As novel biomarkers are identified, emergency physicians should be aware of both the potential clinical usefulness and the limitations of promising biomarkers. Testing should always be guided by a patient's history and physical examination to avoid misusing biomarkers as "screening" tools in critically ill patients. This update focuses on the present and future value of cardiac biomarkers in the care of patients who have suspected cardiac and cardiac-related diseases in the emergency department.

Technical aspects

When incorporating the results of biomarker investigations into clinical practice, it is important to understand a few technical aspects of biomarker assays, such as the type of assay used, precision (especially in point-of-care testing [POCT]), and performance relative to published or local hospital guidelines.

* Corresponding author.
E-mail address: javil001@umaryland.edu (J.M. Aviles).

0733-8627/05/$ - see front matter. Published by Elsevier Inc.
doi:10.1016/j.emc.2005.07.016

Assays

Knowledge of the types of biomarker assays that are performed locally is important. Different assays have different methods of detecting biomarkers and thus different levels of detection, precision, and cutoff values. Therefore, results from different assays for a specific biomarker are not comparable. For example, each troponin I (TnI) assay uses unique antibodies, which are directed at specific epitopes of troponin I to determine the protein concentration. These epitopes degrade at variable rates, resulting in a wide distribution of TnI values and detection limits. In contrast, the detection limit of the troponin T (TnT) assay is lower because, owing to patent rights, only one TnT assay is commercially available [1–3]. Another important issue is the precision and cutoff values used for each troponin assay. Although the European Society of Cardiology and the American College of Cardiology have recommended that the cutoff value for cardiac troponin represent the 99th percentile of a normal reference population with less than 10% imprecision, these guidelines have not been adopted universally [4,5]. Because of the lack of assay standardization, the true cutoff values and sensitivity and specificity of creatine kinase (CK)-MB, TnI, and TnT for myocardial injury are unknown [5].

When evaluating a novel biomarker for clinical use, it is important to evaluate the novel assay in light of the gold standard, the assay characteristics, and the patient population being tested. Often, characteristics of a novel assay are neither reported nor commercially available, making replication impossible. A gold standard that is less sensitive than the novel marker will limit results. For example, early troponin cutoff values were high because studies used CK-MB cutoff values and CK-MB receiver-operating curve characteristics as the gold standard. As troponin assays improved and minimally elevated troponin levels were found to be clinically significant, troponin cutoff values were lowered. However, the combination of lower troponin cutoff values and single versus serial troponin measurements significantly lower the sensitivity of troponin assays, causing new markers to appear stronger than troponin. Moreover, the sensitivity of a new marker, if reported for a selected population, can drop significantly when applied to a general chest pain population [6].

Point-of-care testing

The role of cardiac biomarkers in the diagnosis of acute coronary syndromes (ACS) and the importance of rapid diagnosis and rule-out protocols have led to the development of POCT. Recommended turnaround times for cardiac biomarkers are 30 to 60 minutes [7,8]. Point-of-care testing has been shown to decrease test turnaround times and emergency department (ED) lengths of stay [9]. Central laboratory assays are different from POCT assays. Many commercially available POCT assays use whole blood for analysis because proximity to patient care areas limits thrombosis

[10]. The cutoff values of other troponin POCT assays are higher because they are not as sensitive or precise compared with standard troponin assays. It is unknown whether the increased costs of POCT correlate with improved clinical outcomes or more rapid turnaround times alone [6]. Emergency physicians with access to POCT should consider the relative sensitivity and precision of POCT compared with central laboratory assays.

Biomarker testing guidelines

The testing guidelines for biomarkers of cardiac necrosis have been established by the National Academy of Clinical Biochemistry [8]. Although these guidelines refer specifically to biomarkers of necrosis, some principles may apply to the larger field of biomarkers. Blood collections should be referenced relative to the time of ED presentation, and two different markers should be used, an early marker (ie, myoglobin or CK-MB) and a later, rising definitive marker (TnI or TnT). The testing interval in patients who have diagnostic ECG findings should be shorter to facilitate monitoring of infarct size and complications (ie, infarct expansion or reinfarction). There is considerable variability in chest pain rule-out protocols. Most centers rule patients out within 6 to 9 hours of presentation. In centers without a rapid rule-out protocol, markers such as myoglobin may be unnecessary.

Acute myocardial infarction and unstable angina

Biomarkers of necrosis

Acute myocardial infarction refers to irreversible myocardial necrosis caused by an imbalance between oxygen supply and demand. In 75% of cases, plaque rupture and thrombus formation are the causes of acute coronary syndromes. Early diagnosis and subsequent reperfusion therapies within 4 to 6 hours of onset of symptoms can salvage myocardium at risk. Therefore, optimal markers of myocardial necrosis need to be rapidly detectable in blood.

Historically, markers of cardiac necrosis were measured by an assay of enzymatic activity. Present assays measure protein concentration; therefore, the terms biochemical diagnostic markers or biomarkers are more appropriate than cardiac enzymes [5].

In 2000, the definition of AMI was revised to include cardiac-specific markers of necrosis, troponins, and CK-MB. Older, nonspecific cardiac markers should not be used in the diagnosis of AMI (ie, total CK, aspartate amino transferase, lactate dehydrogenase, or lactate dehydrogenase isoenzymes) [7]. Moreover, the diagnostic threshold for AMI was lowered, considering any elevation in troponin levels to be diagnostic of AMI. The impact of these changes on clinical practice has been a substantial increase in the number of patients diagnosed with AMI [3,11,12].

Cardiac biomarkers have characteristic release and clearance kinetics. Thus, the time to presentation and comorbidities that affect clearance may confound the interpretation of biomarkers. Myoglobin is the earliest biochemical marker of myocardial cell damage, and it is detectable in blood within 1 to 2 hours of myocyte damage. Blood levels of CK-MB may be detectable in blood after 4 to 6 hours of myocardial ischemia [2]. Cardiac troponins are elevated within 4 to 12 hours of symptom onset and remain elevated for 4 to 10 days (Fig. 1) [13].

Based on these patterns of release and clearance, a diagnostic algorithm of serial biomarker measurements has been developed. Serial sampling of multiple cardiac markers beginning at the time of presentation is recommended currently. The sensitivity of serial measurements of multiple markers nears 100%, whereas the sensitivity of a single measurement of any biomarker at the time of presentation is poor. The recommended time between the first and second blood draw is 6 to 7 hours [14]. If cardiac marker levels are not elevated but clinical suspicion remains high, a third set of markers should be drawn at 12 to 24 hours after presentation [7]. The markers currently used in this multimarker approach are myoglobin, CK-MB, and troponin.

Myoglobin

Myoglobin is a heme protein found in the cytoplasm of cardiac and skeletal muscle cells that rises most rapidly after myocardial injury but is not

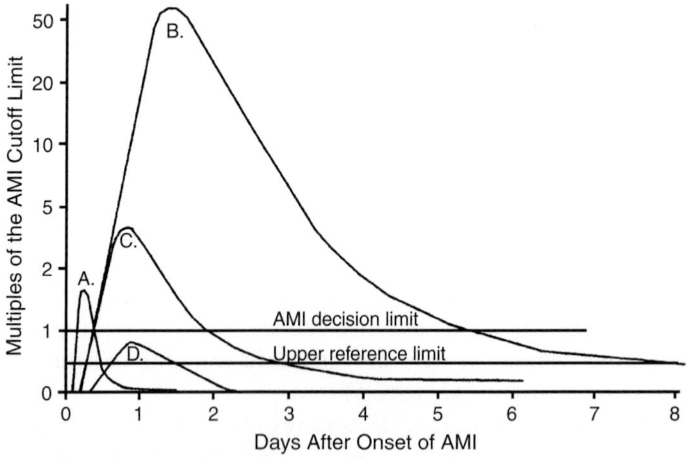

Fig. 1. Timing of release of various biomarkers after acute ischemic myocardial infarction. Peak A, early release of myoglobin or CK-MB isoforms after AMI; peak B, cardiac troponin after AMI; peak C, CK-MB after AMI; peak D, cardiac troponin after unstable angina. Data are plotted on a relative scale, where 1.0 is set at the AMI cutoff concentration. (*From* Wu AH, Apple FS, Gibler WB, et al. National Academy of Clinical Biochemistry Standards of Laboratory Practice: recommendations for the use of cardiac markers in coronary artery diseases. Clin Chem 1999;45:1104–21; with permission.)

cardiac-specific [2]. Myoglobin levels are frequently elevated in patients who have renal failure, skeletal muscle injury, trauma, and other diseases. Myoglobin is not used in most hospital laboratories.

Creatine kinase-MB isoform

CK-MB is an enzyme present primarily in cardiac muscle and active in energy generation. CK-MB is released rapidly after myocardial injury and is more cardiac-specific than myoglobin. However, CK-MB also comprises up to 5% of skeletal muscle and can be elevated in noncardiac disease states. Before the use of troponin, CK-MB was the gold standard for the biochemical diagnosis of AMI. CK-MB is released early during AMI, and it plays an important role in defining infarct size, infarct expansion, and reinfarction [15].

Cardiac troponins

Cardiac troponins and tropomyosin form the thin filament component of the contractile structure in striated muscle. Troponins are released into the blood stream following irreversible ischemic myocardial cell injury and remain elevated for a prolonged time. There is no clinical difference between TnT and TnI for diagnosing cardiac necrosis. There are separate cardiac and skeletal isoforms of both TnI and TnT, allowing for the development of highly cardiac-specific assays [13,16]. Troponin assays can detect as little as 1 g of myocardial tissue necrosis, and even minute elevations in cardiac troponins have been associated with myocardial necrosis and increased rate of short- and long-term mortality [7,17–19].

Cardiac troponins have been studied in symptomatic and asymptomatic patients who have renal dysfunction. It is important that emergency physicians include the patient's history and physical examination when considering an elevated troponin level in patients who have renal dysfunction. In patients in whom acute coronary syndrome is not suspected, renal failure may be associated with chronic elevations of TnI and TnT, without evidence of acute myocardial necrosis. However, an acute increase from baseline troponin levels may be associated with increased mortality [1,20]. Therefore, baseline troponin levels are helpful when differentiating between acute and chronic elevations in cardiac troponins.

Elevated levels of cardiac troponins in patients who have renal dysfunction may be attributable to decreased renal clearance and increased release from cytoplasm because of the loss of membrane integrity. TnT is of higher molecular weight and is more commonly present in the free, unbound form in the cytoplasm, potentially explaining why TnT is more frequently elevated than TnI [1]. A study of asymptomatic patients who had renal failure did not show TnI levels to be elevated in this population. The previously noted false-positive TnI results in patients who have renal failure were measured during acute disease states, including sepsis or pulmonary embolism, which may independently cause elevated troponin levels [21].

In symptomatic patients who have chest pain and renal dysfunction, elevated levels of cardiac troponin predict patients at an increased risk for adverse cardiovascular outcomes. In a study of 7033 patients who had suspected acute coronary syndromes, the elevated levels of TnT were predictive of death or myocardial infarction across the spectrum of creatinine clearance (Fig. 2) [22].

Despite the value of cardiac troponin as a very sensitive marker for myocardial damage, elevated troponin levels do not reflect the mechanism of damage and should not be used alone to diagnose myocardial infarction. Troponin levels may be elevated in patients who have myocarditis, pericarditis, decompensated heart failure, and septic shock. The use of troponin measurements as a screening tool in patients whose conditions have a low suspicion for ACS lowers the sensitivity and positive predictive value to 47% and 19%, respectively [23].

Biomarkers of cardiac ischemia

Infarct versus ischemia

Myocardial ischemia or unstable angina does not by definition cause myocyte necrosis and is not be identified by current markers of myocardial necrosis (CK-MB, TnI, and TnT). Studies using diagnostic criteria for AMI before 2000 may refer to troponin as a marker of ischemia; however, the

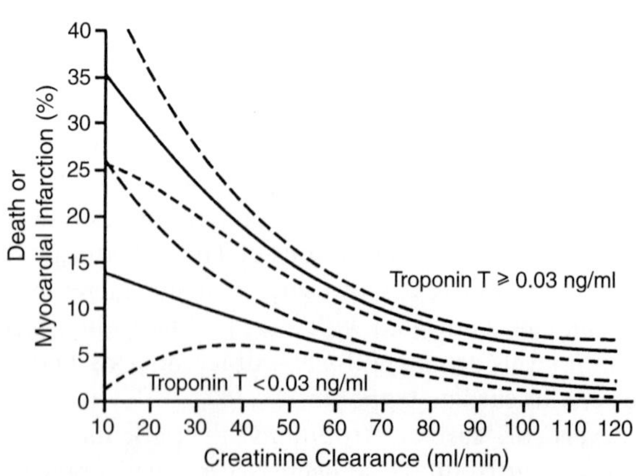

Fig. 2. Incidence of the death or myocardial infarction according to baseline troponin T level and creatinine clearance rate. The rate of death or myocardial infarction was significantly higher among patients who had a baseline troponin T level of 0.03 ng/mL or higher across the entire spectrum of creatinine clearance rates, according to an unadjusted analysis. The dashed lines indicate 95% CI. (*From* Aviles RJ, Askari AT, Lindahl B, et al. Troponin T levels in patients with acute coronary syndromes, with or without renal dysfunction. N Engl J Med 2002;346:2047–52; with permission.)

diagnosis of AMI was redefined in 2000 as any elevation in cardiac troponin coupled with clinical evidence of ACS [7].

Novel markers of ischemia are promising and may play an important role in risk-stratifying patients presenting to the emergency department with suspected ACS and no ECG or troponin/CK-MB evidence of AMI. Markers under study include ischemia-modified albumin (IMA) and key elements of the inflammatory cascade.

Ischemia-modified albumin

Ischemia-modified albumin is a novel marker of ischemia generated by the conformational modification in the N terminus of albumin, induced by the low pH environment during ischemia, and resulting in decreased transitional binding of cobalt to albumin [2]. The Albumin Cobalt Binding test was approved recently for the detection of myocardial ischemia by the US Food and Drug Administration.

IMA is sensitive not only for detecting myocardial ischemia, it also rises rapidly after ischemia onset [24,25]. In patients who are suspected of having ACS and nondiagnostic ECG findings on presentation to the ED, the sensitivity and specificity of IMA for identifying patients who have definite unstable angina are 75% and 75.6%, respectively [26]. Although IMA may be a useful marker for rapid ACS rule-out protocols, further research is needed.

Biomarkers of inflammation associated with cardiac ischemia

Atherosclerosis is an inflammatory disease, and all stages of plaque development and eventual rupture leading to acute coronary syndromes can be considered an inflammatory response to injury [27]. The identification of molecules in the inflammatory cascade with key roles in the pathogenesis of atherosclerosis has allowed investigation into their potential use as biomarkers for diagnosis and prognosis and potentially as targets of therapy in patients who have atherosclerotic disease. C-reactive protein (CRP) is the only inflammatory marker available clinically [28]. All other biomarkers of inflammation require additional study and assay standardization before clinical use. In the future, inflammatory markers may play a role in risk stratification and even early diagnosis of patients who have suspected ACS presenting to the ED [29]. The following overview provides the emergency physician with a mechanistic framework for future applications inflammatory biomarkers.

Normal endothelium resists the adhesion of circulating leukocytes. Early atheroma formation involves endothelial dysfunction and recruitment of leukocytes. Vascular cell adhesion molecule (VCAM)-1 has a particular affinity for monocytes and T lymphocytes. Other less selective molecules involved in endothelial leukocyte adhesion include intracellular adhesion molecule (ICAM)-1, P-selectin, and E-selectin. Clinical studies have shown an association between levels of VCAM-1, ICAM-1, and P-selectin and the prediction of cardiovascular risk [30–33].

The increased expression of VCAM may occur because of inflammation caused by modified lipoproteins, which accumulate in the intima. Low-density lipoprotein (LDL) is modified by many pathways, including oxidation, glycation (diabetes), aggregation, and immune complex formation [34]. Myeloperoxidase (MPO) is one pro-inflammatory enzyme active in LDL oxidation. Preliminary studies show promising results of MPO as a predictor of cardiovascular risk and as a diagnostic tool in patients in the ED who are suspected having ACS [35–37]. Other pro-inflammatory enzymes associated with increased cardiovascular risk are lipoprotein-associated phospholipase-A2 and pregnancy-associated plasma protein-A [38–40].

Leukocyte homing to a growing atheroma in the arterial intima is facilitated by chemoattractant cytokines, such as monocyte chemoattractant protein-1 and, possibly, interleukin (IL)-8. Once in the arterial intima, monocytes undergo a sequence of morphologic changes and become macrophages. Macrophage-colony stimulating factor contributes to inducing these changes. Macrophages take up modified LDL and ultimately become foam cells, the pathologic hallmark of the atherosclerotic plaque.

Atheroma progression occurs in bursts, likely caused by a physical disruption because of superficial erosion, microvascular disruption and hemorrhage, and fracture of the fibrous plaque. Two possible mechanisms of superficial erosion are cell death and disruption of the basement membrane. Cell death may occur because of local inflammatory mediators or cytolytic attack. Inflammatory mediators and oxidated lipoproteins stimulate matrix metalloproteinases (MMP), which degrade the basement membrane. Neovascularization and subsequent hemorrhage are likely promoted by vascular endothelial growth factor.

The fracture of the fibrous cap is perhaps the most important cause of atheromic disruption. Together, the interferon-γ–induced decreased collagen production and increased collagenases activity of MMP-1, -8, and -12 contribute to the fracture of the fibrous cap. The fibrous cap is further weakened by gelatinases, including MMP-2 and -9. MMP-9 has been associated with premature coronary atherosclerosis and cardiovascular disease [29]. Inflammatory mediators in the atheroma that increase MMP expression include IL-1β, tumor necrosis factor-α, and CD40-ligand. Studies of CD40-ligand have shown convincing evidence that it is an early marker of cardiovascular disease and is potentially useful as a diagnostic and prognostic tool [34,41–45].

The triggers for the inflammatory cascade and endothelial dysfunction are not well understood. Possible causes include modified LDL, free radicals released because of tobacco use, diabetes, hypertension, homocysteine, genetic alterations, infection, and lipoprotein (a). Homocysteine and lipoprotein (a) have been investigated for prognosis and as potential therapeutic targets, and early results are encouraging.

Acute-phase reactants, indicators of systemic inflammation, have been associated with an increased cardiovascular risk. The acute-phase reactants that have been studied in cardiovascular disease include CRP, fibrinogen, and serum amyloid-A. Among acute-phase reactants, CRP is the strongest predictor of cardiovascular risk. CRP is produced in the liver in response to IL-6 and is also present in coronary artery smooth muscle cells [46]. Many studies have shown that CRP adds to the prediction of cardiovascular risk above and beyond the prediction by traditional risk factors, although a few investigators recently have questioned this assertion. A joint panel convened by the Centers of Disease Control and the American Heart Association recommends the use of CRP for the risk assessment of patients who have an intermediate risk of cardiovascular disease [28]. Although preliminary research is promising, with the exception of CRP, none of the inflammatory biomarkers has a current diagnostic, prognostic, or therapeutic role in clinical practice.

Congestive heart failure

Brain natriuretic peptide and heart failure

In the current era of thrombolytics and invasive therapy for ACS, a growing number of patients who have left ventricular systolic dysfunction are surviving and presenting to the emergency department with symptoms of decompensated congestive heart failure (CHF). Brain-type natriuretic peptide (BNP) is the first biomarker with promising diagnostic and prognostic properties that may add to the physician's assessment of CHF.

BNP and its analog atrial natriuretic hormone (ANP) are neuroendocrine hormones that participate in fluid homeostasis. BNP is produced and secreted by the ventricles, and together, BNP and ANP increase urine volume and urine sodium excretion, vascular smooth muscle relaxation, and the inhibition of the renin-angiotensin-aldosterone system and sympathetic nervous system (Fig. 3) [47]. BNP is proportionately increased in conditions of high volume states, poor left ventricular function, and ventricular hypertrophy [3].

BNP and N-terminal (NT) pro-BNP, its inactive form, have different clearance kinetics, and both can be measured in serum; this has given rise to the development of multiple assays, each with unique characteristics, which has made comparisons complicated. In fact, an evaluation of the relative performance of the different assays is still necessary [48,49]. Another source of variability is that baseline BNP levels increase with age and are higher in women than in men [48]. To establish appropriate reference ranges, the distribution of BNP in different populations still needs to be determined.

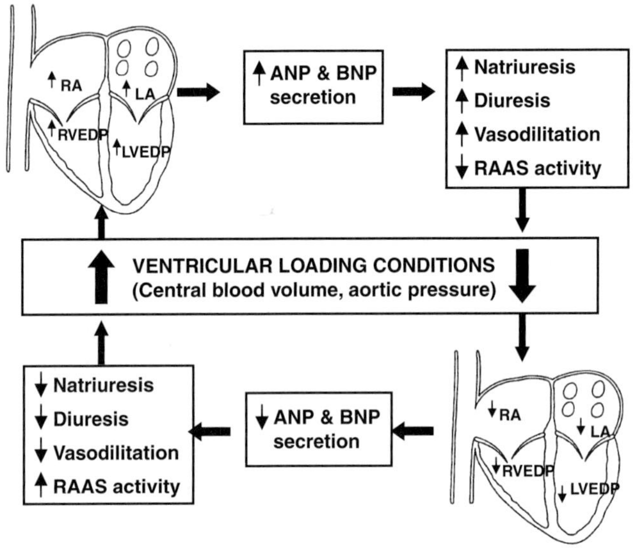

Fig. 3. Mechanism by which cardiac secretion of natriuretic peptides serves to maintain intravascular volume homeostasis. LA, left atrium; LVEDP, left ventricular end-diastolic pressure; RA, right atrium; RAAS, renin-angiotensin-aldosterone system; RVEDP, right ventricular end-diastolic pressure. (*From* Rodeheffer RJ. Measuring B-type natriuretic peptide in heart failure: good to go in 2004? J Am Coll Cardiol 2004;44:740–9; with permission.)

BNP levels have potential diagnostic value in distinguishing between cardiac and pulmonary causes of acute dyspnea. Davis and colleagues [50] first demonstrated that BNP levels differentiate between acutely dyspneic patients who have a primary lung disorder versus patients who have decompensated CHF. Subsequent studies have confirmed these results. In 250 patients who had dyspnea presenting to an urgent care setting, an elevated level of BNP was found to be highly sensitive (96%) and specific (96%) for the diagnosis of CHF. In this study, BNP alone was far more sensitive than the history, symptoms, signs, chest radiography, or ECG in identifying patients who have CHF. However, the specificity of BNP was similar to the history of CHF, signs on physical examination, chest radiography, and EKG [51]. Another study of 321 patients who had acute dyspnea presenting to the ED has shown that BNP is valuable even in patients who have a history of lung disease and current heart failure [52].

The multicenter Breathing Not Properly (BNP) study of 1586 acutely dyspneic patients aimed to confirm the results of previous studies and to characterize the potential clinical use of BNP [53]. BNP not only correlated closely with the severity of CHF by New York Heart Association (NYHA) class, it also predicted patients at an increased risk for CHF (odds ratio 29.6) and added significant information to other clinical indicators of CHF. A subgroup analysis found that BNP was useful in diagnosing new cases of

CHF, even in patients who had chronic obstructive pulmonary disease or reactive airway disease [54]. Moreover, BNP was shown to improve the diagnostic accuracy of CHF in patients who have acute dyspnea from 74% to 81%, particularly in patients who have an intermediate pretest probability [55].

An important limitation of BNP studies is the lack of a gold standard for the diagnosis of CHF. Decompensated CHF is a clinical diagnosis. Studies of BNP or any marker of CHF must choose between using a standard of physician assessment of clinical symptoms versus an echocardiographic standard of left ventricular (LV) dysfunction (systolic or diastolic or both). Both standards are potentially flawed. For example, if BNP is a more sensitive marker for CHF than physician assessment is, BNP can appear worse in performance analyses because additional cases CHF identified by BNP would be considered false-positives. In contrast, patients who have LV dysfunction may not exhibit any clinical signs of decompensated heart failure, yet elevated levels BNP may still be detected.

BNP is also an attractive indicator of prognosis in patients who have CHF. In a population-based study of 3346 asymptomatic patients in whom BNP levels correlated with a preclinical probability of CHF, both BNP and NT-proBNP levels predicted patients at increased risk of death and cardiovascular events, even after adjustment for traditional risk factors [56]. In symptomatic patients who have CHF, elevated levels of BNP also portend a poor prognosis. In a substudy of the Carvedilol Prospective Randomized Cumulative Survival (COPERNICUS) trial [49] of 2289 patients who had severe chronic CHF, elevated levels of NT-proBNP were universally associated with an increased risk for all-cause mortality and hospitalization for heart failure during follow-up. Similarly, in a study of 452 patients who had chronic CHF, BNP was the only predictor of sudden cardiac death [57].

BNP levels drawn in the ED during evaluation for acute dyspnea are also predictive of cardiovascular risk. In a study of 325 patients who had acute dyspnea, elevated BNP levels were associated with progressively worse prognosis over 6 months, including more CHF deaths and hospital admissions or repeat ED visits [58]. In the multicenter Rapid Emergency Department Heart Failure Outpatient Trial (REDHOT) [59], physicians were blinded to BNP levels. Although there was no association between BNP levels and physician decisions to admit patients, NYHA functional class or short-term mortality in this study, BNP was a strong predictor of 90-day outcomes including CHF visits, admissions, and mortality. Moreover, hospitalized patients who had clinically severe disease but lower BNP levels seemed to have a better prognosis than patients who had higher BNP levels, suggesting that BNP may play a role in selecting patients who would benefit from aggressive inpatient management.

Treatment and admission decisions that consider BNP levels have been shown to affect hospital stay and the cost of medical care. In the B-type

Natriuretic Peptide for Acute Shortness of Breath Evaluation study [60] of 452 patients, the diagnostic use of BNP in addition to clinical history and examination resulted in reduced admission rates, from 75% to 85% (P = .008), reduced hospital stays, from 8.0 to 11.0 days (P = .001), decreased intensive care unit admissions, from 15% to 24% (P = .01), and reduced cost of treatment, from $7262 to $5410 ($P$ = .006). These notable differences are presumably attributable to the earlier administration of appropriate therapy, the establishment of timely alternative diagnoses, and the use of BNP results in lieu of other costly diagnostic tests [47]. More study is needed in this area to determine if BNP has an impact on cost-effective outcomes or BNP is primarily a biomarker useful for diagnosis and prognosis.

Despite promising results, emergency physicians should remain cautiously optimistic about the use of BNP in clinical practice. BNP should not be used alone or indiscriminately as a screening tool [3,61]. Instead, the results of BNP measurements need to be evaluated in light of a clinical assessment in patients who have suspected heart failure. Until the impact of BNP on clinical decision making is fully elucidated, the history and physical examination will continue to guide diagnosis, therapy, and disposition in patients who have heart failure.

Troponins and heart failure

Elevated troponin levels have been associated with heart failure. Elevated troponin levels can be found in as many as 15% to 52% of patients who have stable chronic CHF. The mechanism mediating this elevation is not known, but presumably it is associated with chronic cellular injury, remodeling, and release of inflammatory molecules. Although there is a paucity of data assessing troponin levels and heart failure, elevated troponin levels have been associated with worse clinical and functional status and poor long-term prognosis [16]. Further research is necessary before the results of preliminary studies are clinically useful.

Other clinical entities causing elevations in cardiac biomarkers

Pulmonary embolism

The mechanism responsible for elevated troponin, CK-MB, and BNP biomarkers in patients who have pulmonary embolism (PE) relate to right ventricular myocardial injury. Although LV ischemia in patients who have coronary disease theoretically may contribute, studies do not support this notion [16]. The distribution curve for troponin levels in patients who have PE is smaller, with an early peak (4 hours) and return to baseline [1,62]. Elevated levels of cardiac biomarkers may be useful in identifying higher risk patients who have PE [63].

Myocarditis or myopericarditis

Troponin levels are elevated in approximately 50% of patients who have clinically suspected myocarditis [64]. When a histologic diagnosis of myocarditis is confirmed, troponin levels usually are elevated. Clinical studies have shown an association between elevated troponins and onset of heart failure symptoms in patients who have myocarditis [65].

In patients who have acute pericarditis, the elevation in troponin levels has been attributed to injury of the epicardial layer of the myocardium in immediate proximity to an inflamed visceral pericardium [16]. Bonnefoy and colleagues [66] have shown that half of the patients who had idiopathic pericarditis included in their study had elevated troponins. Patients with higher troponin values were more likely to have ST-segment elevation, were younger, and had had a recent episode of systemic infection.

Septic and critically ill patients

The mechanism accounting for elevated troponin levels in patients who have sepsis and critically ill patients relates to stress-induced microvascular ischemic injury and direct myocytotoxic injury by infectious organisms and inflammatory mediators. Studies have identified elevated troponin levels in 50% to 85% of patients who have septic and hypovolemic shock [16].

Cardiac contusion

Patients with trauma and cardiac contusion are at risk for life-threatening arrhythmias and heart failure in the first 24 to 28 hours. Therefore, the early identification of cardiac contusion is of great importance. Cardiac troponins are highly sensitive in identifying patients who have myocardial injury attributable to cardiac contusion. The histologic appearance of myocardial contusion is nearly identical to AMI. Troponin levels peak earlier compared with AMI, and if baseline levels are normal, only a second measurement 4 to 6 hours later is required to exclude a diagnosis of myocardial injury [67].

Summary

The use of cardiac biomarkers in the emergency department continues to evolve. The close link of biomarkers to the pathophysiology of cardiovascular disease makes biomarkers attractive diagnostic and prognostic tools. A few markers have gained wide acceptance in clinical practice, wherease others remain works in progress. Consensus statements have reaffirmed the role of cardiac troponins in patients who are suspected of having acute coronary syndromes, and brain natriuretic peptide has proven useful in the diagnostic work-up of patients who have dyspnea. Other candidate markers, such as members of the inflammatory cascade, remain under active investigation, with limited or no clinical value. Despite these advances, it is important to highlight that the high sensitivities, specificities, and predictive value of novel biomarkers are only applicable when using the patient's history and physical examination to guide biomarker testing.

References

[1] Hamm CW, Giannitsis E, Katus HA. Cardiac troponin elevations in patients without acute coronary syndrome. Circulation 2002;106:2871–2.

[2] Azzazy HM, Christenson RH. Cardiac markers of acute coronary syndromes: is there a case for point-of-care testing? Clin Biochem 2002;35:13–27.

[3] Panteghini M. Role and importance of biochemical markers in clinical cardiology. Eur Heart J 2004;25:1187–96.

[4] Braunwald E, Antman EM, Beasley JW, et al. ACC/AHA guidelines for the management of patients with unstable angina and non-ST-segment elevation myocardial infarction: executive summary and recommendations: a report of the American College of Cardiology/American Heart Association task force on practice guidelines (committee on the management of patients with unstable angina). Circulation 2000;102:1193–209.

[5] Jaffe AS, Ravkilde J, Roberts R, et al. It's time for a change to a troponin standard. Circulation 2000;102:1216–20.

[6] Jaffe AS, Katus H. Acute coronary syndrome biomarkers: the need for more adequate reporting. Circulation 2004;110:104–6.

[7] Alpert JS, Thygesen K, Antman E, et al. Myocardial infarction redefined: a consensus document of The Joint European Society of Cardiology/American College of Cardiology Committee for the redefinition of myocardial infarction. J Am Coll Cardiol 2000;36:959–69.

[8] Wu AH, Apple FS, Gibler WB, et al. National Academy of Clinical Biochemistry Standards of Laboratory Practice: recommendations for the use of cardiac markers in coronary artery diseases. Clin Chem 1999;45:1104–21.

[9] Lee-Lewandrowski E, Corboy D, Lewandrowski K, et al. Implementation of a point-of-care satellite laboratory in the emergency department of an academic medical center: impact on test turnaround time and patient emergency department length of stay. Arch Pathol Lab Med 2003;127:456–60.

[10] Wu AH, Smith A, Christenson RH, et al. Evaluation of a point-of-care assay for cardiac markers for patients suspected of acute myocardial infarction. Clin Chim Acta 2004;346:211–9.

[11] Kontos MC, Fritz LM, Anderson FP, et al. Impact of the troponin standard on the prevalence of acute myocardial infarction. Am Heart J 2003;146:446–52.

[12] Koukkunen H, Penttila K, Kemppainen A, et al. Differences in the diagnosis of myocardial infarction by troponin T compared with clinical and epidemiologic criteria. Am J Cardiol 2001;88:727–31.

[13] Newby LK. Markers of cardiac ischemia, injury, and inflammation. Prog Cardiovasc Dis 2004;46:404–16.

[14] Balk EM, Ioannidis JP, Salem D, et al. Accuracy of biomarkers to diagnose acute cardiac ischemia in the emergency department: a meta-analysis. Ann Emerg Med 2001;37:478–94.

[15] Panteghini M. Acute coronary syndrome: biochemical strategies in the troponin era. Chest 2002;122:1428–35.

[16] Roongsritong C, Warraich I, Bradley C. Common causes of troponin elevations in the absence of acute myocardial infarction: incidence and clinical significance. Chest 2004;125:1877–84.

[17] Cantwell RV, Aviles RJ, Bjornsson J, et al. Cardiac amyloidosis presenting with elevations of cardiac troponin I and angina pectoris. Clin Cardiol 2002;25:33–7.

[18] Aviles RJ, Wright RS, Aviles JM, et al. Long-term prognosis of patients with clinical unstable angina pectoris without elevation of creatine kinase but with elevation of cardiac troponin i levels. Am J Cardiol 2002;90:875–8.

[19] Antman EM, Tanasijevic MJ, Thompson B, et al. Cardiac-specific troponin I levels to predict the risk of mortality in patients with acute coronary syndromes. N Engl J Med 1996; 335:1342–9.
[20] Apple FS, Murakami MM, Pearce LA, et al. Predictive value of cardiac troponin I and T for subsequent death in end-stage renal disease. Circulation 2002;106:2941–5.
[21] Donnino MW, Karriem-Norwood V, Rivers EP, et al. Prevalence of elevated troponin I in end-stage renal disease patients receiving hemodialysis. Acad Emerg Med 2004;11:979–81.
[22] Aviles RJ, Askari AT, Lindahl B, et al. Troponin T levels in patients with acute coronary syndromes, with or without renal dysfunction. N Engl J Med 2002;346:2047–52.
[23] Polanczyk CA, Lee TH, Cook EF, et al. Cardiac troponin I as a predictor of major cardiac events in emergency department patients with acute chest pain. J Am Coll Cardiol 1998;32: 8–14.
[24] Quiles J, Roy D, Gaze D, et al. Relation of ischemia-modified albumin (IMA) levels following elective angioplasty for stable angina pectoris to duration of balloon-induced myocardial ischemia. Am J Cardiol 2003;92:322–4.
[25] Sinha MK, Gaze DC, Tippins JR, et al. Ischemia modified albumin is a sensitive marker of myocardial ischemia after percutaneous coronary intervention. Circulation 2003;107: 2403–5.
[26] Roy D, Quiles J, Aldama G, et al. Ischemia modified albumin for the assessment of patients presenting to the emergency department with acute chest pain but normal or non-diagnostic 12-lead electrocardiograms and negative cardiac troponin T. Int J Cardiol 2004;97:297–301.
[27] Libby P. Inflammation in atherosclerosis. Nature 2002;420:868–74.
[28] Smith SC Jr, Anderson JL, Cannon RO III, et al. CDC/AHA workshop on markers of inflammation and cardiovascular disease: application to clinical and public health practice: report from the clinical practice discussion group. Circulation 2004;110:e550–3.
[29] Ridker PM, Brown NJ, Vaughan DE, et al. Established and emerging plasma biomarkers in the prediction of first atherothrombotic events. Circulation 2004;109:IV6–19.
[30] Hwang SJ, Ballantyne CM, Sharrett AR, et al. Circulating adhesion molecules VCAM-1, ICAM-1, and E-selectin in carotid atherosclerosis and incident coronary heart disease cases: the Atherosclerosis Risk In Communities (ARIC) study. Circulation 1997;96:4219–25.
[31] Blake GJ, Ridker PM. Inflammatory bio-markers and cardiovascular risk prediction. J Intern Med 2002;252:283–94.
[32] Ridker PM, Hennekens CH, Roitman-Johnson B, et al. Plasma concentration of soluble intercellular adhesion molecule 1 and risks of future myocardial infarction in apparently healthy men. Lancet 1998;351:88–92.
[33] Ridker PM, Hennekens CH, Buring JE, et al. C-reactive protein and other markers of inflammation in the prediction of cardiovascular disease in women. N Engl J Med 2000;342: 836–43.
[34] Ross R. Atherosclerosis–an inflammatory disease. N Engl J Med 1999;340:115–26.
[35] Brennan ML, Penn MS, Van Lente F, et al. Prognostic value of myeloperoxidase in patients with chest pain. N Engl J Med 2003;349:1595–604.
[36] Zhang R, Brennan ML, Fu X, et al. Association between myeloperoxidase levels and risk of coronary artery disease. JAMA 2001;286:2136–42.
[37] Baldus S, Heeschen C, Meinertz T, et al. Myeloperoxidase serum levels predict risk in patients with acute coronary syndromes. Circulation 2003;108:1440–5.
[38] Packard CJ, O'Reilly DS, Caslake MJ, et al for the West of Scotland Coronary Prevention Study Group. Lipoprotein-associated phospholipase A2 as an independent predictor of coronary heart disease. N Engl J Med 2000;343:1148–55.
[39] Bayes-Genis A, Conover CA, Overgaard MT, et al. Pregnancy-associated plasma protein A as a marker of acute coronary syndromes. N Engl J Med 2001;345:1022–9.
[40] Lund J, Qin QP, Ilva T, et al. Circulating pregnancy-associated plasma protein a predicts outcome in patients with acute coronary syndrome but no troponin I elevation. Circulation 2003;108:1924–6.

[41] Freedman JE. CD40 ligand: assessing risk instead of damage? N Engl J Med 2003;348: 1163–5.
[42] Aggarwal A, Schneider DJ, Terrien EF, et al. Increased coronary arterial release of interleukin-1 receptor antagonist and soluble CD40 ligand indicative of inflammation associated with culprit coronary plaques. Am J Cardiol 2004;93:6–9.
[43] Schonbeck U, Varo N, Libby P, et al. Soluble CD40L and cardiovascular risk in women. Circulation 2001;104:2266–8.
[44] Heeschen C, Dimmeler S, Hamm CW, et al. Soluble CD40 ligand in acute coronary syndromes. N Engl J Med 2003;348:1104–11.
[45] Varo N, de Lemos JA, Libby P, et al. Soluble CD40L: risk prediction after acute coronary syndromes. Circulation 2003;108:1049–52.
[46] Pearson TA, Mensah GA, Alexander RW, et al. Markers of inflammation and cardiovascular disease: application to clinical and public health practice: a statement for healthcare professionals from the Centers for Disease Control and Prevention and the American Heart Association. Circulation 2003;107:499–511.
[47] Mark DB, Felker GM. B-type natriuretic peptided: a biomarker for all seasons? N Engl J Med 2004;350:718–20.
[48] Redfield MM, Rodeheffer RJ, Jacobsen SJ, et al. Plasma brain natriuretic peptide concentration: impact of age and gender. J Am Coll Cardiol 2002;40:976–82.
[49] Hartmann F, Packer M, Coats AJ, et al. Prognostic impact of plasma N-terminal pro-brain natriuretic peptide in severe chronic congestive heart failure: a substudy of the Carvedilol Prospective Randomized Cumulative Survival (COPERNICUS) trial. Circulation 2004;110: 1780–6.
[50] Davis M, Espiner E, Richards G, et al. Plasma brain natriuretic peptide in assessment of acute dyspnoea. Lancet 1994;343:440–4.
[51] Dao Q, Krishnaswamy P, Kazanegra R, et al. Utility of B-type natriuretic peptide in the diagnosis of congestive heart failure in an urgent-care setting. J Am Coll Cardiol 2001;37: 379–85.
[52] Morrison LK, Harrison A, Krishnaswamy P, et al. Utility of a rapid B-natriuretic peptide assay in differentiating congestive heart failure from lung disease in patients presenting with dyspnea. J Am Coll Cardiol 2002;39:202–9.
[53] Maisel AS, Krishnaswamy P, Nowak RM, et al. Rapid measurement of B-type natriuretic peptide in the emergency diagnosis of heart failure. N Engl J Med 2002;347: 161–7.
[54] McCullough PA, Hollander JE, Nowak RM, et al. Uncovering heart failure in patients with a history of pulmonary disease: rationale for the early use of B-type natriuretic peptide in the emergency department. Acad Emerg Med 2003;10:198–204.
[55] McCullough PA, Nowak RM, McCord J, et al. B-type natriuretic peptide and clinical judgment in emergency diagnosis of heart failure: analysis from Breathing Not Properly (BNP) Multinational Study. Circulation 2002;106:416–22.
[56] Wang TJ, Larson MG, Levy D, et al. Plasma natriuretic peptide levels and the risk of cardiovascular events and death. N Engl J Med 2004;350:655–63.
[57] Berger R, Huelsman M, Strecker K, et al. B-type natriuretic peptide predicts sudden death in patients with chronic heart failure. Circulation 2002;105:2392–7.
[58] Harrison A, Morrison LK, Krishnaswamy P, et al. B-type natriuretic peptide predicts future cardiac events in patients presenting to the emergency department with dyspnea. Ann Emerg Med 2002;39:131–8.
[59] Maisel A, Hollander JE, Guss D, et al. Primary results of the Rapid Emergency Department Heart Failure Outpatient Trial (REDHOT): a multicenter study of B-type natriuretic peptide levels, emergency department decision making, and outcomes in patients presenting with shortness of breath. J Am Coll Cardiol 2004;44:1328–33.
[60] Mueller C, Scholer A, Laule-Kilian K, et al. Use of B-type natriuretic peptide in the evaluation and management of acute dyspnea. N Engl J Med 2004;350:647–54.

[61] Packer M. Should B-type natriuretic peptide be measured routinely to guide the diagnosis and management of chronic heart failure? Circulation 2003;108:2950–3.
[62] Konstantinides S, Geibel A, Olschewski M, et al. Importance of cardiac troponins I and T in risk stratification of patients with acute pulmonary embolism. Circulation 2002;106:1263–8.
[63] Fedullo PF, Tapson VF. Clinical practice: the evaluation of suspected pulmonary embolism. N Engl J Med 2003;349:1247–56.
[64] Lauer B, Niederau C, Kuhl U, et al. Cardiac troponin T in patients with clinically suspected myocarditis. J Am Coll Cardiol 1997;30:1354–9.
[65] Smith SC, Ladenson JH, Mason JW, et al. Elevations of cardiac troponin I associated with myocarditis: experimental and clinical correlates. Circulation 1997;95:163–8.
[66] Bonnefoy E, Godon P, Kirkorian G, et al. Serum cardiac troponin I and ST-segment elevation in patients with acute pericarditis. Eur Heart J 2000;21:832–6.
[67] Sybrandy KC, Cramer MJ, Burgersdijk C. Diagnosing cardiac contusion: old wisdom and new insights. Heart 2003;89:485–9.

ELSEVIER
SAUNDERS

Emerg Med Clin N Am
23 (2005) 977–998

EMERGENCY
MEDICINE
CLINICS OF
NORTH AMERICA

Noninvasive Imaging Techniques to Aid in the Triage of Patients with Suspected Acute Coronary Syndrome: A Review

Katrina Barnett, MD, James A. Feldman, MD*

Department of Emergency Medicine, Boston Medical Center/ Boston University School of Medicine, 1 BMC Place, Boston, MA 02118, USA

Evaluating patients who present with symptoms suggestive of acute coronary syndrome (ACS) to the Emergency Department (ED) remains one of the greatest clinical challenges in emergency medicine. The emergency physician must consider this diagnosis in patients who present with a broad range of symptoms, including chest pain and chest pain equivalents (shoulder, jaw, epigastric, or back pain) as well as any acute cardiovascular complaint (dyspnea, syncope, or palpitations). Furthermore, many patient subgroups with ACS will present either with "atypical features," including weakness or confusion in elderly or diabetic patients, or as a secondary process in patients with an acute medical condition such as sepsis or shock. Patients also can present at varying intervals from symptom onset or symptom resolution to the ED. They may have previous cardiac disease or baseline EKG abnormalities that further complicate the initial triage decision-making.

The approach to patients who are clinically unstable or have diagnostic EKG abnormalities is well defined. Cardiac biomarkers play an important role in the evaluation of patients with suspected ACS who have EKGs that are considered nondiagnostic. However, biomarkers often require serial measurement over 6 to 8 hours [1]. Although shorter intervals have been reported (presentation and 90 minutes) [2,3], and efforts are in progress to identify new biomarkers, such as activated platelets, that could potentially identify ACS before myocardial necrosis occurs [4–6], these measures have not been examined in well-controlled clinical trials [7,8]. The present approach in many chest pain centers is to, first, exclude myocardial necrosis

* Corresponding author.
E-mail address: jfeldma@bu.edu (J.A. Feldman).

doi:10.1016/j.emc.2005.07.011

with serial EKG and biomarker sampling and, second, to unmask or identify cardiac ischemia with some provocative test. These provocative tests are briefly reviewed in this article.

It is worth noting that there are some reports that advocate an early invasive diagnostic strategy with the liberal use of coronary angiography to definitively complete the triage evaluation [9]. Given the evidence favoring an early interventional approach for both ST-segment elevation myocardial infarction (STEMI) and non-STEMI patients [10,11], many centers may start to divide chest-pain patients into high-risk and low-risk categories and undertake an early invasive approach for all patients in the high-risk group. However, the ideal diagnostic test would rapidly, accurately, and non-invasively answer two key questions at the time of the initial evaluation: (1) whether there is evidence of myocardial ischemia; and (2) whether there is significant obstruction of coronary blood flow, which is the most common cause of cardiac ischemia.

This article reviews the use of noninvasive tests to aid in the triage of patients with suspected ACS. Discussion describes available noninvasive imaging modalities for the rapid evaluation of suspected ACS (listed below). The provocative tests used after a "rule out MI" observation is made to identify clinically significant symptomatic coronary artery disease.

- Transthoracic echocardiography
- Acute radioisotope perfusion imaging
    - CT scanning
    - Calcium scoring
- CT coronary angiography
- Magnetic resonance imaging or magnetic resonance angiography

Transthoracic echocardiography

Transthoracic echocardiography is a noninvasive diagnostic modality that can be used in the triage of patients who have active symptoms suggestive of ACS but a nondiagnostic EKG. When limited to those studies performed in the ED, a systematic review indicated that rest echocardiography had excellent sensitivity (93%; 95% CI, 81%-97%) and good specificity (66%; 95% CI, 43%-83%) [12]. The American College of Cardiology (ACC)/American Heart Association (AHA) Guidelines on the Clinical Use of Echocardiography [13] note that the absence of segmental wall motion abnormalities has a high negative predictive value ("weighted mean negative predictive value as high as 98% in suspected myocardial infarction"). However, only three of the published studies on rest echocardiography have evaluated patients strictly in the ED setting for acute myocardial infarction (AMI) (total number of subjects, 397) [12].

Although it is noninvasive, echocardiography is highly dependent on the operator and reader and may be less useful in patients whose symptoms have resolved before ED arrival or who have pre-existing wall motion abnormalities. The actual clinical impact of rest echocardiography has not been carefully studied in a well-designed clinical trial, and its clinical effect was considered "not known" in a systematic review [8]. However, the AHA/ACC Guidelines on Echocardiography [13] do list the use of echocardiography as a class I indication in the diagnosis of chest pain in patients with suspected acute myocardial ischemia when baseline EKG and other laboratory markers are nondiagnostic and the study can be obtained either during pain or within minutes after the abatement of pain. Ioannidis and colleagues [12] state that "the existing evidence suggests that rest echocardiography can have a very good and probably excellent performance in the diagnosis of AMI and ACI in selected groups of patients" and that "the data pertain mostly to low risk patients who have normal or nondiagnostic EKGs."

There are no well-designed prospective trials of ED-based echocardiography (ECHO) studies that include diverse practice settings and a broad population of patients being evaluated for possible ACS, in which patients with negative studies are discharged directly from the ED. Furthermore, the definition of a "positive study" has varied in the cohort studies available. Kontos and colleagues [14], for example, have considered a positive ECHO to have any of the following: (1) abnormal wall motion of two or more contiguous segments; (2) abnormal wall motion of one segment visible in two different views; or (3) global hypokinesis with an estimated ejection fraction of less than 40%. Lim and colleagues [15] have defined a positive ECHO as segmental wall motion abnormalities or global myocardial dysfunction, and patients who had negative ECHOs underwent graded exercise EKG testing before discharge.

Newer techniques such as harmonic imaging and the use of myocardial contrast agents may enhance the utility of transthoracic ECHO in the ED [16], but the clinical impact of these methods must be demonstrated in prospective clinical trials. Both pressure within the myocardium and exposure to ultrasound destroys microbubbles. The development of lower energy imaging methods that can image microbubbles without destroying them and advances in the development of microbubbles that can be injected intravenously may soon allow noninvasive assessment of myocardial perfusion at the bedside [17,18]. Fig. 1 demonstrates the use of contrast-enhanced echocardiography to demonstrate failed and successful thrombolysis in patients with acute myocardial infarction.

Myocardial perfusion imaging

For more than 25 years, investigators have explored the use of radioactive isotopes as a means of noninvasively evaluating coronary perfusion in patients who are evaluated in the ED for suspected ACS. In 1979, Wackers and colleagues [19] described the use of thallium, a potassium analog, to aid

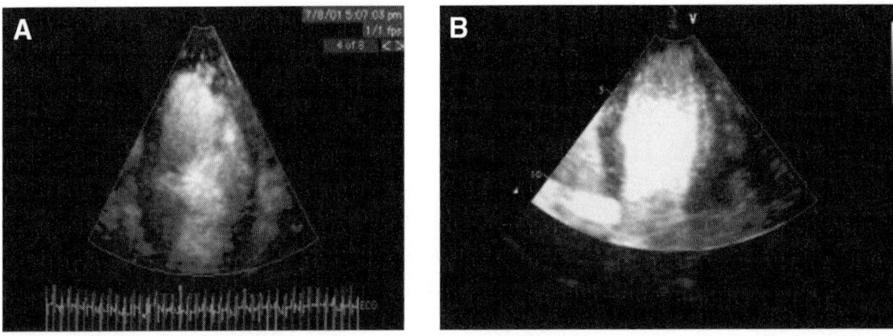

Fig. 1. Apical four-chamber view of myocardial contrast echocardiography using intermittent power Doppler imaging triggered at end systole after injection of a 0.5 mL bolus of erflutren Protein-Type A Microspheres for Injection, USP. (*A*) Patient with recent anteroseptal myocardial infarction treated with thrombolysis but no clinical evidence of reperfusion. Absence of perfusion in septum and apex (*black*) compared with apical lateral segment (*brown*) is readily appreciated. There is some dropout in the basal lateral segment caused by attenuation from apical contrast. (*B*) Patient with anterseptal myocardial infarction treated successfully with thrombolysis (ventricular walls brown). Normal contrast uptake is noted in the septum with minor apical defect only. (*From* Stewart MJ. Contrast echocardiography. Heart 2003;89:342–8; with permission from BMJ Publishing Group.)

in the triage of patients who had chest pain. Many centers have incorporated perfusion imaging into risk stratification protocols with or without cardiac biomarker testing. The clinical impact of this technology also has been described in a multicenter controlled clinical trial [20].

The strength of acute perfusion imaging is its ability to demonstrate specific abnormalities in myocardial perfusion. Some evidence suggests that studies remain abnormal even when performed in patients whose symptoms have resolved before arrival in the ED. The newer technetium agents provide higher quality images, have minimal redistribution after the initial injection, and allow imaging at a time point up to several hours after the initial injection [20].

Several excellent reviews have described the evolution of the use of acute perfusion imaging techniques [16,21,22]. Thallium (Tl)-201, a potassium analog that is taken up by viable myocardial cells in direct proportion to coronary blood flow [21], has been replaced largely by the use of technetium Tc-99m-labeled agents for evaluating patients in the ED setting because thallium requires rapid imaging with little delay from the time of injection.

As summarized by Gibbons [21], several technetium Tc-99m-labeled agents have been developed, including teboroxime, tetrofosmin, and sestamibi. Teboroxime, like thallium, requires rapid image acquisition. Sestamibi, the most widely used agent, and tetrofosmin are distributed to the myocardium in relation to blood flow. Their uptake requires a viable myocardial cell and an intact cell membrane. Both of these agents are bound within the myocardial cell in a nearly irreversible fashion, which allows time from the injection to image acquisition. The use of single photon emission-computed tomography (SPECT) with gated image acquisition has largely replaced multiple view planar images. SPECT is superior from the standpoint of localization, quantification, and image quality. Similar to the principles underlying CT, images acquired in an arc around the patient are then recreated into a three-dimensional image of regional perfusion [21,22].

Cardiac perfusion studies using agents such as technetium Tc-99m sestamibi have been shown to accurately identify myocardial infarction or ischemia in patients with chest pain who have nondiagnostic EKGs. Bilodeau and colleagues [23] have reported the use of perfusion imaging in 45 patients who were injected with sestamibi during a chest pain episode. The sensitivity was 96% for the detection of coronary artery disease (CAD). Hilton and colleagues [24] also have demonstrated a sensitivity for sestamibi of 94% and a specificity of 85% for the detection of CAD in a study of 102 patients. Varetto and colleagues [25] have reported a sensitivity of 100% (95% CI, 80%-100%) even when patients were injected with sestamibi after the acute chest pain had resolved. In clinical studies, technetium Tc-99m tetrofosmin has been shown to be as sensitive and specific as thallium and angiography in detecting cardiac ischemia and infarction [26,27].

There have been several observational cohort reports and one large prospective clinical trial that have provided data on the use of perfusion imaging as a triage aid. A systematic review in 2001 of the five studies that have examined rest perfusion scanning determined the following test characteristics: the sensitivity for detecting AMI was 91.5% to 100%, with a specificity of 49.3% to 84.4%; and the sensitivity for detecting any form of ACS was 89% (95% CI, 73%-96%), with a specificity of 77% (95% CI, 63%-89%) [12].

Udelson and colleagues [20] studied the clinical impact of acute sestamibi perfusion imaging at seven academic medical centers among 2475 patients who presented with chest pain or other symptoms suggestive of ACS. Among patients without ACS, the incorporation of perfusion imaging reduced the hospitalization rate by 10% (52% without to 42% with ACS). This study also has confirmed the prognostic value of a normal resting scan in the ED: among patients with normal scans, the risk of acute MI was 0.6%, and the relative risk at 30 days of an acute cardiac event (death, revascularization, AMI) was 3%.

Some centers have incorporated acute rest perfusion imaging into algorithms that complement serial cardiac biomarker sampling [28] or as a diagnostic aid in patients who have been placed into a particular risk stratification group based on clinical and EKG variables. The Virginia Commonwealth University Medical Center five-level protocol includes perfusion imaging for patients stratified as level 3 (probable ACS) and level 4 (possible unstable angina). Patients in level 4 include those with nonischemic EKG and either typical symptoms less than 30 minutes in duration or atypical symptoms, and they are discharged following a negative perfusion study with outpatient stress testing [29]. Several cohort studies have reported very high negative predictive values for AMI among low-risk patients who have negative rest scans [16].

There are several problems that limit the use of acute perfusion imaging, including technical, patient, and system factors. Technical aspects include the problem of differentiating diaphragm and breast shadows from pathologic perfusion defects. To offset these difficulties, some authors suggest obtaining prone and supine images [30] and having the emergency physician discuss the patient's clinical assessment and scan interpretation directly with the physician who is interpreting the scan. Patient factors include whether patients have a history of MI and whether pain (or equivalent symptom) presents at the time of injection. Udelson and colleagues [20], for example, excluded patients with a history of myocardial infarction because the detection of new perfusion abnormalities in such patients, even with a reference scan, can be difficult. System issues include the need to be able to access imaging tracers around the clock and to have experienced readers available to interpret scan results.

The role of acute perfusion imaging in patients whose symptoms have resolved remains controversial, although various guidelines have been published [31]. Some experts suggest that the injection of radioactive tracers must be performed while the patient is experiencing ischemic symptoms to maximize sensitivity. Other investigators have suggested there is evidence that the injection of a tracer soon after symptom resolution is still sensitive [25,32]. Some centers that use routine rest perfusion imaging in the ED require tracer injection before therapeutic interventions such as nitrate administration (Emergency Room Assessment of Sestamibi for the Evaluation of (ERASE) Chest Pain Trial investigators, personal communication, 1998), whereas other practitioners image patients within 2 to 6 hours of symptom resolution. The American Society of Nuclear Cardiology [31] suggests that patients be injected within 2 hours of symptom resolution. Possible physiologic explanations for residual perfusion abnormalities include impaired cell membrane function or collateral flow, myocardial stunning leading to wall motion abnormalities, or the return of coronary blood flow to a level that resolves pain but is still below normal [19].

Many institutions have demonstrated that despite barriers, acute perfusion imaging can be successfully and cost effectively incorporated into decision making in the ED [33–35]. However, recent advances in CT and magnetic resonance imaging (MRI) suggest that these techniques may replace nuclear imaging in the same way that perfusion lung scanning has been replaced by CTPA at many centers, as part of the evaluation for suspect pulmonary embolism. Additionally, CT and MRI are technologies that increasingly are routinely available around the clock in many ED settings.

Fig. 2 shows the acute perfusion scan of a patient who presented to the ED with atypical chest pain and a normal EKG. The white arrows point to an acute inferolateral perfusion defect. The patient was taken to immediate percutaneous coronary intervention where an occluded left

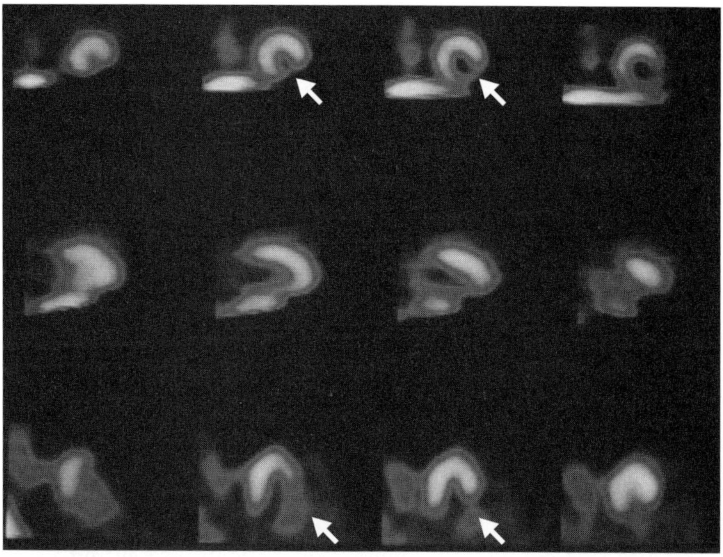

Fig. 2. Acute resting myocardial perfusion image in the acute perfusion scan of a patient who presented to the ED with atypical chest pain and a normal EKG. The white arrows point to an acute inferolateral perfusion defect. (Courtesy of James Udelson, MD, Boston, MA).

circumflex artery was identified and successfully stented. Occlusion of the circumflex artery is especially difficult to identify on EKG and often is silent on electrocardiography [36].

Computerized tomography and angiography

There are several CT-based techniques that have been developed to assess cardiac status. One technique is coronary calcium assessment, which depends on the premise that calcium deposits in the coronary vessels are almost always caused by coronary atherosclerotic disease. There have been many studies showing that coronary calcium scoring can be used to assess the burden of coronary atherosclerosis and has both a high sensitivity and negative predictive value for CAD ($\geq$80%), although it cannot specifically identify a culprit lesion or rule out an unstable noncalcified plaque [16]. Both electron beam (EB)CT (or ultrafast CT) and multidetector (MD)CT can be used to assess the quantity of calcium in the coronary arteries within a matter of minutes. EBCT has been studied more extensively and validated because the technology has been applied to cardiac imaging for over 20 years. MDCT scanners, however, are more widely available and have been shown to correlate well with EBCT in regard to coronary calcium scoring [37]. Neither EBCT nor MDCT suffer much from motion artifact caused by their capability for rapid image acquisition.

The original scoring system, described by Agatson and colleagues [38] in 1990, was based on a combination of the number of calcium deposits and deposit density (based on x-ray attenuation in Hounsfield units) and area, as detected by EBCT. This system has correlated well with fluoroscopic and pathologic data [39]. The generally accepted cutoff values for calcium scoring are a score of 0 indicates no coronary calcium; 1 to 100 indicates mild atherosclerosis; 101 to 400 indicates moderate atherosclerosis; and greater than 400 indicates extensive coronary calcium deposition.

Although most coronary calcium scoring has been studied in an elective or nonacute setting, there are a few small studies that have examined the value of calcium scoring as a triage tool for the chest pain patient in the Emergency Department. Laudon and colleagues [40] have shown that in 105 patients presenting to the ED with chest pain, negative enzymes, and an indeterminate EKG (without previous CAD and strictly within age limits), EBCT calcium scoring could reliably rule out CAD with a sensitivity and negative predictive value of 100% (95% CI, 77%-100%), although a specificity of only 63% (95% CI, 54%-75%). In addition, McLaughlin and colleagues [41] studied 137 consenting patients presenting with chest pain, a nondiagnostic EKG, negative enzymes, and no history of CAD or current pregnancy. There were no age limits, and the mean age was 53 ± 2 years. Of the 48 negative studies, only one patient had a cardiac event, a creatine kinase (CK) concentration of 453 U/L in a 45-year-old man with a positive cocaine level at the time of admission, which gives a negative predictive value of 98%.

Coronary calcium scoring, however, does have several limitations. This technique cannot assess for noncalcified plaques, which may occur in younger patients. In addition, it cannot identify specific culprit or vulnerable lesions. Also, because the strength of coronary calcium scoring in the acute setting lies predominately in its negative predictive value, given a low calcium score, the technique is much less helpful in patients who are known to have CAD. McLaughlin and colleagues [41] have noted lower reliability in cocaine users, young women, and active smokers. Finally, even in the asymptomatic population referred for testing, 50% of men over 50 and women over 65 have detectable coronary calcium, and the numbers increase dramatically as the age increases. Hence, the technique loses some of its negative predictive value in older patients [42].

Another CT-based technique that has promise in the arena of the acute coronary syndrome is CT coronary angiography, which has been attempted with both MDCT and EBCT. To date, coronary angiography has been tested in an elective patient population, for example, in patients who are scheduled for elective invasive catheterization, as opposed to patients in an emergent setting. In 125 such patients, however, Achenbach and colleagues [43] showed CT angiography to be useful in identifying stenoses in the proximal and mid segments of the coronary arteries, with a sensitivity of up to 92% (95% CI, 84.1%-96.7%) and a specificity of up to 94% (95% CI,

90.5%-96%) in the patients who could be evaluated. In this study, the investigators determined the time needed for a contrast bolus from a peripheral vein to reach the aortic root. They then injected a second bolus and acquired images according to the projected transit time, with EKG triggering during a breath hold. EBCT angiography with intravenous contrast (Fig. 3) shows the left main coronary artery bifurcating into the left anterior descending and the circumflex coronary arteries in both transaxial imaging (*A*) and three-dimensional reconstruction (*B*).

Presently, CT angiography has several limitations. Image quality, which rendered 37% of the scans in this study at least partially nonevaluable, is a large hurdle. This problem with obtaining adequate image quality is based on a number of factors, especially respiratory motion artifact, severe calcification, and coronary motion. Image quality improves greatly if patients are in a slow, regular rhythm during image acquisition, and some investigators routinely premedicate patients with β-blockers and exclude

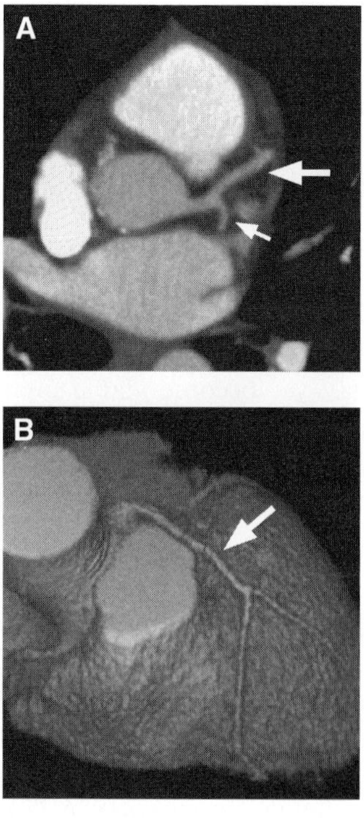

Fig. 3. (*A*) Transaxial EBCT image after intravenous injection of contrast agent shows the left main coronary and bifurcation into the left anterior descending coronary artery (*large arrow*) and circumflex coronary artery (*small arrow*). (*B*) Three-dimensional shaded surface display (*arrow*, left anterior descending coronary artery). (*From* Achenbach S, Ropers D, Pohle K, et al. Clinical results of minimally invasive coronary angiography using computed tomography. Cardiol Clin 2003;21(4):549–59; with permission.)

patients in irregular rhythms, such as atrial fibrillation. In addition, some investigators have recommended premedicating with sublingual nitroglycerin to increase coronary blood flow during the examination [44]. Although these may be viable steps in a symptom-free elective population, they may be more difficult to achieve with a more acute population. Stents and severe calcifications both cause artifacts on CT angiography, and patients with either cannot be adequately evaluated and are generally excluded, as are patients who have previously undergone coronary artery bypass graft surgery.

In summary, coronary calcium scoring can be helpful in assessing the atherosclerotic burden in a younger ED chest pain population, although it is important to remember that it cannot rule out noncalcified plaques. Larger studies must confirm its reliability in this setting. CT angiography has not been studied in an ED population, but if the technological difficulties can be overcome, this technique offers a minimally invasive assessment of the proximal and mid coronary arteries for specific obstructing lesions. In addition to calcified obstructing lesions, there also has been preliminary work looking at the ability of CT angiography to evaluate noncalcified plaques. This technique may become useful in coronary risk assessment, similar to calcium scoring, but is currently in early stages [44].

Magnetic resonance imaging and angiography

Cardiac imaging with MRI and MR angiography (MRA) has been studied extensively, although to date it has not become applied widely. It suffers from similar limitations as CT, foremost of which are motion artifact and acquisition time [45]. However, the technology continues to advance, and MRI and MRA may yet become viable imaging alternatives. If the technical difficulties are solved, MRI and MRA offer the possibility of noninvasive, nonionizing, high-resolution imaging that can assess the heart from multiple perspectives at the same time.

MRI

Cardiac MRI encompasses a variety of techniques and approaches, including perfusion imaging, gated wall motion assessment, plaque characterization, angiography, and the assessment of myocardial and plaque inflammation [16]. Myocardial infarct imaging generally uses several of these modalities simultaneously to confirm diagnoses. Infarcts can be imaged without contrast because the pathologic changes in the myocardium caused by ischemia and necrosis alter the imaging properties of the tissue, but most studies focus on contrast-enhanced perfusion imaging of infarcts. Gadolinium, a popular contrast agent, leaves the vasculature and distributes into the tissues, thereby enhancing the images, and helps to detect infarcts earlier in their course. In an intriguing study of patients with hypertrophic obstructive cardiomyopathy who were undergoing elective septal embolization to intentionally infarct part of the obstructing septum and decrease its size, Schulz-Menger and colleagues [46] were able to image and follow myocardial infarcts out from a known time of onset, comparing enhanced and nonenhanced imaging techniques. They found that T1-weighted gadolinium-enhanced MRI could distinguish infarcted myocardium at 1 hour out, which noncontrast T2-weighted imaging was unable to do reliably until 24 hours later.

The standard sequence of MRI infarct imaging has two stages. Early imaging, during the first pass of the contrast agent through the myocardium, will reveal a hypoenhanced area. This is the core of the infarct, in which the microvasculature is plugged or damaged to the point that it allows little if any blood flow to the tissue. A larger hypoenhanced core predicts complications and poor outcome. Rescanning minutes later reveals hyperenhancement of a much larger area of tissue than the hypoenhanced core and generally corresponds to the area of infarct. The pathophysiology of what these different regions represent is not entirely clear. Early hypoenhanced regions represent nonviable tissue, but they do not comprise its full extent. Hyperenhanced tissue includes some tissue that is nonviable but also some that can show the potential for functional improvement [47]. This may be because hyperenhancement, in addition to representing necrosis, may also represent peri-infarct edema [46].

One strength of MRI infarct imaging is that it provides extremely high-resolution images. Wagner and colleagues [48] imaged 91 patients with contrast-enhanced MRI within 2 months of SPECT imaging with thallium and sestamibi to electively assess patients with known or suspected CAD. Of the 181 cardiac segments in which MRI was able to identify subendocardial infarction, 85 were undetectable by SPECT imaging. This meant that there were six patients who had subendocardial infarcts on MRI and no infarct visible on rest SPECT imaging. However, four of these six patients had inducible ischemia visible on SPECT during stress imaging. Contrast enhanced MRI (Fig. 4) shows delayed hyperenhancement of the right ventricle (RV) free wall 48 hours after isolated RV infarction.

In addition to imaging infarcts, MRI can be used as a single test to evaluate overall cardiac function. Chui and colleagues [49] were able to evaluate wall motion, perfusion, and ejection fraction with MRI alone in 13 patients admitted and medically stabilized for non-ST-elevation ACS. In this small study, Chui and colleagues showed that the information provided by a single MRI scan performed within 12 days of admission showed a good correlation with conventional angiography, with an overall sensitivity of 92% (95% CI, 74.8%-99%) and a specificity of 94% (95% CI, 65%-99.8%).

Although most cardiac MRI studies are performed on inpatients or elective patients, one study has examined its feasibility in the emergency

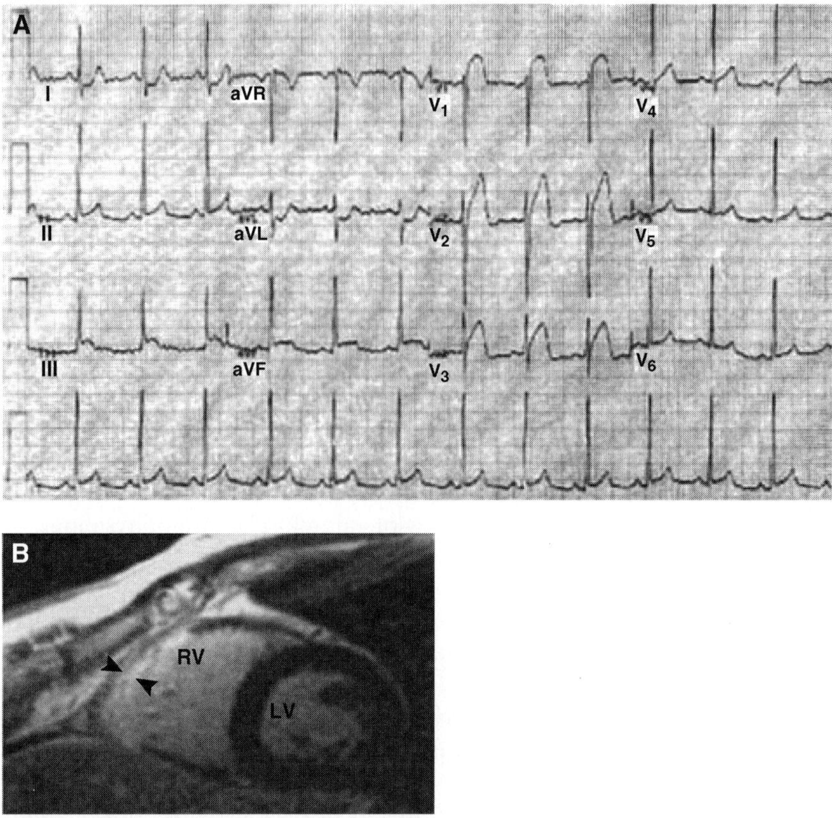

Fig. 4. A standard 12-lead electrocardiogram (*A*) showed marked ST-segment elevation in leads V_1, V_2, and V_3 and slight ST-segment elevation in leads II, III, and aVF. Contrast-enhanced MRI (*B*) shows delayed hyperenhancement of the RV free wall 48 hours after isolated RV infarction. (*From* Finn, AV, Antman EM. Isolated right ventricular infarction. Images in Clinical Medicine. N Engl J Med 2003;349(17):1636; with permission.)

department. Kwong and colleagues [50] evaluated 161 stable patients presenting to the ED with greater than 30 minutes of chest pain, a nondiagnostic EKG, the ability to lie flat, and no contraindications to MRI. Patients were studied within 12 hours of presentation, the scans lasted 38 ± 12 minutes, and patients were away from the ED for 58 ± 10 minutes. The sensitivity and specificity of MRI for ACS (including unstable angina) in this setting were 84% (95% CI, 65.8%-94.7%) and 85% (95% CI, 78.6%-90.5%), respectively, which was more sensitive than an abnormal EKG, a peak troponin level, or a Thrombolysis in Myocardial Infarction (TIMI) risk score, although both peak troponin and TIMI risk were more specific. Importantly, however, this protocol was feasible in the setting of the Emergency Department. More research will be needed to assess the feasibility and reliability of ED-based cardiac MRI.

MR angiography

Magnetic resonance technology is being applied to imaging both coronary arteries and plaques. Currently, however, similar to the limitations of CT angiography, MRA can assess only the proximal and mid segments of the coronary tree. MRA has been studied both with and without contrast, but as yet, there is no standardized protocol. Kim and colleagues [51] performed an international multicenter study of free-breathing noncontrast MR coronary angiography of 109 patients presenting for elective conventional x-ray coronary angiography catheterization, in which their overall accuracy was 72% (95% CI, 63%-81%) but improved for left main or three-vessel disease to 87% (95% CI, 81%-93%). As these authors note, however, there is still a significant portion of cardiac segments that cannot be assessed because of difficulties with image quality, and as yet there is no consensus on the best technique for MR coronary angiography.

MRI has been used for some time to image and characterize atherosclerotic plaques in noncardiac sites, such as the carotids and the aorta. The coronary vasculature, however, is more challenging because it is much smaller and more mobile than either of those sites is. During the last few years, a number of studies have attempted to image coronary plaque, both invasively and noninvasively and with and without contrast enhancement. New invasive technologies such as intravascular and transesophageal MRI allow a high-resolution closer look at the coronary vessels. A number of new contrast agents are being tested that might be able to target unstable plaques. Two examples include paramagnetic lipid-encapsulated nanoparticles that bind to fibrin on the surface of an unstable plaque and superparamagnetic iron oxides that can be phagocytosed by plaque macrophages [52,53]. Such techniques might someday allow us to image an actively unstable coronary plaque in real time but currently require a great deal of further research and development.

Provocative tests to identify ACS following a rule-out protocol

A variety of provocative noninvasive test strategies can be used to identify ischemia, following a rule-out approach. These strategies include graded exercise testing with EKG, nuclear perfusion imaging or echocardiography and pharmacologic stress testing, and stress imaging with an inotrope such as dobutamine or a vasodilator such as adenosine. To date there are some limited data on tests such as exercise testing performed without a period of observation and cardiac biomarker testing [54], and a few reports on direct stress ECHO or stress perfusion imaging as the initial triage aide performed in the ED, where patients with negative test results are discharged directly. In addition, each of the available provocative techniques has tradeoffs in terms of sensitivity, specificity, reported reliability, and limitations in certain populations such as women or the elderly.

Table 1
Provocative tests

Exercise stress testing (full bruce, modified bruce protocol)	Vasodilator imaging dipyridamole or adenosine	Inotrope imaging
EKG monitoring Perfusion Imaging ECHO imaging	Radioisotope perfusion imaging ECHO	Dobutamine ECHO

Emergency physicians routinely evaluate patients who may have "negative" results from one of the available provocative tests (Table 1). Failure to appreciate the limitations of these tests can lead to adverse outcomes from missed disease in patients in whom a negative test is incorrectly assumed to mean the absence of clinically significant disease [55].

Exercise stress testing

Exercise Tolerance Testing with EKG monitoring

The Bruce protocol is the most widely adopted protocol and has been validated extensively [56]. The protocol has seven stages, each lasting 3 minutes, resulting in 21 minutes' exercise for a complete test. In stage 1, the patient walks at 1.7 mph up a 10% incline. The speed and incline increase with each stage. Accepted goals are completing 9 to 12 minutes of exercise or reaching 85% of the maximum predicted changes in heart rate (220 bbm-age). A normal test result or a result that indicates a low probability of coronary artery disease is one in which 85% of the maximum predicted heart rate is achieved with a physiologic response in blood pressure and no associated ST segment depression.

Calculation of the Duke prognostic treadmill score can be used to provide additional information about the probability of severe CAD [57] and prognosis [57–61]. The Duke score is equal to exercise time (minutes based on the Bruce protocol) minus (5 × ST-segment deviation in millimeters) minus (4 × treadmill angina index). An angina index of 2 is defined as limiting angina, 1 as nonlimiting angina, and 0 as no angina. Duke treadmill scores range from −25 (high risk) to +15 (low risk). A score of +5 or higher is associated with a 4-year survival of 98% to 99%, whereas a score of less than −10 is associated with a 4-year survival of only 71% to 79% [58,59].

Exercise testing has a sensitivity of 78% and a specificity of 70% for detecting coronary artery disease [56]. A negative test result, therefore, cannot be used to rule in or rule out ischemic heart disease, unless the probability of coronary artery disease is taken into account. Although the use of stress testing has become part of standard chest pain unit algorithms, the lack of well-controlled interventional trials limits the strength of evidence regarding its role in the ED. Chan and colleagues [62] demonstrated that there was no statistical difference in outcome among chest pain patients admitted to telemetry who received inpatient, outpatient, or no ETT within 30 days. Hollander [63] notes "it is not logical to mandate stress testing on lower risk patients released from the ED when only one quarter of admitted patients even receive a stress test." A recent evidence-based review of direct ETT testing concluded that the clinical impact of this technology has a "clinical effect unknown, quality of evidence rated C (subject to significant bias)" [8]. The AHA/ACC guidelines on exercise stress testing recognize its acceptance in structured chest pain protocols [1].

Emergency physicians also must be aware that ETT, although considered safe and widely incorporated into testing strategies in patients who are already considered to be at very low risk of having significant disease, can have complications. It is also quite possible that adverse events associated with stress tests performed in the ED setting are under-reported. Tandy and colleagues [64] have described a case report in which an ETT obtained in a patient with an EKG considered by the emergency physician to be nondiagnostic that in retrospect demonstrated Wellens' syndrome led to a fatal outcome. Other complications associated with ETT have included AMI during testing or following a normal ETT, related possibly to plaque rupture [65,66].

Recent reviews and a meta-analysis have discussed the limitations of EKG monitored stress testing in women [33,67]. The sensitivity and specificity in exercise EKG in women is moderate, with a mean weighted sensitivity of 61% (95% CI, 54%-68%) and a mean weighted specificity of 70% (95% CI, 68%-77%) [33,67]. The report of the ACC/AHA Practice Guidelines Committee states that: "because of the increased incidence of false-positive exercise EKG tests in women, stress imaging has been recommended as the initial test. The optimal strategy for detecting CAD in women remains to be defined. The ACC/AHA Committee to Update Guidelines for the Management of Chronic Stable Angina believes that the data available at present are insufficient to justify replacing standard exercise testing with stress imaging when evaluating women for CAD" [68].

Exercise EKG testing also can be problematic in the elderly. Authors have noted that the elderly population may be unable to perform exercise stress test caused by the higher prevalence of pulmonary airway, degenerative joint and peripheral vascular diseases, and exercise capacity and baseline EKG abnormalities [69–71].

Exercise perfusion imaging

Exercise perfusion imaging is performed with image acquisition after peak stress using treadmill or bicycle exercise and rest image acquisition or redistribution imaging at a later time. A negative stress perfusion scan is predictive of very low risk [72]. In a study of patients referred for stress thallium scans, the cardiac event rate (nonfatal MI or cardiac death) was only 0.88% after a negative stress thallium test [73]. It is important to note that the event rate in the study population was low (1.51%/y); subjects who were more than 75 years of age, had undergone revascularization 3 months before or after study scans, or had previous MI were excluded, and 3.8% of subjects were lost to follow-up. Iskander and Iskandrian [74] have reported that the average annual rate of death or nonfatal MI in patients with stable chest pain who had a negative stress sestamibi SPECT scan was 0.6% based on a review of studies published between 1994 and 1997. The authors note that although this estimate was based on 12,000 patients who were followed for an average of 20 months, several reports came from the same site, and there may have been multiple reports that included the same patients.

Redberg and Shaw [75] performed a meta-analysis of nuclear imaging studies in women. They have reported that the sensitivity of exercise thallium Tl 201 in women was 78% (95% CI, 72%-83%), and the specificity was 64% (95% CI, 51%-77%). Technetium Tc 99m sestamibi improves specificity and reduces false-positive studies by providing a brighter signal intensity and reducing breast attenuation artifacts in women. In a study that used random order to compare imaging agents, the false-positive rate was reduced by more than 50% [76].

Exercise ECHO

Exercise ECHO combines exercise on a treadmill or a bicycle and ECHO imaging. Images are acquired within 1 minute of completing the maximum workload or during an upright or within supine cycle exercise before the resolution of ischemia to maximize sensitivity [77]. The mean weighted sensitivity for exercise ECHO is 81%, specificity is 86%, and the overall accuracy is 83% [13]. Sensitivity of this modality is lower for patients with single-vessel disease and in those who have less than 70% stenosis.

The role of exercise ECHO in low-risk patients, such as those who would most often be evaluated in an ED chest pain setting, remains uncertain. Elhendy and colleagues [78] studied 571 men and 1047 women who were referred for exercise ECHO evaluation. Patients were followed for a median of 3 years. The authors have concluded that among patients with low pretest probability of coronary artery disease by clinical criteria, exercise ECHO identified some but not all future events and did not appear to be cost effective in low-risk patients.

Pharmacologic imaging

Pharmacologic methods are used when patients are unable to achieve adequate exercise stress. Intravenous vasodilators such as adenosine or dipyridamole are often combined with submaximal exercise. Cardio-specific vasodilators such as α_2-adrenergic receptor agonists are undergoing clinical trials [71]. These agents may allow specific coronary vasodilation and improved imaging techniques. Kim and colleagues [79] performed a meta-analysis comparing the performance of different pharmacologic stress imaging techniques for the diagnosis of coronary artery disease. The authors have reported that maximum sensitivity was achieved with vasodilator and nuclear perfusion, with dipyridamole and adenosine giving similar vasodilatory performance. The overall weighted mean sensitivity of adenosine SPECT was 90% (95% CI, 89%-92%), and specificity was 75% (95% CI, 70%-79%). Dobutamine echocardiography had a higher specificity than pharmacologic perfusion imaging did. In designing ED-based evaluation protocols, tests that have greater sensitivity often are more desirable to minimize the risk of failing to identify significant disease.

Inotrope-enhanced echocardiography (dobutamine echocardiography) is another pharmacologic imaging technique that has been extensively studied. The mean weighted values for sensitivity, specificity, and overall accuracy for dobutamine stress echocardiography are 82%, 84%, and 83%, respectively [13]. For purposes of analysis, the left ventricle usually is divided into a 16-segment model with rest-, low-, and high-dose image analysis [80]. Although the test is considered accurate, the assessment of improvement or deterioration of wall motion abnormalities is subjective and, thus, so is the test interpretation [81,82]. It is important for emergency physicians to be aware that, although agreement among within-institution interpretations has been reported to be high, inter-institutional agreement has lower agreement (κ 0.37 among five centers for abnormal or normal dobutamine stress ECHO) [82]. Tripi and colleagues [83] have reported the results of a small, select cohort study of patients who had negative CK levels ($\leq$170 U/L) and negative dobutamine ECHOs, who were discharged from the ED following a negative study. The investigators reported that 54 of 58 patients with negative studies were discharged safely. Larger controlled trials are still needed to demonstrate the safety and effectiveness of this approach.

Summary

There are several noninvasive imaging methods that are available to aid in the evaluation and triage of patients who present to the Emergency Department with symptoms suggestive of acute cardiac ischemia. Although the clinical evaluation and EKG interpretation remain fundamental tools for risk stratification and risk assessment, rapid advancements in noninvasive technologies will soon provide high quality visualization of the coronary anatomy and allow rapid identification of ischemic myocardium. Some of the presently available noninvasive techniques such as acute nuclear perfusion imaging have been studied in large prospective clinical trials, whereas other techniques such as CT calcium scoring and MRI have been examined only in small cohort studies without formal evaluation of the safety and effectiveness of the use of these techniques to aid clinical decision making in the ED setting. Emergency physicians should be aware of the strengths and limitations of the noninvasive methods available to identify symptomatic coronary artery disease. Patients and providers can anticipate rapid progress in this exciting area.

Acknowledgments

We thank Ms. Kathleen Shea for her expert preparation of this manuscript.

References

[1] Braunwald E, Antman EM, Beasley JW, et al. ACC/AHA 2002 guideline update for the management of patients with unstable angina and non–ST-segment elevation myocardial infarction: a report of the American College of Cardiology/American Heart Association task force on practice guidelines (Committee on the Management of Patients with Unstable Angina). 2002. Available at: http:www.acc.org/clinical/guidelines/unstable/incorporated/index.htm.

[2] Fesmire FM, Percy RF, Bardoner JB, et al. Serial creatinine kinase (CK) MB testing during the emergency department evaluation of chest pain: utility of a 2-hour deltaCK-MB of + 1.6 ng/ml. Am Heart J 1998;136(2):237–44.

[3] Fesmire FM. Delta CK-MB outperforms delta troponin I at 2 hours during the ED rule out of acute myocardial infarction. Am J Emerg Med 2000;18(1):1–8.

[4] Freedman JE. CD40 ligand–assessing risk instead of damage? N Engl J Med 2003;348(12): 1163–5.

[5] Heeschen C, Dimmeler S, Hamm CW, et al. Soluble CD40 ligand in acute coronary syndromes. N Engl J Med 2003;348(12):1104–11.

[6] Manolio T. Novel risk markers and clinical practice. N Engl J Med 2003;349(17):1587–9.

[7] Balk EM, Ioannidis JP, Salem DN, et al. Accuracy of biomarkers to diagnose acute cardiac ischemia in the emergency department: a systematic review. Ann Emerg Med 2001;37(5): 453–61.

[8] Lau J, Ioannidis J, Balk E, et al. Diagnosing acute cardiac ischemia in the emergency department: a systematic review of the accuracy and clinical effect of current technologies. Ann Emerg Med 2001;37(5):453–60.

[9] Forrester JS Jr, Liebson PR, Parrillo JE, et al. Risk stratification post-myocardial infarction: is early coronary angiography the more effective strategy? Prog Cardiovasc Dis 2002;45(1): 49–66.

[10] Cannon CP, Turpie AG. Unstable angina and non-ST-elevation myocardial infarction: initial antithrombotic therapy and early invasive strategy. Circulation 2003;107(21):2640–5.

[11] Neumann FJ, Kastrati A, Pogatsa-Murray G, et al. Evaluation of prolonged antithrombotic pretreatment ("cooling-off" strategy) before intervention in patients with unstable coronary syndromes: a randomized controlled trial. JAMA 2003;290(12):1593–9.

[12] Ioannidis J, Salem D, Chew P, et al. Accuracy of imaging technologies in the diagnosis of acute cardiac ischemia in the emergency department: a meta-analysis. Ann Emerg Med 2001; 37(5):471–7.

[13] Cheitlin MD, Armstrong WF, Aurigemma GP, et al. ACC/AHA/ASE 2003 guideline update for the clinical application of echocardiography: a report of the American College of Cardiology/American Heart Association task force on practice guidelines (ACC/AHA/ASE Committee to uptake the 1997 guidelines for the clinical application of Echocardiography). Available at: http:www.acc.org/clinical/guidelines/echo/index.pdf. J Am Coll Cardiol 2003; 42(5):954–70.

[14] Kontos MC, Arrowood JA, Paulsen WH, et al. Early echocardiography can predict cardiac events in emergency department patients with chest pain. Ann Emerg Med 1998;31(5): 550–7.

[15] Lim SH, Sayre MR, Gibler WB. 2-D echocardiography prediction of adverse events in ED patients with chest pain. Am J Emerg Med 2003;21(2):106–10.
[16] Kontos MC, Tatum JL. Imaging in the evaluation of the patient with suspected acute coronary syndrome. Semin Nucl Med 2003;33(4):246–58.
[17] Sieswerda GT, Yang L, Boo MB, et al. Real-time perfusion imaging: a new echocardiographic technique for simultaneous evaluation of myocardial perfusion and contraction. Echocardiography 2003;20:545–55.
[18] Stewart MJ. Contrast echocardiography. Heart 2003;89(3):342–8.
[19] Wackers FJ, Lie KI, Liem KL, et al. Potential value of thallium-201 scintigraphy as a means of selecting patients for the coronary care unit. Brit Heart J 1979;41(1):111–7.
[20] Udelson JE, Beshansky JR, Ballin DS, et al. Myocardial perfusion imaging for evaluation and triage of patients with suspected acute cardiac ischemia: a randomized controlled trial. JAMA 2002;288(21):2693–700.
[21] Gibbons RJ. Myocardial perfusion imaging. Heart 2000;83(3):355–60.
[22] Kim SC, Adams SL, Hendel RC. Role of nuclear cardiology in the evaluation of acute coronary syndromes. Ann Emerg Med 1997;30(2):210–8.
[23] Bilodeau L, Theroux P, Gregoire J, et al. Tc-99M sestamibi tomography in patients with spontaneous chest pain: correlations with clinical, electrocardiographic and angiographic findings. J Am Coll Cardiol 1991;18(7):1684–91.
[24] Hilton TC, Thompson RC, Williams HJ, et al. Tc-99M sestamibi myocardial perfusion imaging in the emergency room evaluation of chest pain. J Am Coll Cardiol 1994;23(5): 1016–22.
[25] Varetto T, Cantalupi D, Altieri A, et al. Emergency room Tc-99M sestamibi imaging to rule out acute myocardial ischemic events in patients with nondiagnostic electrocardiograms. J Am Coll Cardiol 1993;22(7):1804–8.
[26] Sridhara BS, Braat S, Rigo P, et al. Comparison of myocardial perfusion imaging with Tc-99M tetrofosmin versus tl-201 in coronary-artery disease. Am J Cardiol 1993;72(14): 1015–9.
[27] Zaret BL, Rigo P, Wackers FJT, et al. Myocardial perfusion imaging with Tc-99M tetrofosmin - comparison to (tl)-t-201 imaging and coronary angiography in a phase-iii multicenter. Circulation 1995;91(2):313–9.
[28] Fesmire FM, Hughes AD, Stout PK, et al. Selective dual nuclear scanning in low-risk patients with chest pain to reliably identify and exclude acute coronary syndromes. Ann Emerg Med 2001;38(3):207–15.
[29] Jesse RL, Kontos MC, Roberts CS. Diagnostic strategies for the evaluation of the patient presenting with chest pain. Prog Cardiovasc Dis 2004;46(5):417–37.
[30] Stowers SA, Umfrid R. Supine-prone SPECT myocardial perfusion imaging: the poor man's attenuation compensation. J Nucl Cardiol 2003;10(3):338.
[31] Wackers FJ, Brown KA, Heller GV, et al. American Society of Nuclear Cardiology position statement on radionuclide imaging in patients with suspected acute ischemic syndromes in the emergency department or chest pain center. J Nucl Cardiol 2002;9(2): 246–50.
[32] Varetto T, Cantalupi D, Altieri A, Orlandi C. Emergency room technetium-99m sestamibi imaging to rule out acute myocardial ischemic events in patients with nondiagnostic electrocardiograms. J Am Coll Cardiol 1993;22:1804–8.
[33] Radensky PW, Hilton TC, Fulmer H, et al. Potential cost effectiveness of initial myocardial perfusion imaging for assessment of emergency department patients with chest pain. Am J Cardiol 1997;79(5):595–9.
[34] Stowers SA, Eisenstein EL, Th Wackers FJ, et al. An economic analysis of an aggressive diagnostic strategy with single photon emission computed tomography myocardial perfusion imaging and early exercise stress testing in emergency department patients who present with chest pain but nondiagnostic electrocardiograms: results from a randomized trial. Ann Emerg Med 2000;35(1):17–25.

[35] Weissman IA, Dickinson CZ, Dworkin HJ, et al. Cost-effectiveness of myocardial perfusion imaging with SPECT in the emergency department evaluation of patients with unexplained chest pain. Radiology 1999;(2):353–7.
[36] O'Keefe JH Jr, Gibbons RJ. Left circumflex occlusion–underrecognized and undertreated. J Thromb Thrombolysis 2000;10(3):221–5.
[37] Rumberger JA. Clinical use of coronary calcium scanning with computed tomography. Cardiol Clin 2003;21(4):535–47.
[38] Agatston AS, Janowitz WR, Hildner FJ, et al. Quantification of coronary artery calcium using ultrafast computed tomography. J Am Coll Cardiol 1990;15(4):827–32.
[39] Wexler L, Brundage B, Crouse J, et al. Coronary artery calcification: pathophysiology, epidemiology, imaging methods, and clinical implications: a statement for health professionals from the American Heart Association Writing Group. Circulation 1996; 94(5):1175–92.
[40] Laudon DA, Vukov LF, Breen JF, et al. Use of electron-beam computed tomography in the evaluation of chest pain patients in the emergency department. Ann Emerg Med 1999;33(1): 15–21.
[41] McLaughlin VV, Balogh T, Rich S. Utility of electron beam computed tomography to stratify patients presenting to the emergency room with chest pain. Am J Cardiol 1999;84(3): 327–8.
[42] Mitchell TL, Pippin JJ, Devers SM, et al. Age- and sex-based nomograms from coronary artery calcium scores as determined by electron beam computed tomography. Am J Cardiol 2001;87(4):453–6.
[43] Achenbach S, Moshage W, Ropers D, et al. Value of electron-beam computed tomography for the noninvasive detection of high-grade coronary-artery stenoses and occlusions. N Engl J Med 1998;339(27):1964–71.
[44] Achenbach S, Ropers D, Pohle K, et al. Clinical results of minimally invasive coronary angiography using computed tomography. Cardiol Clin 2003;21(4):549–59.
[45] Slater J, Rill V. Coronary artery disease: new insights into the pathophysiology, prevalence and early detection of a monster menace. Semin Ultrasound CT MR 2003;24(2):114–22.
[46] Schulz-Menger J, Gross M, Messroghli D, et al. Cardiovascular magnetic resonance of acute myocardial infarction at a very early stage. J Am Coll Cardiol 2003;42(3):513–8.
[47] Gerber BL, Lima JA, Garot J, et al. Magnetic resonance imaging of myocardial infarct. Top Magn Reson Imaging 2000;11(6):372–82.
[48] Wagner A, Mahrholdt H, Holly TA, et al. Contrast-enhanced MRI and routine single photon emission computed tomography (SPECT) perfusion imaging for detection of subendocardial myocardial infarcts: an imaging study. Lancet 2003;361(9355):374–9.
[49] Chiu CW, So NM, Lam WW, et al. Combined first-pass perfusion and viability study at MR imaging in patients with non-ST segment-elevation acute coronary syndromes: feasibility study. Radiology 2003;226(3):717–22.
[50] Kwong RY, Schussheim AE, Rekhraj S, et al. Detecting acute coronary syndrome in the emergency department with cardiac magnetic resonance imaging. Circulation 2003;107(4): 531–7.
[51] Kim WY, Danias PG, Stuber M, et al. Coronary magnetic resonance angiography for the detection of coronary stenoses. N Engl J Med 2001;345(26):1863–9.
[52] Kramer CM. Magnetic resonance imaging to identify the high-risk plaque. Am J Cardiol 2002;90(10C):15L–7L.
[53] Pennell D. Cardiovascular magnetic resonance. Heart 2001;85(5):581–9.
[54] Kirk JD, Turnipseed S, Lewis WR, et al. Evaluation of chest pain in low-risk patients presenting to the emergency department: the role of immediate exercise testing. Ann Emerg Med 1998;32(1):1–7.
[55] Duseja R, Feldman JA. Missed acute cardiac ischemia in the ED: limitations of diagnostic testing. Am J Emerg Med 2004;22(3):219–25.
[56] Hill J, Timmis A. Exercise tolerance testing. BMJ 2002;324(7345):1084–7.

[57] Shaw LJ, Peterson ED, Shaw LK, et al. Use of a prognostic treadmill score in identifying diagnostic coronary disease subgroups. Circulation 1998;98(16):1622–30.
[58] Mark DB. Risk stratification in patients with chest pain. Primary Care; Clinics in Office Practice 2001;28(1):99–118.
[59] Mark DB, Shaw L, Harrell FE Jr, et al. Prognostic value of a treadmill exercise score in outpatients with suspected coronary artery disease. N Engl J Med 1991;325(12):849–53.
[60] Mark DB, Hlatky MA, Harrell FE Jr, et al. Exercise treadmill score for predicting prognosis in coronary artery disease. Ann Intern Med 1987;106(6):793–800.
[61] Pryor DB, Shaw L, Harrell FE Jr, et al. Estimating the likelihood of severe coronary artery disease. Am J Med 1991;90(5):553–62.
[62] Chan GW, Sites FD, Shofer FS, et al. Impact of stress testing on 30-day cardiovascular outcomes for low-risk patients with chest pain admitted to floor telemetry beds. Am J Emerg Med 2003;21(4):282–7.
[63] Hollander JE. Evaluation of the patient with chest pain: are the bells and whistles evidence based? Ann Emerg Med 2003;41(3):352–4.
[64] Tandy TK, Bottomy DP, Lewis JG. Wellens' syndrome. Ann Emerg Med 1999;33(3):347–51.
[65] Capezzuto A, Achilli A, Pontillo D, et al. Acute myocardial infarction shortly after a normal exercise stress test: case reports. Angiology 1995;521–6.
[66] Fertels SH, Heller DR, Maniet A, et al. Acute myocardial infarction due to exercise-induced plaque rupture. Clin Cardiol 1998;21(10):767–8.
[67] Kwok Y, Kim C, Grady D, et al. Meta-analysis of exercise testing to detect coronary artery disease in women. Am J Cardiol 1999;83(5):660–6.
[68] Gibbons RJ, Abrams J, Chatterjee K, et al. ACC/AHA 2002 guideline update for the management of patients with chronic stable angia: a report of the American College of Cardiology/American Heart Association Task Force on Practice Guidelines (Committee to update the 1999 Guidelines for the Management of Patients with Chronic Stable Angia). 2002. Available at: www.acc.org/clinical/guidelines/stable/stable.pdf. Accessed August 26, 2005.
[69] Fleg JL. Stress testing in the elderly. Am Geriatr Cardiol 2001;10(6):308–13 [quiz: 313–15].
[70] Fleischmann KE, Hunink MG, Kuntz KM, et al. Exercise echocardiography or exercise SPECT imaging? a meta-analysis of diagnostic test performance. JAMA 1998;280(10): 913–20.
[71] Lateef F, Gibler WB. Provocative testing for chest pain. Am J Emerg Med 2000;18(7): 793–801.
[72] Sabharwal NK, Lahiri A. Role of myocardial perfusion imaging for risk stratification in suspected or known coronary artery disease. Heart 2003;89(11):1291–7.
[73] Vanzetto G, Ormezzano O, Fagret D, et al. Long-term additive prognostic value of thallium-201 myocardial perfusion imaging over clinical and exercise stress test in low to intermediate risk patients: study in 1137 patients with 6-year follow-up. Circulation 1999; 100(14):1521–7.
[74] Iskander S, Iskandrian AE. Risk assessment using single-photon emission computed tomographic technetium-99m sestamibi imaging. J Am Coll Cardiol 1998;32(1):57–62.
[75] Redberg RF, Shaw LJ. Diagnosis of coronary artery disease in women. Prog Cardiovasc Dis 2003;46(3):239–58.
[76] Taillefer R, DePuey EG, Udelson JE, et al. Comparative diagnostic accuracy of Tl-201 and Tc-99m sestamibi SPECT imaging (perfusion and ECG-gated SPECT) in detecting coronary artery disease in women. J Am Coll Cardiol 1997;29(1):69–77.
[77] Marwick TH. Stress echocardiography. Heart 2003;89(1):113–8.
[78] Elhendy A, Shub C, McCully RB, et al. Exercise echocardiography for the prognostic stratification of patients with low pretest probability of coronary artery disease. Am J Med 2001;111(1):18–23.
[79] Kim C, Kwok YS, Heagerty P, et al. Pharmacologic stress testing for coronary disease diagnosis: a meta-analysis. Am Heart J 2001;142(6):934–44.

[80] Geleijnse ML, Fioretti PFP, Roelandt PFJ. Methodology, feasibility, safety and diagnostic accuracy of dobutamine stress echocardiography. J Am Coll Cardiol 1997;30(3):595–606.
[81] Hoffmann R, Lethen H, Marwick T, et al. Standardized guidelines for the interpretation of dobutamine echocardiography reduce interinstitutional variance in interpretation. Am J Cardiol 82(12):1520–4.
[82] Hoffmann R, Lethen H, Marwick T, et al. Analysis of interinstitutional observer agreement in interpretation of dobutamine stress echocardiograms. J Am Coll Cardiol 1996;27(2): 330–6.
[83] Trippi JA, Lee KS, Kopp G, et al. Dobutamine stress tele-echocardiography for evaluation of emergency department patients with chest pain. J Am Coll Cardiol 1997;30(3):627–32.

ELSEVIER
SAUNDERS

Emerg Med Clin N Am
23 (2005) 999–1025

EMERGENCY
MEDICINE
CLINICS OF
NORTH AMERICA

ECG Patterns Confounding the ECG Diagnosis of Acute Coronary Syndrome: Left Bundle Branch Block, Right Ventricular Paced Rhythms, and Left Ventricular Hypertrophy

William J. Brady, MD[a,*], Brian Lentz, MD[b], Kevin Barlotta, MD[b], Richard A. Harrigan, MD[c], Theodore Chan, MD[d]

[a]*Department of Emergency Medicine and Internal Medicine, University of Virginia, Charlottesville, VA 22908, USA*
[b]*Department of Emergency Medicine, University of Virginia, Charlottesville, VA 22908, USA*
[c]*Department of Emergency Medicine, Temple University, Philadelphia, PA 19140, USA*
[d]*Department of Emergency Medicine, University of California San Diego, San Diego, CA 92103, USA*

Acute myocardial infarction (AMI) is reliably diagnosed using the patient's history and examination, serum markers, and 12-lead ECG. Although these tools are powerful in the evaluation of the chest-pain patient, each of these diagnostic investigations has its limitations—recognizing these limitations empowers the clinician in in the patient evaluation. The descriptive history of the event may be obscured by many factors, including patient age, comorbid states, language barriers, and other factors. Serum marker analysis, although useful in the diagnosis of AMI, do not offer significant sensitivity in the early evaluation of the chest-pain patient who is experiencing potential acute infarction.

As the history and serum marker analysis are compromised, the ECG also has limitations in this setting—an important area of diagnostic limitation is the presence of confounding ECG patterns. Several ECG patterns confound the diagnosis of AMI, including left bundle branch block (LBBB), ventricular paced rhythms (VPR), and left ventricular hypertrophy

* Corresponding author.
E-mail address: wb4z@virginia.edu (W.J. Brady).

doi:10.1016/j.emc.2005.07.004 *emed.theclinics.com*

(LVH). These patterns produce new ST-segment/T-wave abnormalities, which are the new normal findings in these patients. The clinician may be led astray by these findings in two distinct instances: (1) diagnosing ECG change related to acute coronary syndromes (ACS) when the abnormality results solely from the confounding pattern; and (2) not acknowledging the confounding nature of these ECG patterns in the evaluation of potential ACS, thereby placing excessive diagnostic confidence in the ECG.

ST-segment and T-wave abnormalities are frequently encountered in the emergency department (ED) chest-pain patient. These abnormalities result from a range of clinical syndromes, including AMI and non-AMI entities. In particular, ST-segment elevation is not an uncommon finding on the ECG in these patients; this abnormality, however, is less commonly related to AMI. Only 15% to 25% of such patients who experience ST-segment elevation have AMI.–The remainder have noninfarction diagnoses [1,2]. In a review of adult ED chest-pain patients who experience ST-segment elevation on the ECG, ST-segment elevation resulted from AMI in only 15% to 33% of this population; once again, LVH and LBBB were frequently seen and were the most common causes of the ST-segment elevation [1,2]. In the coronary care unit population, Miller and colleagues [3] demonstrated that ST-segment elevation was diagnostic for acute infarct in only half of the cases with a past history of ischemic heart disease. These confounding syndromes are not infrequently misdiagnosed as acute infarction, which then may subject the patient to unnecessary and potentially dangerous interventions. For instance, Sharkey and colleagues reported that 11% of patients receiving fibrinolysis did not suffer from AMI. The ECG syndromes producing this noninfarction ST-segment elevation included LVH (30%) and intraventricular conduction abnormalities, including LBBB (30%) [4].

The following review highlights the diagnostic dilemma encountered in these confounding ECG patterns; the discussion focuses on the expected ECG abnormalities seen in these patients and the findings seen in ACS.

Left bundle branch block

LBBB is a significant ECG finding in ED chest-pain patients because it identifies a potentially ill patient while simultaneously reducing the diagnostic sensitivity of the ECG. The left bundle branch is anatomically composed of two distinct groupings or fasicles: the anterior and posterior fasicles; a LBBB is, therefore, a bifasicular block involving dysfunction of two segments of the intraventricular conduction system. The diagnostic criteria (Figs. 1–4) for LBBB include a widened QRS complex with a duration of greater than 0.12 seconds. The right precordial leads (V1 and V2) demonstrates a QS or rS complex; a monophasic R wave is seen in the lateral leads I, aVl, V5, and V6. In the normal, anticipated LBBB pattern (Figs. 1–4), the appropriate position of the ST segment and T wave is predicted based on its relationship with the major, terminal segment of the QRS complex. The

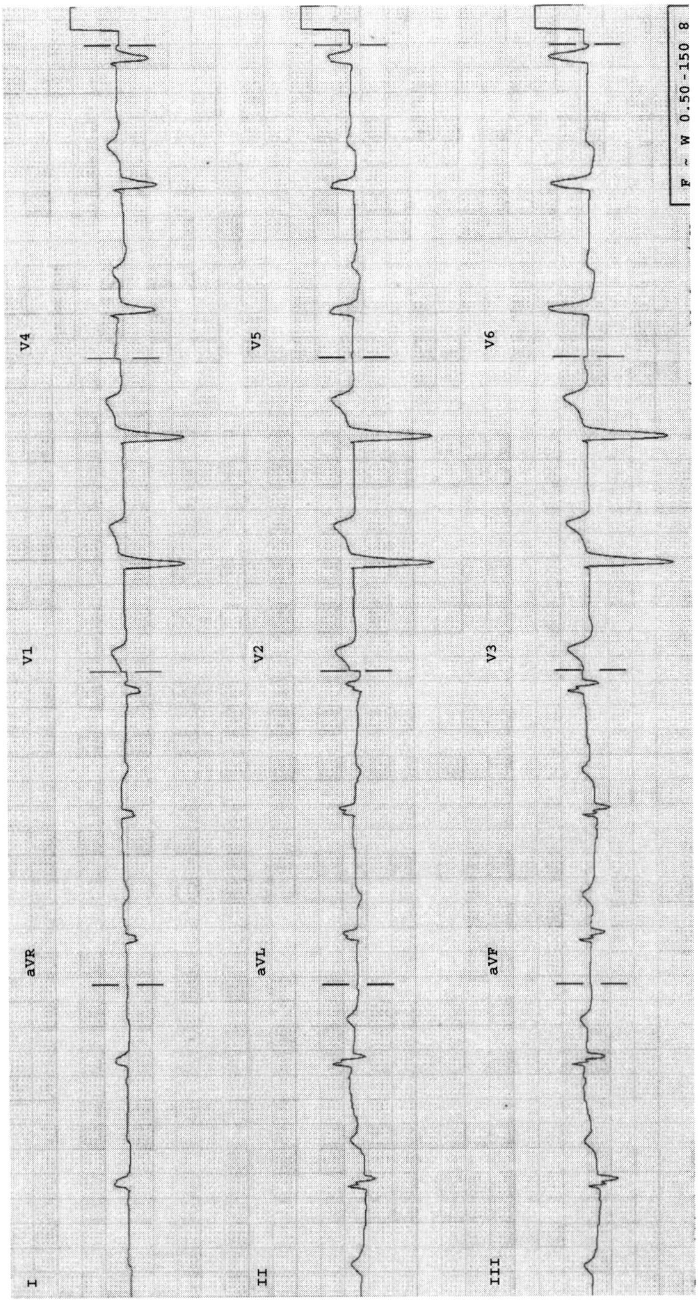

Fig. 1. 12-lead ECG with LBBB pattern. Note that ST segments and T wave are appropriately located and configured.

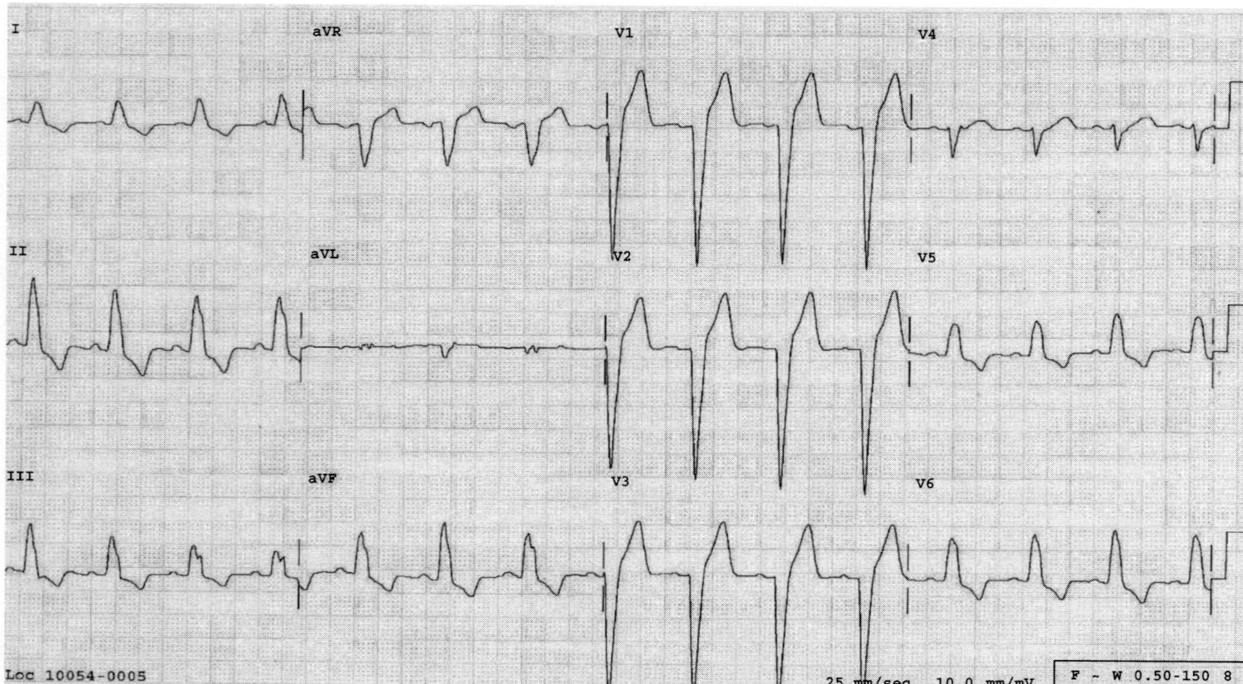

Fig. 2. 12-lead ECG with LBBB pattern. Note that patient presented with cardiogenic shock and positive serum troponin, consistent with AMI. Also note that ST segments and T wave are appropriately located and configured. This patient is example of confounding nature of the ECG in LBBB presentations. This ECG demonstrated ST-segment and T-wave configurations appropriate for a LBBB.

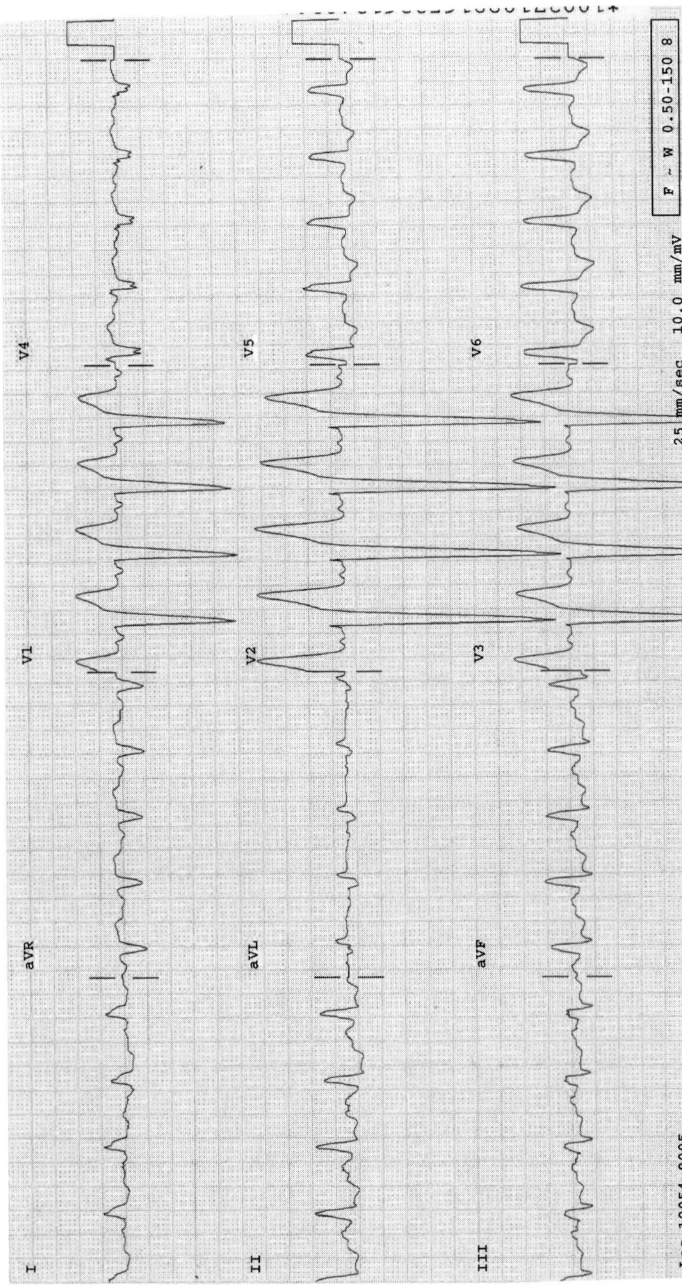

Fig. 3. Sinus tachycardia with LBBB pattern.

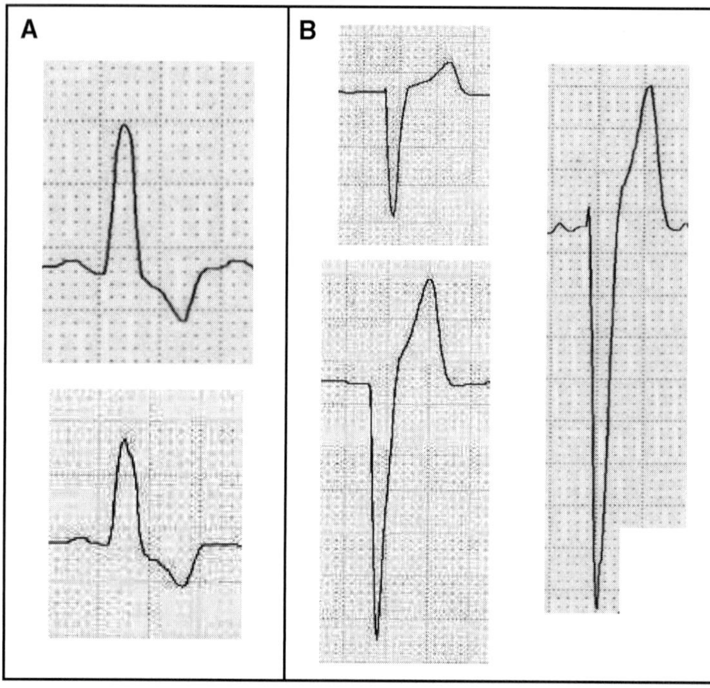

Fig. 4. (*A*) ECG examples of leads I, aVl, V5, and V6 in LBBB. Note large monophasic R wave with appropriate, concordant ST-segment depression and T-wave inversion. (*B*) ECG leads (inferior and anterior) with predominantly negative QRS complexes. The ST segments are elevated with upright T wave. Waveforms are appropriate for LBBB pattern in this distribution.

QRS complex may be located on the opposite side of the isoelectric baseline from the ST segment and T wave—this relationship is termed discordant. For instance, in leads with predominantly negative QRS complexes, such as the right precordial leads V1, V2, and V3, the ST segment is elevated with an upright T wave (Fig. 4B); conversely, if leads such as the lateral leads I, aVl, V5, and V6, the ST segment is depressed with an inverted T wave caused by the primarily positive nature of the QRS complex (Fig. 4A). This relationship can be described as the "concept of appropriate discordance" (Fig. 4).

Because of the abnormal pattern of ventricular depolarization in the LBBB pattern, reliable interpretation of the ST segment and T wave is compromised. Many authorities might state that the ECG is invalidated as a diagnostic tool in the evaluation of potential ACS. Other clinicians believe the ECG continues to represent a reliable investigation in these complicated patients. The likely answer lies in between these two extreme views. The LBBB pattern markedly reduces the diagnostic value of the ECG in this instance. The diagnostic pitfall may occur in one of two situations: (1) the pattern may reduce the diagnostic sensitivity of the ECG for AMI, or (2) the pattern may masquerade as an ACS event when, in reality, none is occurring.

AMI patients who have developed LBBB experience a greatly increased risk for acute cardiovascular complication and death [5]. Because of this increased risk, the presence of a new LBBB pattern—new onset or not known to be old—on the ECG of a patient suspected of AMI, represents an indication for emergent revascularization with percutaneous coronary intervention. The clinical presentation must be strongly suggestive of an ACS event in this presentation scenario. In the setting of a presumed ACS event, the new development of a LBBB is most often associated with a large amount of myocardium in jeopardy with a pronounced risk for cardiogenic shock, complete heart block, and death. In patients who have developed pre-existing LBBB, markedly decreased left ventricular function is the rule; an additional injury to the heart may result in further loss of myocardium, which would likely be devastating.

Another clinical variable that LBBB AMI patients possess is a tendency toward a chest-pain free presentation. Reportedly, approximately half of patients have developed AMI and LBBB present with anginal equivalent complaints (ie, lack chest discomfort). Certainly adding a second diagnostic confounder to the presentation understandably increases the opportunity for a missed or delayed diagnosis. Shlipack and colleagues have explored this issue, finding that LBBB patients who experience presumed AMI who presented with chest pain were more than five times more likely to receive reperfusion therapy compared with similar patients lacking chest discomfort. These LBBB AMI chest-pain patients were also more likely to receive the appropriate, primary treatments of aspirin, β-adrenergic blockade, heparin, and nitrates. The patients who have developed LBBB lacking chest pain had a 50% greater risk for death during hospitalization. The primary reason for this increased mortality was medical undertreatment [6].

Over the past several decades, numerous investigators have attempted to develop ECG criteria for the diagnosis of AMI in the setting of LBBB, but most have been unsuccessful. The suggested decision tools have lacked sensitivity and specificity while also being cumbersome in application. Wackers reported on findings of 96 patients who experience LBBB and suspected AMI [7]. Fifty-five patients were diagnosed as AMI. ST-segment changes were considered significant if they demonstrated a concordance of 2 mm or more or a discordance of 7 mm or more with the direction of QRS deflection. The sensitivity, specificity, and positive predictive value of these findings for AMI were 54%, 97%, and 96%, respectively. Hands and colleagues [8] described 35 patients who have developed suspected AMI in the presence of LBBB; AMI was diagnosed in 20 patients. ST-segment concordance had a sensitivity for AMI of 16.7% with a specificity and positive predictive value of 90.9% and 80%, respectively. Hands and colleagues [8] did not study discordance of ST segments. Sgarbossa and colleagues are perhaps the first group of clinicians to tackle this issue with some degree of success. They have developed and validated a clinical prediction rule based on a set of ECG criteria for the diagnosis of AMI in patients who experience chest pain and LBBB [9]. The basis of this rule is assessment of the degree of ST-segment changes. Using the subset of patients in the GUSTO-1 trial who had enzyme-confirmed AMI with LBBB, the investigators were able to develop three ECG criteria of diagnostic value. To understand and apply these rules in clinical practice, the clinician must be comfortable with the terms "discordant" and "concordant" (Fig. 5). Discordant is the normal, expected position of the ST segment and T wave in relation to the major, terminal portion of the QRS complex relative to the isoelectric baseline. Concordant, most often an abnormal finding in this presentation, describes the ECG relationship when the major portion of the QRS complex and ST segment/T wave are located on the same side of the isoelectric baseline, whether it be concordant ST-segment depression (Fig. 5A) or condordant ST-segment elevation (Fig. 5A). The Sgarbossa criteria [9] include: (1) ST-segment elevation of 1 mm or more concordant with the QRS complex (Fig. 5A); (2) ST-segment depression of 1 mm or more in leads V1, V2, or V3 concordant with the QRS complex (Fig. 5B); and (3) ST-segment elevation of 5 mm or more that was discordant with the QRS complex (Fig. 5C) [9]. The investigators noted that criterion 1 and 2 were powerful diagnostic findings, strongly supportive of ECG AMI. Criterion 3 was weakly associated with AMI; the investigators stressed that this finding should be supported by other diagnostic findings in the potential ACS patient who has developed LBBB. Refer to Figs. 6 and 7

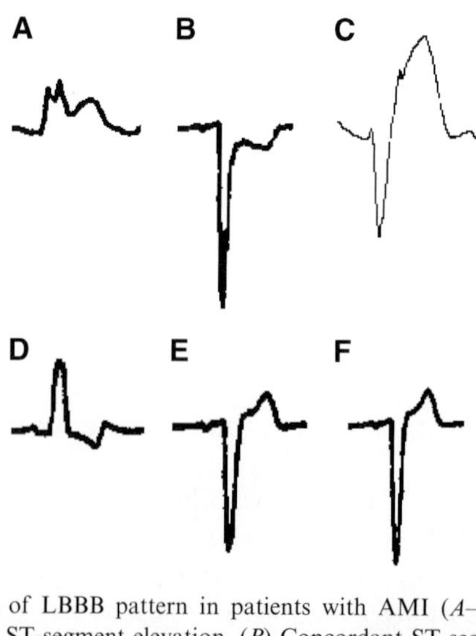

Fig. 5. ECG examples of LBBB pattern in patients with AMI (*A–C*) and non-ECG AMI (*D–F*). (*A*) Concordant ST-segment elevation. (*B*) Concordant ST-segment depression in lead V2. (*C*) Excessive, discordant ST-segment elevation. (*D*) Discordant ST-segment depression with T wave inversion, a normal ECG finding in the bundle branch block presentation. (*E,F*) Discordant ST-segment elevation with upright T wave, normal ECG findings in the bundle branch block presentation.

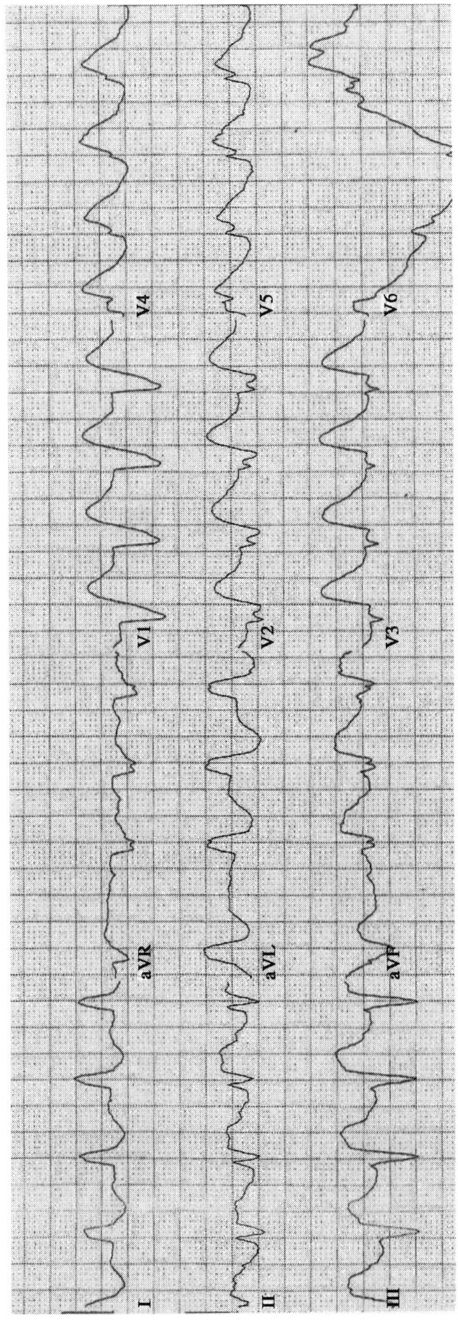

Fig. 6. 12-lead ECG with ECG AMI and LBBB pattern. Note concordant ST-segment elevation in leads V3, V4, V5, and aVf. Also note excessive discordant ST-segment elevation in lead III.

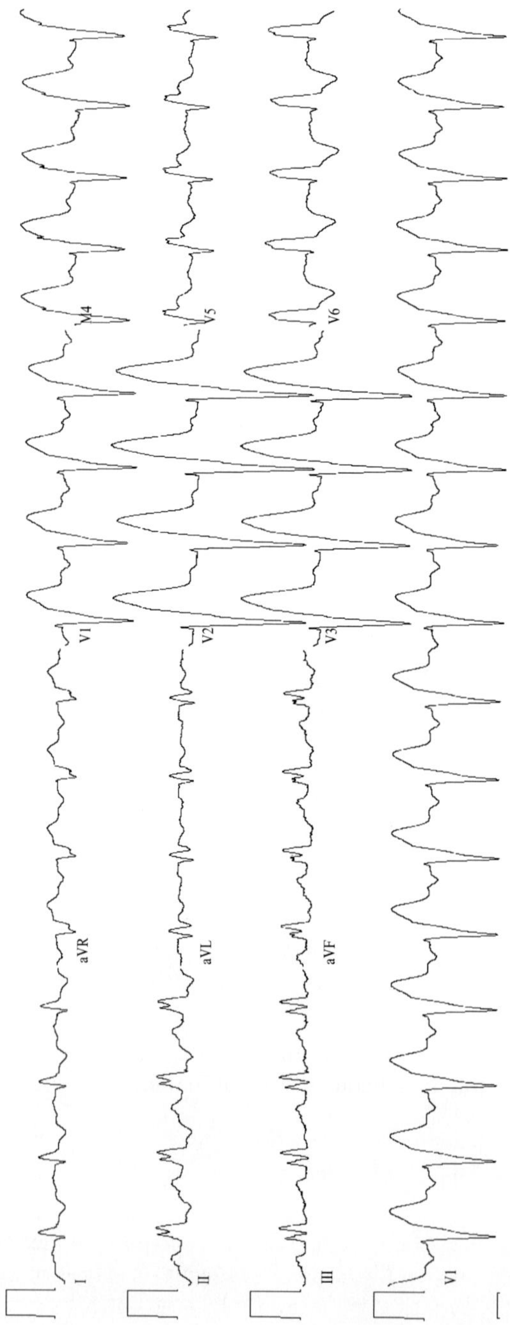

Fig. 7. 12-lead ECG with ECG AMI and LBBB pattern. Note excessive discordant ST-segment elevation in leads V2, V3, and V4; also note the concordant ST-segment elevation in Lead V5.

for examples of LBBB with ECG AMI. Also note that the ECG in Fig. 2, although ECG-appropriate for the LBBB pattern, was performed in the setting of hypotension, pulmonary edema, and positive serum troponin—essentially, a clinical diagnosis of AMI with an ECG demonstrating a "normal" LBBB pattern [9].

A recent critique of the Sgarbossa criteria [9] refined the decision rule. Investigators challenged the validity of the Sgarbossa findings, noting that similar ECG observations could be made in clinically stable (ie, non-ACS) patients who have developed LBBB, raising questions about the specificity. The investigators considered the patients in their clinical practice and found the criteria appropriate with the following exception: ST-segment elevation greater than 5 mm is occasionally found in leads with predominantly negative QRS complexes, particularly of large amplitude, in the absence of AMI; if the ST segment is temporally stable (ie, not dynamic), the investigators suggested excluding this criterion [10].

When a complex set of clinical criteria is suggested, a question regarding the application of the material by other practitioners, essentially an analysis of the external validity and interobserver reliability. Using these criteria, Skolove and colleagues compared the interobserver agreement between cardiologists and emergency physicians. They found an excellent agreement between the two groups when the Sgarbossa criteria [9] were applied [11].

Knowing this clinical decision rule may not be adequate enough itself to affect treatment, a recent study explored the issue, finding that less than 10% of AMIs would have been detected using the Sgarbossa [9] ECG criteria. If these criteria were to be used as a screening tool for fibrinolysis, then most patients may be refused treatment. Because of the high rate of mortality in this subset of patients, it was recommended that all patients who have developed LBBB and chest pain receive fibrinolytic agents [6].

This treatment strategy has been challenged by Kontos and colleagues [12]. Their study showed that the proposed criteria for identifying patients who experience AMI in the setting of LBBB occurred too infrequently or had a predictive value too low to identify most patients. They recognized that patients who have developed LBBB and presumed AMI who received fibrinolytic therapy had a 24% reduction in mortality, but most studies did not differentiate between RBBB and LBBB. Because RBBB does not obscure ischemia, the beneficial effects in patients who have developed LBBB may be overestimated. The actual prevalence of AMI in patients who have developed LBBB is low and, therefore, treating all chest-pain patients may mean giving a potentially dangerous drug to patients who do not need it [12].

In response to the critics of the Sgarbossa clinical decision rule [9], Edhouse and colleagues performed a retrospective analysis of LBBB and the ability to diagnose AMI electrocardiographically. In this study, all patients who do not experience AMI had clinical prediction rule scores not suggestive of AMI; approximately 80% of those patients who experience biochemically proven AMI had scores supporting the diagnosis of AMI. The researchers concluded that the diagnosis of AMI in the chest-pain patient who has developed LBBB is difficult yet noted that the clinical decision rule was useful in the suspected AMI patient who has developed LBBB [13].

A debate remains whether or not the Sgarbossa criteria [9] are always useful to diagnose AMI in LBBB. Although imperfect, the criteria do give the clinician some guidelines on which to base initiation of treatment. The ECG is not completely invalid if a patient has LBBB as was previously believed. Critics of the Sgarbossa criteria [9] note that the decision tool lacks significant diagnostic power to identify reliably AMI in LBBB patients. Although correct, this observation must be considered in light of the confounding nature of LBBB and the status of the existing literature base. Until publication of this material, clinicians considered the LBBB a confounding pattern in the consideration of ECG AMI. Although the Sgarbossa criteria [9] do not provide a complete, total answer to this diagnostic challenge, they do provide the clinician with one ECG tool to evaluate these complicated patients.

The chest-pain patient who has developed LBBB represents a significant challenge to the clinician. Currently, no single or combination diagnostic approach exists that reliably reveals AMI in a timely fashion in these LBBB patients. Even if the Sgarbossa clinical prediction rule [9] is found to be less useful in the objective evaluation of the ECG in the patient who has developed LBBB, this initial report has merit; it has forced the clinician to review the ECG in detail and cast some degree of doubt on the widely taught belief that the ECG is invalidated in the search for AMI in the LBBB patient.

Right ventricular paced rhythm

The intraventricular conduction system rapidly and efficiently transmits the electrical impulse of depolarization throughout the ventricle. The ECG is essentially a graph of voltage relative to time, a sophisticated voltmeter. With impulse propagation throughout the ventricles occurring less efficiently in patients who have implanted ventricular pacemakers, the total time of depolarization is greater; therefore, the QRS complex width is greater than that encountered in situations of normal intraventricular conduction. In right VPRs, activation of the ventricular tissues occurs initially from the right and subsequently to the left: the right ventricle, followed the interventricular septum, ending with the left ventricle. A pacer spike, a narrow negative or positive deflection immediately preceding the QRS complex, is seen in some ECG leads; in certain leads, a pacer spike may not be apparent, necessitating multilead analysis to determine the true nature of the wide-complex rhythm. In right VPRs, the ventricular depolarization pattern partially resembles a LBBB pattern with the primary difference encountered in leads V5 and V6, with a monophasic R wave seen in LBBB and a QS complexes in right ventricular paced patterns.

In the patient who experience a right VPR, the ECG (Figs. 8–10) displays a wide QRS complex. Leads I and aVl (Fig. 10A) are frequently the only ECG leads with a predominantly positive QRS complex. The remainder of the ECG leads demonstrate a broad, negative QRS complex with a QS configuration; these leads include the inferior (II, III, and aVf), lateral (V5 and V6), and anterior (V1–V4) anatomic segments (Fig. 10B). In certain instances, the right precordial leads may demonstrate a partially negative QRS complex with an rS or RS configuration.

The appropriate position and configuration of the ST segment and T wave can be predicted by the "concept of appropriate discordance" as described in the LBBB presentation. The major, terminal portion of the QRS complex and the ST segment/T wave are located on opposite sides of the isoelectric baseline. In the ECG leads with a predominantly positive QRS complex, such as leads I and aVl, the ST segment is depressed with an inverted T wave (Figs. 8, 9, and 10A). In leads with a primarily negative QRS complex such as the inferior (II, III, and aVf) and precordial (V1–V6) leads, ST segment elevation with a prominent, upright T wave is usually observed (Figs. 8, 9, and 10B). These findings (ST segment and T wave abnormalities) are the expected, normal findings in a right VPR. The ECG must be interpreted in the chest-pain patient with particular attention given to the ST segment and T wave, looking for a loss of this QRS complex ST-segment/T-wave discordance. Loss of this discordance, or in the extreme case, the development of concordance in chest-pain patients may indicate an acute coronary event, including AMI. Certainly, the lack of these findings does not rule out an ACS.

As with the LBBB presentation, numerous investigators have attempted to develop a reliable set of ECG rules to assist the clinician with ECG interpretation in these complicated presentations. In the early 1960s, Sodi-Palles proposed a range of abnormalities potentially suggestive of ACS; this system, however, was plagued by many issues, including poor sensitivity, cumbersome application of numerous potential abnormalities, and an inability to recognize acute findings [14]. Additional work, performed by Cardenas and colleagues, reported yet another range of ECG findings suggestive of MI in the right ventricular paced pattern. As with the Sodi-Palles proposal, this material did not focus on acute events; furthermore, no consideration of the ST segment and T wave was made. The worrisome findings for infarction in this study included an initial R wave in leads aVR and V1, a QR complex in leads V5 and V6, and a RS complex in leads V5 and V6 [14]. Castellanos and colleagues described further ECG changes reportedly associated with MI. As with the two previous reports, little emphasis is placed on the acute event; further, these findings are not consistent when applied across the spectrum of chest-pain patients who experience a right ventricular paced and possible ACS [15]. Niremberg and

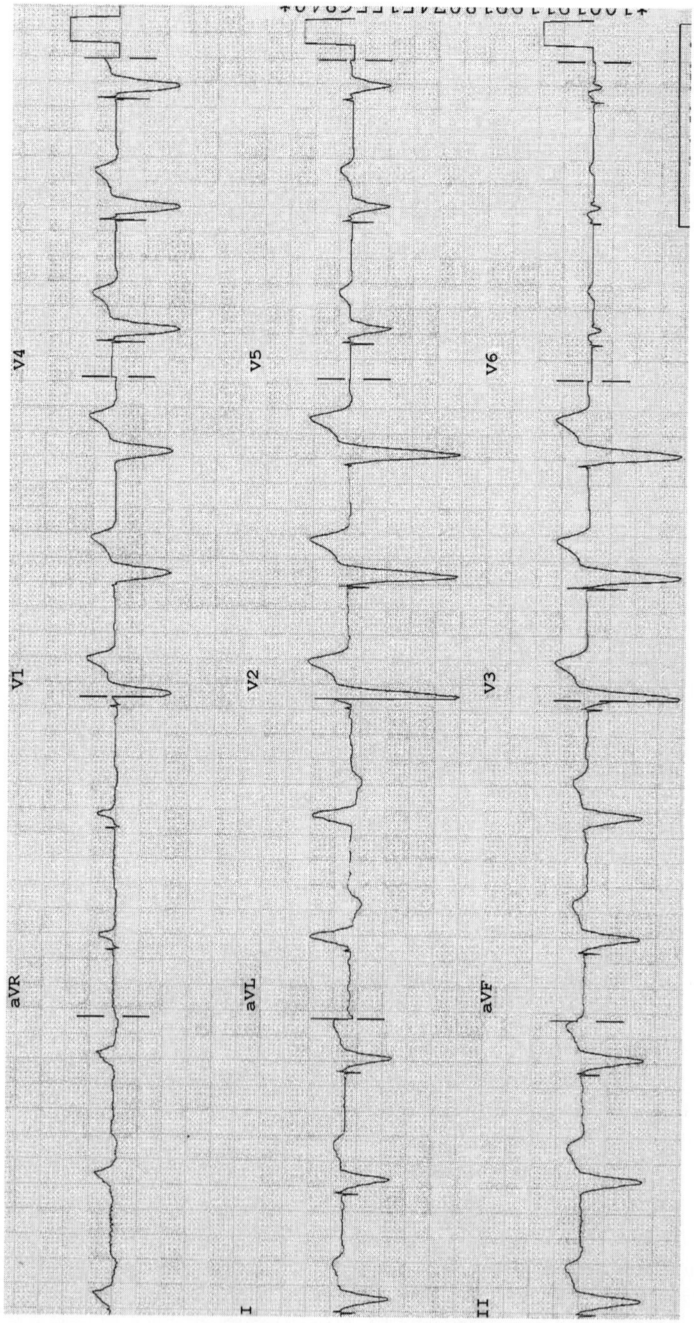

Fig. 8. Right VPR with appropriate ST-segment and T-wave locations and configurations.

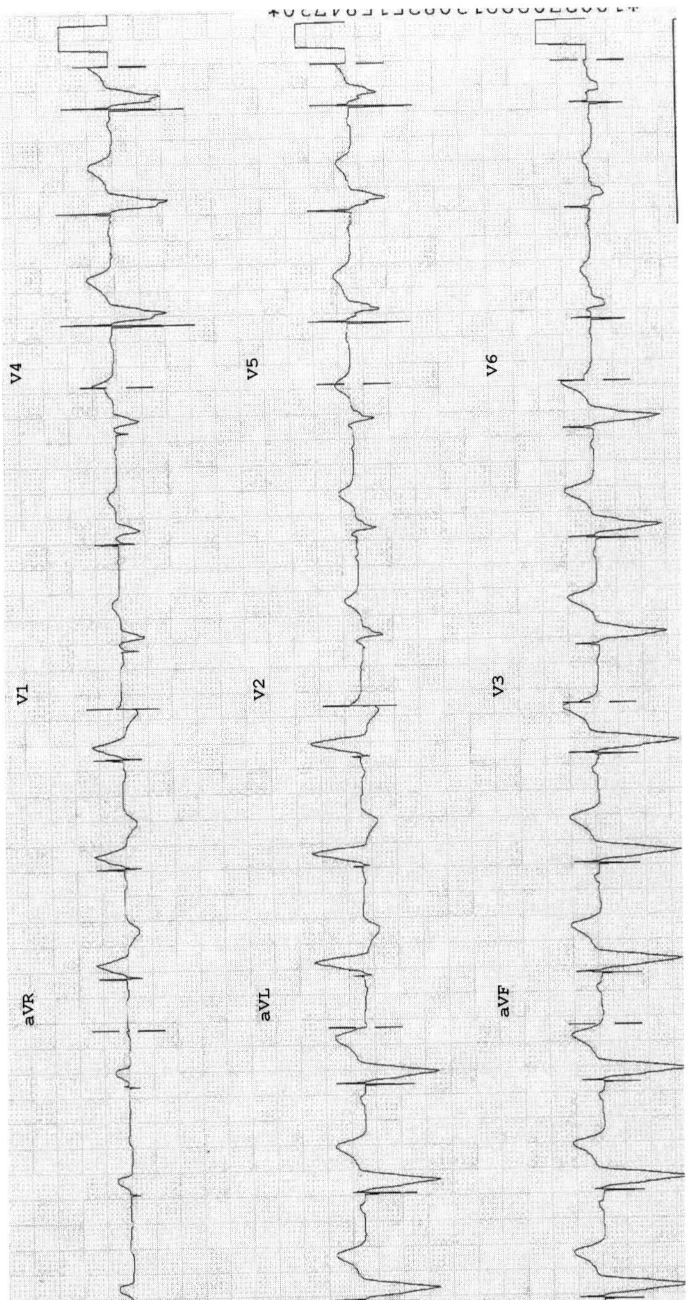

Fig. 9. Right VPR with appropriate ST-segment and T-wave locations and configurations.

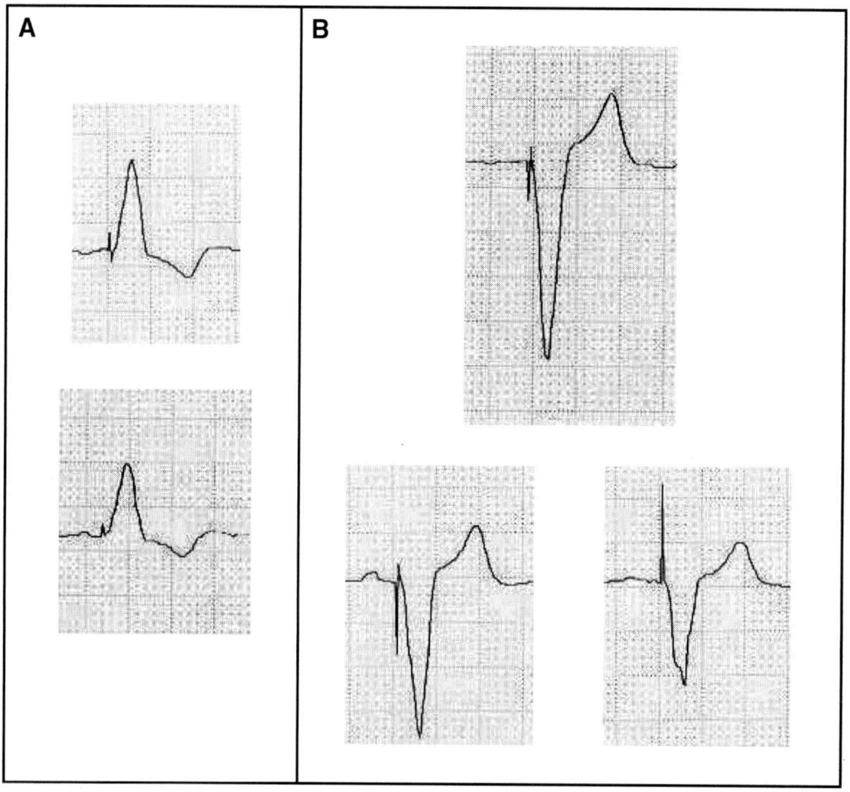

Fig. 10. Right VPR with appropriate ST-segment and T-wave locations and configurations. (*A*) Lateral leads (I and aVl) demonstrate monophasic R wave with discordant ST-segment depression. (*B*) Representative precordial leads with QS complexes reveal discordant ST-segment elevation.

colleagues reported that the abnormal ST segments and T wave were seen in most paced patients who have ACS. This clinical material, however, is highly dependent on past ECGs for comparison, significantly limiting its usefulness in the acute phase of ED management [16]. These investigators did not offer a significant advantage to the acute care clinician in the evaluation of the chest-pain patient who experiences right VPR and possible ACS.

As with the LBBB presentation, Sgarbossa and colleagues performed an analysis focusing on the immediate diagnosis of AMI in patients who experience right ventricular paced patterns, work in marked contrast to previous investigators in this area of ECG [17]. The import of this work is reduced somewhat by the small number of patients (totaling 17) in this subset analysis of the GUSTO trail [18]. Three ECG criteria were found to be useful in the early diagnosis of AMI, including: (1) discordant ST-segment elevation greater than 5 mm (Figs. 11A and 12 [leads V3 to

V4]); (2) concordant ST-segment elevation greater than 1 mm (Figs. 11B and 12 [leads II, III, aVf]); and (3) ST-segment depression greater than I mm in leads V1, V2, or V4 (Fig. 11C). The reader should note that the T wave is not mentioned in this analysis. These three criteria were all associated with low sensitivities for AMI; the specificities, however, were more robust [17]. As with most ECG criteria, this tool is likely helpful in ruling in an AMI and has no value in ruling out an AMI by way of the ECG. Refer to Fig. 12 for an example of a patient who has antero-inferior ECG abnormality in an ACS presentation.

Note that the most statistically powerful ECG predictor of AMI in this study does not violate the concept of appropriate discordance in obvious fashion [17]. Yet it does. If one considers that the appropriate position and configuration of the ST segment in leads with a primarily negative QRS complex is one of minimal to modest elevation, this criterion is more understandable. Although the appropriate position of the ST is elevated above the isoelectric baseline, the degree or magnitude of the elevation is excessive and, therefore, potentially abnormal.

These presentations are complicated in the patient's history, the ECG, and the outcome. Although the Sgarbossa paper [17] provides some ECG guidance in this setting, the true incidence of these findings is unknown. Furthermore, the clinician must realize, however, that these ST-segment changes are only suggestions of AMI in patients who produce complicated ECGs; by themselves, the criteria are not diagnostic of AMI. Their absence does not rule out the possibility of AMI. Therapeutic decisions must be made while considering these limitations.

Left ventricular hypertrophy

Left ventricular hypertrophy (LVH) develops from the compensatory response of the myocardium to the excessive workload imposed by increased

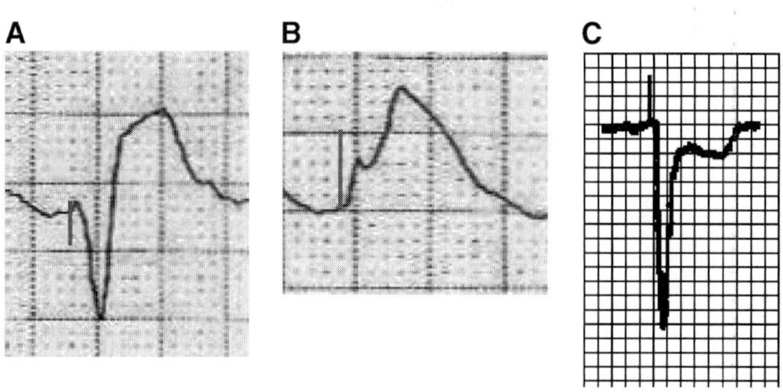

Fig. 11. Right VPR with abnormal ST-segment position and configuration suggestive of AMI. (*A*) Excessive, discordant ST-segment elevation. (*B*) Concordant ST-segment elevation. (*C*) Concordant ST-segment depression in lead V1, V2, or V3.

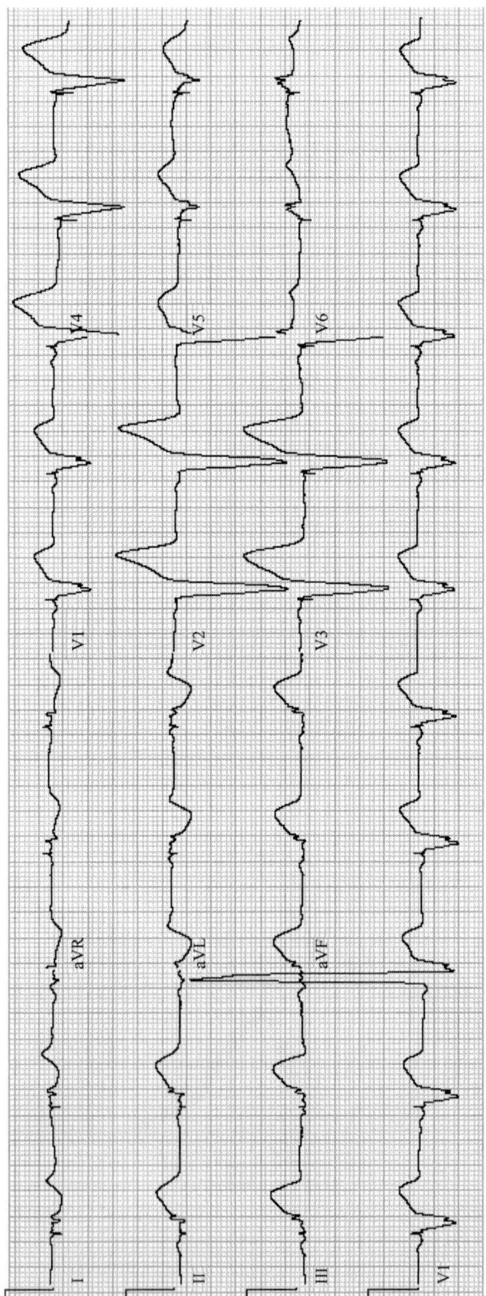

Fig. 12. Right VPR with AMI. Note concordant ST-segment elevation in leads II, III, and aVf and excessive, discordant ST-segment elevation in leads V3 and V4.

systemic pressure and by mechanical and neurohormonal stimuli that accompany hypertension. LVH is associated with an increase in the risk for cardiovascular mortality, including MI [19]. The prevalence of LVH by ECG criteria (2.9% for men and 1.5% for women) is much lower than that reported by echocardiography (15%–20%), demonstrating that the ECG is not a sensitive marker for this anatomical abnormality.

The LVH pattern is not an uncommon finding on the ECG in patients who experience chest pain in the ED [1,2]. The ECG changes associated with LVH can complicate the interpretation and diagnosis of patients who have potential ACS [20,21], underscoring the importance of the emergency physician's ability to recognize the ECG pattern of LVH and differentiate these changes from those attributed to ACS.

Many different diagnostic criteria have been proposed to diagnose LVH on the ECG including the Sokolow-Lyon Index (S-wave amplitude in V1 coupled with the R-wave amplitude in V5 or V6 > 35 mm), the Cornell Voltage Criteria (S wave in V3 plus the R wave in aVL > 28 mm for men and > 20 mm for women), and the Romhilt and Estes Point Score System [22]. These criteria reflect the presence of tall, left precordial R waves (I, aVL, V5, and V6) and deep, right precordial S waves (V1 and V2), consistent with the increased left ventricular mass and close proximity to the anterior chest wall (Figs. 13–16). LVH is also associated with poor R-wave progression and the presence of a QS pattern (no R wave) in leads V1 and V2 (rarely beyond lead V3). Two additional findings include widening of QRS complex (> 0.11 seconds) and QRS complex notching (delay in the intrinsicoid deflection to ≥ 0.05 seconds in leads V5 and V6) have been described [23,24].

Repolarization abnormalities resulting from LVH can produce changes in the ST-segment/T-wave morphology that may be suggestive of AMI and may confound the early evaluation of the chest-pain patient (Figs. 14, 15B, 15C, and 16A). These changes are present in over 70% of patients who have developed LVH; a significant minority of these individuals, however, do not demonstrate change (Figs. 13 and 15A) [25]. In a retrospective study investigating interobserver variability with regard to the ST-segment waveform, Erling and colleagues reported that the rate of disagreement involving LVH was significantly more than any other ECG pattern studied [20]. In addition, Larsen and colleagues have described misinterpretation of LVH related repolarization change in greater than 70% of patients believed initially to have ACS [25].

The repolarization abnormalities associated with LVH can be divided into those associated with ST-segment elevation coupled with prominent, "hyperacute" T waves and those associated with ST-segment depression and T-wave inversions. In the former situation, ST-segment elevation and prominent T waves can be identified in the right to midprecordial leads (Figs. 14, 15B, 15C, and 16A). As described earlier, the QS pattern that develops in these leads can produce ST elevation consistent with the concept of appropriate discordance. Although ST segment is usually 2 to 4 mm in

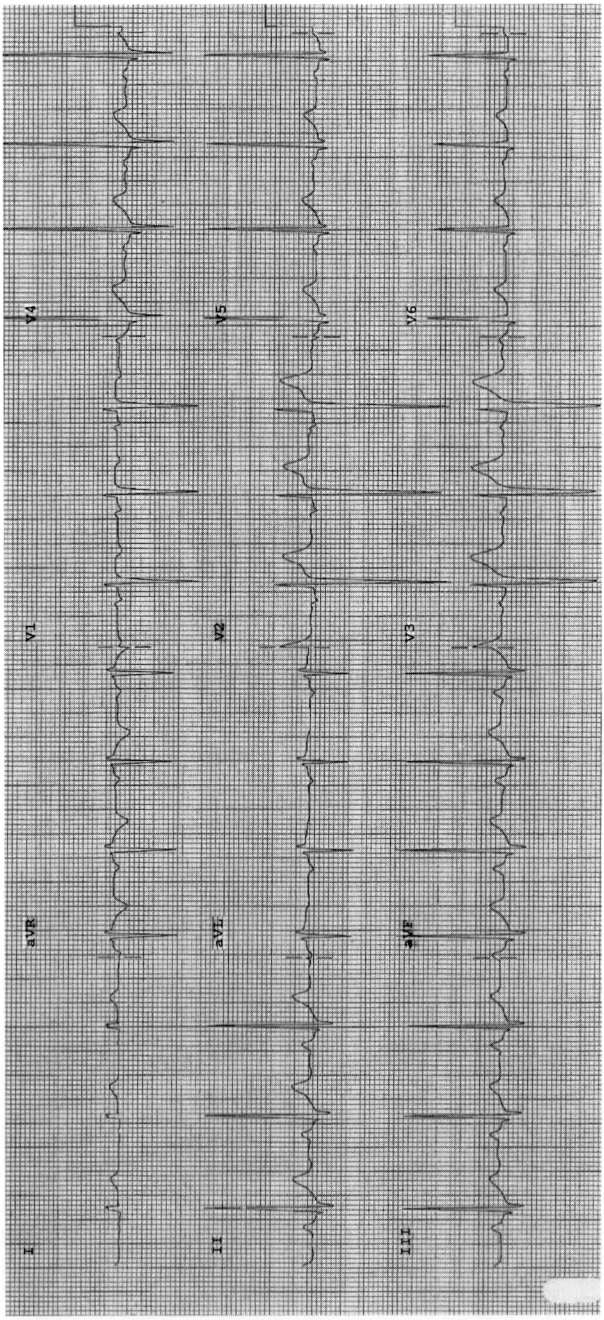

Fig. 13. 12-lead ECG with left ventricular hypertrophy pattern. Note absence of ST-segment and T-wave changes.

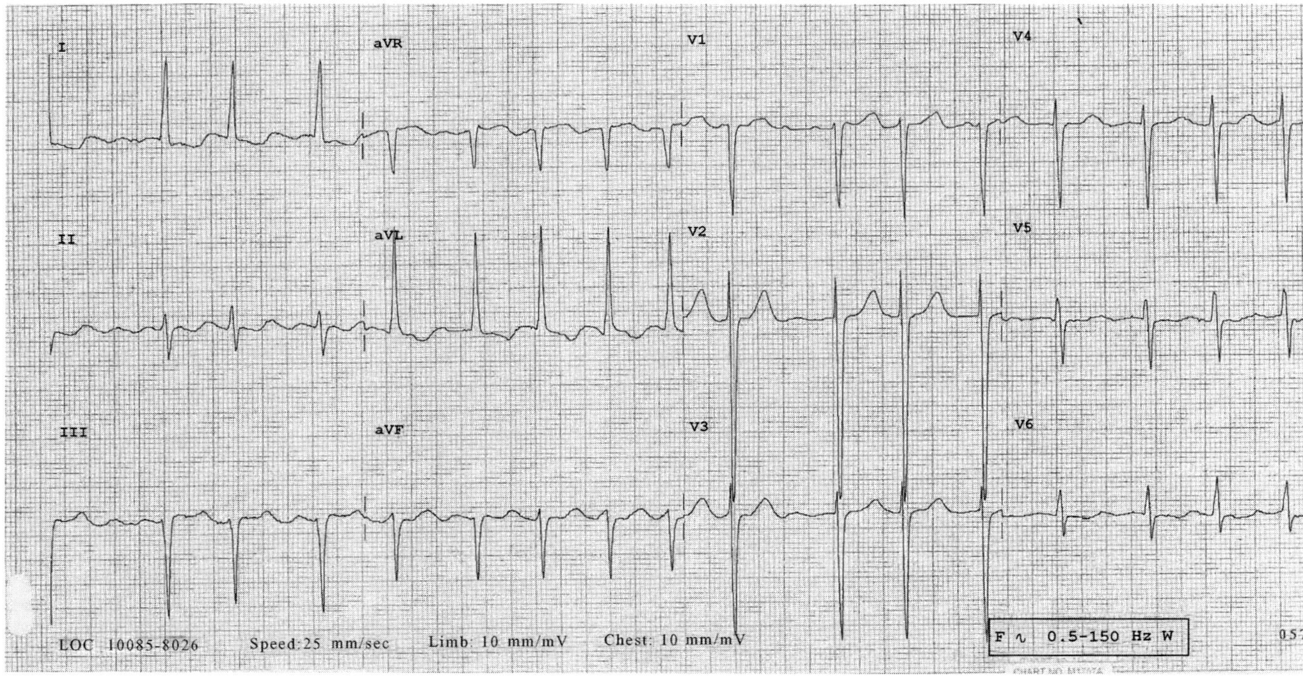

Fig. 14. 12-lead ECG with left ventricular hypertrophy pattern. Note presence of minimal ST-segment and T-wave changes in the anterior (ST-segment elevation) and lateral (ST-segment depression with T-wave inversion) leads.

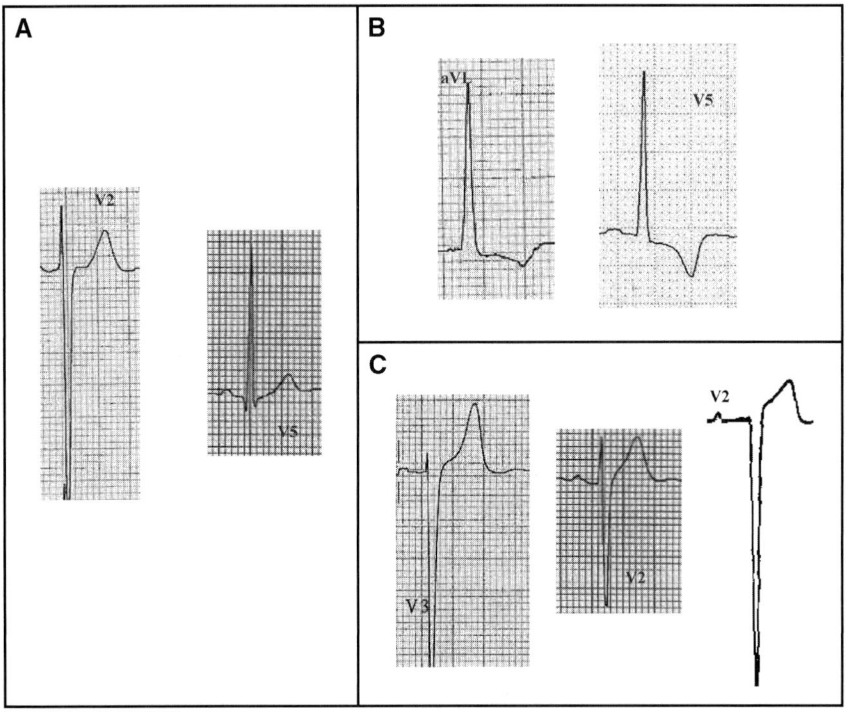

Fig. 15. ECG structures in left ventricular hypertrophy pattern. (*A*) Note absence of ST-segment and T-wave changes. (*B*) Predominantly positive QRS complexes with ST-segment depression and T-wave inversion. (*C*) Predominantly negative QRS complexes with ST-segment elevation and upright T wave.

height, it can be greater than 5 mm, making it difficult to distinguish from AMI. However, the initial upsloping of the ST segment in LVH is usually concave, in contrast to the flattened or convex pattern associated with AMI. Although helpful, this morphologic distinction is imperfect as the ST segment in early AMI can also possess a concave appearance [2]. In the latter situation, an "LVH strain" pattern can be identified in leads with prominent R waves, (ie, the lateral leads [I, aVL, V5, and V6]). The morphology of the ST segment/T waves are described as an initially convex, downsloping ST segment extending into a gradual downsloping inverted, asymmetric T wave with an abrupt return to baseline. Other characteristic findings suggestive of LVH-associated repolarization change include depression of the J point, an "overshoot" or terminal positivity of the T wave as it abruptly returns toward baseline, a T-wave inversion in V6 greater than 3 mm and greater than T wave inversion in V4. The asymmetric nature of the T-wave inversion coupled with the other ECG findings described earlier can aid in distinguishing between LVH and ACS, wherein symmetric T-wave inversions are more common [22]. Although diagnostic criteria and morphologic patterns can aid the emergency physician in the evaluation and interpretation of the ECG, the ECG should always be interpreted in the context of an individual patient.

Another feature of LVH-related ST segment/T wave change is its relative permanence. The ECG changes resulting from acute coronary ischemia are dynamic in nature; they are likely to change over the short-term in the early phase of evaluation in the ED. Conversely, the ST-segment/T-wave abnormalities related to LVH are constant or fixed; these changes are unlikely to change during the initial ED evaluation. This difference in the longevity of the ST segment/T wave changes in the two syndromes lends itself to differentiation using serial ECG monitoring or ST-segment trend analysis–evolution of the ST-segment/T-wave abnormalities in the ED is suggestive of ACS.

The ECG diagnosis of an ACS event is made more challenging in this ECG LVH scenario. With the pre-existing ST-segment and T-wave abnormalities encountered in three quarters of patients who have the LVH pattern, superimposed ECG change of an ACS is often not apparent. Refer to Figs. 16A, 16B, and 17 for an example of anterior-wall AMIs developing in the setting of two patients who have the ECG LVH strain pattern.

Medical decision-making and clinical strategies

Patients suspected of AMI who present with a confounding ECG pattern are at an extreme diagnostic disadvantage, a major diagnostic tool has been partially or entirely invalidated. Certainly, an ACS event, not AMI, is likely diagnosed by a review of the clinical history; many treatment strategies, including disposition, can be established based on patient history. Yet fibrinolysis cannot be offered based solely on historical issues. Serum marker analysis provides confirmation of AMI in certain patients. Serum markers are insensitive early in the course of AMI, a time during which reperfusion strategies, such as PCI or fibrinolysis, have the most benefit to offer. Other investigations, such as echocardiography and nuclear imaging are also of benefit in establishing AMI yet are not available in many institutions on a continuous basis.

An awareness of the confounding nature of these patterns coupled with a sound knowledge of the "new normal" ECG patterns assist the clinician in ECG interpretation in these complicated patients. Based on an understanding of the electrophysiological consequences of these conduction disturbances, the ECG suspicion—if not actual diagnosis—of AMI is possible in a significant minority of patients. A diagnostic approach provides the physician with the information necessary to offer the patient early revascularization therapy.

Other diagnostic strategies may also assist the clinician in evaluating these complicated ECGs. Serial ECGs, ST-segment trend monitoring, and

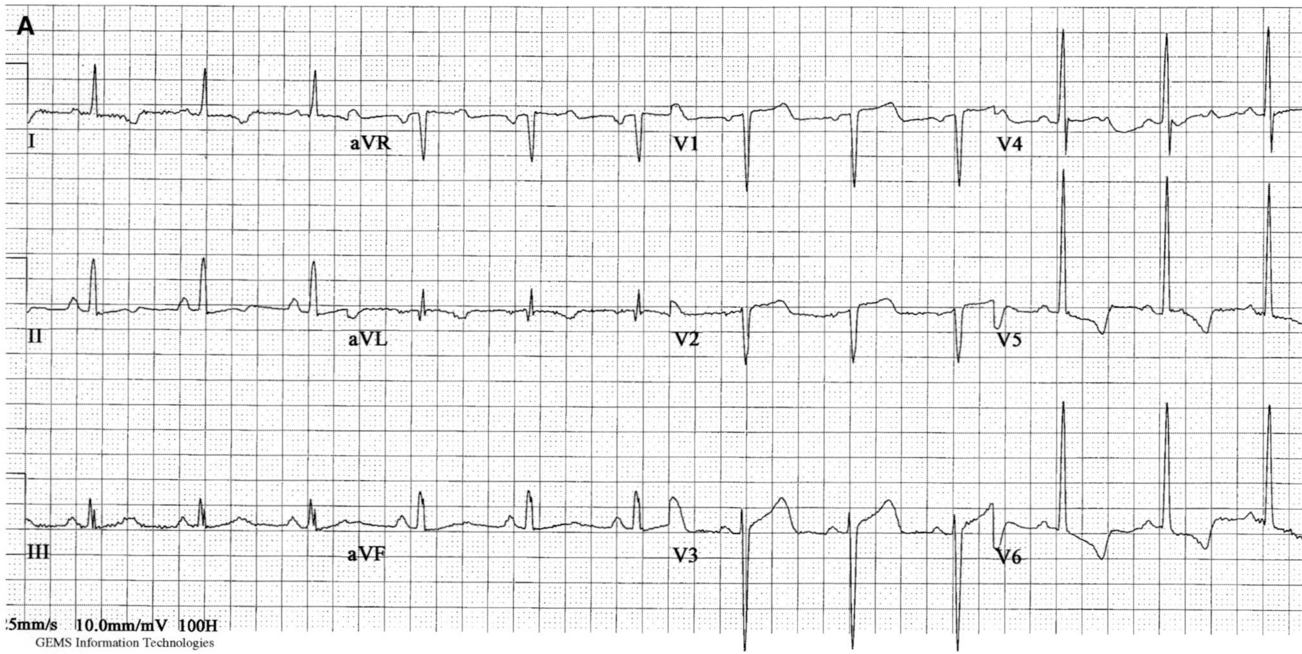

Fig. 16. (*A*) 12-lead ECG with left ventricular hypertrophy pattern. Note presence of significant ST- segment and T-wave changes particularly in anterior (ST-segment elevation) and lateral (ST-segment depression with T-wave inversion) leads. (*B*) Note development of pronounced ST-segment elevation in leads V2 and V3 with obliquely straight form of ST segment, consistent with ST-segment elevation AMI of the anterior wall.

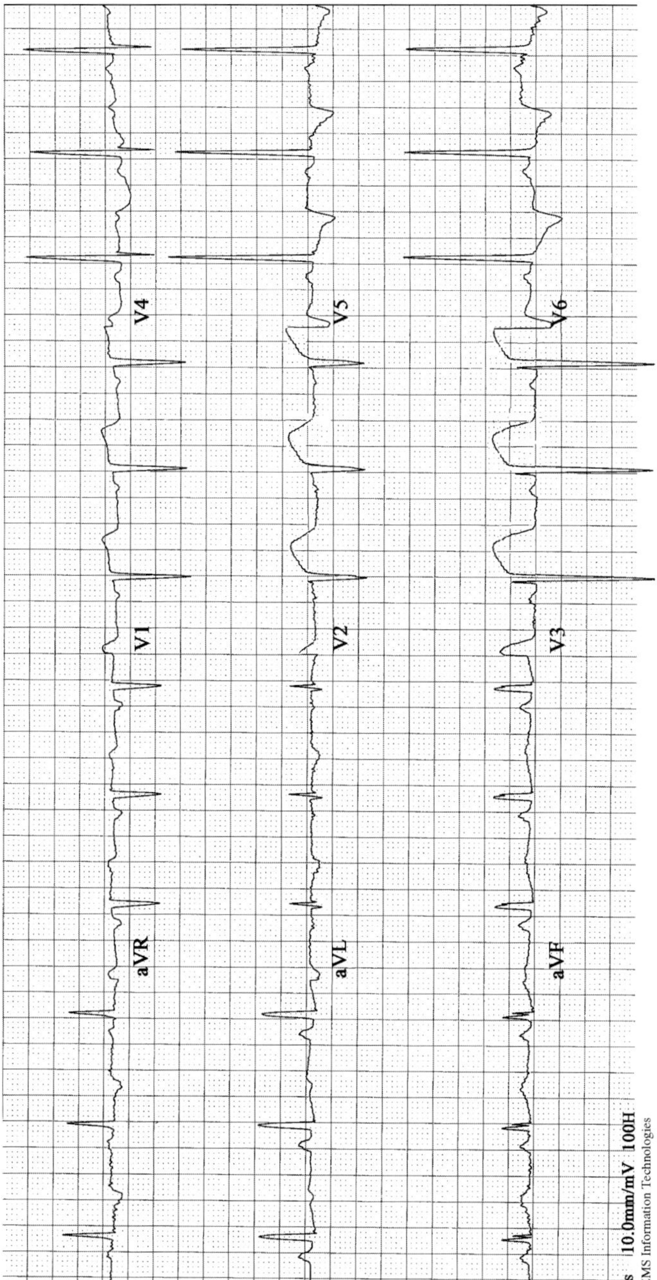

Fig. 16 *(continued)*

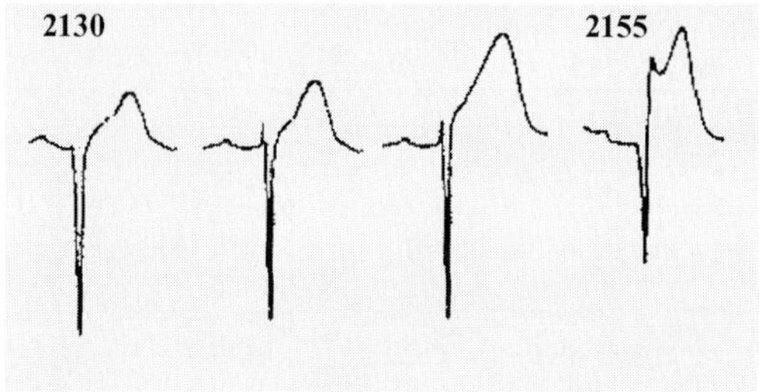

Fig. 17. Lead V2 in a patient with ECG LVH pattern with progressive abnormality demonstrating increasing ST-segment elevation and changing morphology of elevated ST segment.

a comparison with prior ECGs, if available, are potentially of diagnostic value. ST-segment trend monitoring can provide the physician with a powerful tool in this evaluation: the chest-pain patient who has developed confounding patterns, such as LBBB, VPR, and LVH. ST-segment variability may be encountered in these patients with ACS; continuous ST-segment monitoring is potentially useful in detecting dynamic change. For instance, Fesmire [26] was able to diagnose five patients with AMI and LBBB based on dynamic ST segments in the early phase of ED monitoring, resulting in alterations in their care and more appropriate therapy.

References

[1] Brady WJ, Perron AD, Martin ML, et al. Electrocardiographic ST segment elevation in emergency department chest pain center patients: etiology responsible for the ST segment abnormality. Am J Emerg Med 2001;19:25–8.

[2] Brady WJ, Syverud SA, Beagle C, et al. Electrocardiographic ST segment elevation: the diagnosis of AMI by morphologic analysis of the ST segment. Acad Emerg Med 2001;8: 961–7.

[3] Miller DH, Kligfield P, Schreiber TL, et al. Relationship of prior myocardial infarction to false-positive electrocardiographic diagnosis of acute injury in patents with chest pain. Arch Intern Med 1987;147:257–61.

[4] Sharkey SW, Berger CR, Brunette DD, et al. Impact of the electrocardiogram on the delivery of thrombolytic therapy for acute myocardial infarction. Am J Cardiol 1994;73:550–3.

[5] Hindman MC, Wagner GS, JaRo M, et al. The clinical significance of bundle branch block complicating acute myocardial infarction. 1. Clinical characteristics, hospital mortality, and one year followup. Circulation 1978;58:679–88.

[6] Shlipak MG, Go AS, Frederick PD, et al, for the National Registry of Myocardial Infarction 2 Investigators. Treatment and outcomes of left bundle-branch block patients with myocardial infarction who present without chest pain. J Am Col Cardiol 2000;36:706–12.

[7] Wackers FJ. The diagnosis of myocardial infarction in the presence of left bundle branch block. Cardiol Clin 1987;5:393–401.

[8] Hands ME, Cook EF, Stone PH, et al. Electrocardiographic diagnosis of myocardial infarction in the presence of complete left bundle branch block. Am Heart J 1988;116:23–31.

[9] Sgarbossa EB, Pinski SL, Barbagelata A, et al. Electrocardiographic diagnosis of evolving acute myocardial infarction in the presence of left bundle-branch block. N Engl J Med 1996; 334:481–7.

[10] Madias JE, Sinha A, Ashtiani R, et al. A critique of the new ST-segment criteria for the diagnosis of acute myocardial infarction in patients with left bundle-branch block. Clin Cardiol 2001;24:652–5.

[11] Skolove PE, Sgarbossa EB, Amsterdam EA, et al. Interobserver agreement in the electrocardiographic diagnosis of acute myocardial infarction in patients with left bundle branch block. Ann Emerg Med 2000;36:566–71.

[12] Kontos MC, McQueen RH, Jesse RL, Tatum JL, Ornato JP. Can myocardial infarction be rapidly identified in emergency department patients who have left bundle-branch block. Ann Emerg Med 2001;37:431–8.

[13] Edhouse JA, Sakr M, Angus J, et al. Suspected myocardial infarction and left bundle branch block: electrocardiographic indicators of acute ischemia. J Accid Emerg Med 1999;16:331–5.

[14] Soli-Pallares D, Cisnersos F, Medrano GA, et al. Electrocardiographic Diagnosis of Myocardial Infarction in the Presence of Bundle-Branch Block (right and left), Ventricular Premature Beats, and Wolff-Parkinson-White Syndrome. Prog Cardiovasc Dis 1963;6: 107–21.

[15] Castellanos A, Zoble R, Procacci PM, et al. St-qR pattern: new sign for diagnosis of anterior myocardial infarction during right ventricular pacing. Br Heart J 1973;35:1161–6.

[16] Niremberg V, Amikam S, Roguin N, et al. Primary ST changes. diagnostic aid in patients with acute myocardial infarction. Br Heart J 1977;39:502–7.

[17] Sgarbossa EB, Piniski SL, Gates KB, et al. Early electrocardiographic diagnosis of acute myocardial infarction in the presence of ventricular paced rhythm. Am J Cardiol 1996;77: 423–4.

[18] The GUSTO Investigators. An international randomized trial comparing four thrombolytic strategies for acute myocardial infarction. N Engl J Med 1993;329:673–82.

[19] Vakili BA, Okin PM, Devereux RB. Prognostic implications of left ventricular hypertrophy. Am Heart J 2001;141:334–41.

[20] Erling BF, Perron AD, Brady WJ. Disagreement in the interpretation of electrocardiographic ST segment elevation: a source of error for emergency physician? Am J Med 2004; 22:65–70.

[21] Pope JH, Auferheide TP, Rutzhazer R, et al. Missed diagnoses of acute cardiac ischemia in the emergency department. N Engl J Med 2000;342:1163–70.

[22] Gazoni PM, Evans TC. Ventricular hypertrophy in Chan et al's ECG in emergency medicine and acute care. 1st edition. Philadelphia: Elsevier/Mosby; 2005.

[23] Mirvis DM, Goldberger AL. Electrocardiography. In: Braunwald E, editor. Heart disease: a textbook of cardiovascular medicine. Philadelphia: WB Saunders; 2001. p. 1301–21.

[24] Surawicz B, Knilans TK. Chou's electrocardiography in clinical practice: adult and pediatric. 5th edition. Philadelphia: WB Saunders; 2001.

[25] Larsen GC, Griffith JL, Beshansky JR, et al. Electrocardiographic left ventricular hypertrophy in patients with suspected acute cardiac ischemia: its influence on diagnosis, treatment and short-term prognosis. J Gen Intern Med 1994;9:666–73.

[26] Fesmire FM. ECG diagnosis of acute myocardial infarction in the presence of left bundle-branch block in patients undergoing continuous ECG monitoring. Ann Emerg Med 1995;26: 69–82.

ELSEVIER
SAUNDERS

Emerg Med Clin N Am
23 (2005) 1027–1042

EMERGENCY
MEDICINE
CLINICS OF
NORTH AMERICA

Treatment of Patients with Unstable Angina and Non-ST Elevation Myocardial Infarction

Jeffrey Tabas, MD*, Erin McNutt, MD

University of California San Francisco School of Medicine, San Francisco, CA, USA

Determining how and when to treat patients who experience suspected unstable angina (UA) and non-ST elevation myocardial infarction (NSTEMI) is never simple. One of the greatest challenges comes from the distinction between patients who have developed a suspected disease and those who experience a proven disease and how this distinction affects treatment choices. In this article, the authors review the current literature and recommendations from the American College of Cardiology and American Heart Association for treatment of patients who present with UA/NSTEMI. A class 1 recommendation is given when there is evidence or general agreement that a given procedure or treatment is useful and effective. A Class 2a recommendation is given when conflicting evidence or a divergence of opinion exists, but the weight of evidence/opinion is in favor of usefulness/efficacy. This article puts treatment selection into perspective by reviewing benefits and risks of these therapies.

Understanding treatment benefit

Treatment selection for patients who have suspected acute coronary syndrome (ACS) must be based on risk assessment. Benefit from treatment should be considered as the number needed to treat (NNT) to prevent one adverse outcome, such as mortality or myocardial infarction (MI), derived from the *absolute* (not the relative) decrease in adverse outcomes. If a treatment decreases *relative* mortality/MI by 50%

* Corresponding author. Emergency Services, San Francisco General Hospital, 1001 Potero Avenue, Room 1E21, San Francisco, CA 94117.

E-mail address: jtabas@sfghed.ucsf.edu (J. Tabas).

doi:10.1016/j.emc.2005.07.008

and baseline mortality/MI is 20%, the *absolute* decrease is 10% and the NNT is 10. If baseline mortality/MI is only 2%, however, mortality/MI is decreased to 1% and the NNT is 100. Generally, patients who have more severe disease have higher rates of adverse events and, therefore, treatment is more beneficial.

The accuracy of patient selection is another factor that is more subtle but has a major impact on the NNT to benefit from a given therapy. If the NNT is 100, but only half of the treated patients prove to have disease, the NNT is 200. In clinical practice, the accuracy of patient selection and the severity of disease are closely related. The presence of ischemic ECG changes or elevated cardiac markers is by far the most predictive for disease severity and presence of disease in patients who develop suspected UA and NSTEMI.

The number needed to harm (NNH) from a given therapy, however, is less impacted by accuracy of patient selection or disease severity. If the NNH (eg, to cause one intracranial hemorrhage) is 100, it may remain 100 whether or not the treated patient has the disease. Because a therapy is only indicated when treatment benefit outweighs harm, patients need to be selected more carefully for therapies that cause more severe untoward effects; thus, therapies which prove beneficial in patients who present with diagnostic findings of UA/NSTEMI (ischemic ECG changes or elevated cardiac markers) may not be beneficial when applied more broadly to patients who have suspected disease without these findings. Box 1 describes a treatment approach based on these concepts.

Therapies in unstable angina/non-ST elevation myocardial infarction

Aspirin

Aspirin (ASA) at a dose of 160 to 325 mg, should be administered immediately to all patients who have developed suspected UA/NSTEMI and who do not have a life-threatening allergy. The benefits of ASA far outweigh bleeding risks associated with its use. By preventing the formation of thromboxane A_2 through its irreversible inhibition of cyclooxygenase-1 within platelets, ASA decreases platelet aggregation and thrombus propagation. In the ISIS-2 trial, ASA was given at doses of 160 mg on presentation and continued for 1 month in patients who experience suspected MI [1]. The NNT was 40 to prevent one death. Pooled data from four trials involving 2448 patients who present with UA/NSTEMI reveals the NNT to prevent death or MI is 16 [2–6]. When used alone, ASA causes no increase in bleeding requiring transfusion or hemorrhagic stroke [1]. Contraindications to ASA include intolerance and allergy (primarily manifested as asthma), active bleeding, hemophilia, active retinal bleeding, severe untreated hypertension, an active peptic ulcer, or another serious

Box 1. Emergency department treatment approach based on risk assessment

Possible unstable angina/non-ST elevation myocardial infarction

This category represents most patients who may present with symptoms of chest pain, shortness of breath, weakness, upper abdominal pain, or other complaints consistent with ACS but lacking 1) elevation of cardiac markers, 2) ST-depression diagnostic of ischemia on ECG, or 3) shock or heart failure as a result of acute ischemia. Treat with:

- Aspirin (ASA) (or clopidogrel if ASA-allergic)
- Oxygen, nitrates, and beta-blockers if there are no contraindications and the history is compelling

Likely or definite unstable angina/non-ST elevation myocardial infarction

These patients present with symptoms of ACS and 1) elevation of cardiac markers, 2) ST- depression diagnostic of ischemia on ECG, or 3) shock or heart failure as a result of acute ischemia. Treat with:

- ASA
- Oxygen (if hypoxic or in first 6 hours of symptoms)
- Nitrates
- Beta-blockers (if contraindications, then use Calcium Channel Blockers)
- Morphine
- UFH or LMWH
- Clopidogrel if PCI is not planned

If ischemia is ongoing with findings on ECG or cardiac markers, consider adding:

- GP 2b3a antagonist

If PCI is planned add:

- GP 2b3a antagonist (may be given in the cardiac catheterization lab)
- UFH or LMWH or bivalirudin
- Clopidogrel (may be given in the cardiac catheterization laboratory once indications for CABG are determined to be absent)

source of gastrointestinal or genitourinary bleeding. Administration and proper dosing should be confirmed in patients who have received ASA at home or in the prehospital setting. For ASA-allergic patients, give clopidogrel (see later discussion).

American College of Cardiology/American Heart Association Recommendations
Class 1:

- ASA should be administered as soon as possible after presentation and continued indefinitely.

Oxygen

It is common to administer to 2 L of oxygen by nasal cannula to all patients who develop suspected UA/NSTEMI, although little evidence of benefit exists other than in those with hypoxemia ($SaO_2 < 90\%$) or respiratory compromise. In patients who develop likely or definite UA/NSTEMI, oxygen should be delivered during the first 6 hours. Patients who experience severe respiratory distress or hypoxemia may need higher flow rates of oxygen administration or even intubation. Pulse oximetry is also recommended in patients who have developed likely or definite UA/NSTEMI to document oxygenation.

American College of Cardiology/American Heart Association Recommendations
Class 1:

- Supplemental oxygen for patients who experience cyanosis or respiratory distress: finger pulse oximetry or arterial blood gas determination to confirm adequate arterial oxygen saturation ($SaO_2 > 90\%$) and continued need for supplemental oygen in the presence of hypoxemia.

Beta-blockers

In addition to ASA, beta-blocking agents decrease mortality in patients who develop suspected MI. Though no trial has looked specifically at beta blockade in patients who experience UA/NSTEMI alone, data from trials including this patient population suggest a NNT of 140 to 160 to prevent one death at 7 to 14 days [7,8]. By selectively blocking β1 receptors located primarily in the myocardium, agents, such as metoprolol, atenolol, and esmolol, decrease myocardial oxygen demand by reducing heart rate, systemic arterial pressure, and myocardial contractility. As a consequence of reducing heart rate, diastole is prolonged, augmenting flow within the coronary vessels; therefore, beta-blocking agents may reduce mortality by decreasing infarct size and frequency of life-threatening arrhythmias.

Choices of commonly used selective beta-blockers and their dosing regimens are listed in Table 1. Contraindications to the use of beta-blockers include cardiogenic shock, active airway compromise caused by reactive airway disease—asthma or COPD—acute congestive heart failure (CHF), first-degree Atrioventricular (AV) block with a PR interval greater than 0.24

Table 1
Commonly used selective β1-receptor antagonists

Drug	Loading dose	Maintenance dose
Metoprolol	5 mg IV q 5 min × 3 doses	25–50 mg PO 15 min afterload and then q 6 h
Esmolol	0.5 mg/kg IV over 2–5 min	Titrate 0.05 mg/kg/min IV q 10–15 min until max drip of 0.3 mg/kg/min
Atenolol	5 mg IV q 5 min × 2 doses	50–100 mg PO 1–2 hours afterload and then q day

Abbreviations: IV, intravenous; PO, per os (by mouth); q, every.

seconds, second- or third-degree AV block in the absence of a functioning pacemaker, bradycardia less than 50 beats per minute, and systolic blood pressure (BP) less than 90 mm Hg [2]. If potential side effects from beta blockade are a concern, esmolol, an ultra short-acting cardioselective β1 antagonist may be used. Alternatively, smaller doses of metoprolol, starting at 2.5 mg IV may also be administered in this setting. Beta-selective-blocking agents should not be administered to patients who have ACS precipitated by use of cocaine because of the risk for exacerbating coronary spasm by unopposed alpha effect.

American College of Cardiology/American Heart Association Recommendations
Class 1

- Administer a beta-blocker, with the first dose administered intravenously (IV) if there is ongoing chest pain, followed by oral administration, in the absence of contraindications.

Nitrates

Although not shown to affect mortality in patients who experience UA/NSTEMI [9,10], nitrates are recommended based on pathophysiologic principles and uncontrolled clinical observations. In a pooled analysis composed largely of patients from the Fourth International Study of Infarct Survival Collaborative Group (ISIS-4) trial, the NNT to prevent death (MI was not included) was 260 (not statistically significant), although the NNH was 120 to cause profound hypotension in the initial 24 hours [10]. Nitrates vasodilate coronary vessels and may decrease myocardial oxygen consumption through peripheral vasodilatation, leading to a decrease in preload and a more modest decrease in afterload [11]. This decrease in oxygen consumption may be offset by reflex tachycardia and contractility unless a beta-blocker is used concurrently. Nitroglycerin is administered routinely and immediately to patients who experience chest pain at doses of 0.4 mg sublingually every 5 minutes for a total of three doses.

Given the lack of clear benefit from the use of nitrates, caution should be used in patients at risk for hypotensive events, including those who develop suspected right ventricular (RV) infarct or low systolic BPs. Significant bradycardia (<50 beats per minute) or tachycardia are also contraindications, although these recommendations are based on scant evidence [2,12]. IV access should be established before the use of nitrates in these patients to anticipate the need for volume resuscitation. Use of the agents for erectile dysfunction, sildenafil, or vardenafil within 24 hours, or tadalafil within 48 hours, is an absolute contraindication because of the risk for prolonged and exaggerated vasodilatation [13].

In patients who develop likely or definite ischemia, initial treatment consists of 0.4 mg of nitroglycerin sublingual tablet or spray repeated every 5 minutes for three doses. Treatment may be continued with 1 to 2 inches of 2% topical nitropaste applied to the chest wall. Indications for IV therapy include the first 24 to 48 hours for patients who develop likely or definite UA/NSTEMI and experience ongoing or recurrent ischemic discomfort, hypertension, or signs of CHF or for controlled titration of therapy. Recommended dosing starts at 10 to 20 μg/min and is titrated by 10 to 20 μg/min every few minutes. Aggressive titration is reasonable in a patient who has tolerated given an estimated dose of 80 μg/min for five minutes from sublingual dosing. Titration should continue until an effect is seen, or a decrease occurs in systolic pressure to 90 mm Hg, or a decrease in mean arterial pressure of greater than 30% in hypertensive patients or 10% in normotensive patients [2]. Tachyphylaxis develops with the use of nitrates, and recurrence of symptoms may mandate increasing dosages.

American College of Cardiology/American Heart Association Recommendations

Class 1:

- Administer nitroglycerin, sublingual tablet or spray, for the immediate relief of ischemia and associated symptoms.
- Adminster IV in patients who experience continuing or frequently occurring ischemia.

Morphine

Morphine is recommended to relieve pain and discomfort believed to be caused by acute myocardial infarction (AMI). Although no randomized trials have defined its role or dosing regimen, morphine is recommended for pain relief in patients who experience ongoing ischemic discomfort despite treatment with ASA, beta-blockers, and nitroglycerin. Relief of pain and anxiety is believed to decrease adrenergic outflow thereby decreasing myocardial oxygen demand. In the absence of hypotension, morphine may be started at doses of 1 to 5 mg IV [2]. Morphine's major side effects include hypotension, respiratory depression, and nausea, sometimes requiring the use of antiemetics.

Angiotensin-converting enzyme inhibitors

Angiotensin-converting enzyme (ACE) inhibitors are recommended during initial hospitalization for all patients who develop AMI, especially those who experience anterior wall MI or CHF with BP greater than 100 mm Hg [14]. The NNT is 200 to prevent one death. Evidence to support treatment with these agents in the emergency department (ED) is lacking, and therapy should be initiated after the patient has demonstrated hemodynamic stability, usually within the first 36 hours. Generally, a short-acting ACE inhibitor, such as captopril, is started first, allowing titration according to BP.

American College of Cardiology/American Heart Association recommendations for angiotensin-converting enzyme inhibitors
Class 1:

- In patients who experience left ventricular systolic dysfunction, CHF, or diabetes when hypertension persists despite treatment with nitroglycerin and a beta-blocker.

Class 2:

- All patients post UA/NSTEMI.

Calcium channel blockers

Calcium channel blockers reduce cellular membrane influx of calcium, but have variable effects on peripheral arterial vasodilatation, inotropy, chronotropy and atrioventricular conduction. Their role in UA/NSTEMI seems primarily limited to symptom control when contraindications to beta-blockers are present, such as patients who experience cocaine-induced chest pain and coronary vasospasm.

Rapid-release short-acting dihydropyridines, such as nifedipine, nisoldipine, and nicardipine, cause greater peripheral arterial vasodilatation than conduction-slowing effects and have been shown to be detrimental in the setting of UA [15,16]—their use is to be avoided [2]. The nondihydropyridines, such as verapamil and diltiazem, have more effect on slowing atrioventricular and sinus node conduction, thereby decreasing oxygen demand by decreasing contractility, heart rate, and afterload, which may impart benefit [17,18].

American College of Cardiology/American Heart Association recommendations for calcium channel blockers
Class 1:

- In patients who experience frequent or continuing ischemia when beta-blockers are contraindicated in the absence of severe systolic dysfunction or other contraindications.

Class 2a:

- In addition to beta-blockers and nitrates when ischemia persists.

Heparin

The significant benefit shown from heparin use in patients who develop UA/NSTEMI was largely from the pre-ASA era. A meta-analysis of all six randomized controlled trials in UA patients receiving heparin plus ASA versus ASA alone revealed a trend to benefit, with a NNT of 20 to prevent death or MI and a NNH of 90 to cause major bleeding, although neither of these reached statistical significance [19].

Heparin exerts its anticoagulant effect by accelerating the action of circulating antithrombin, which prevents thrombus propagation but does not lyse existing thrombi. Low molecular weight heparins (LMWH) are degradation products of unfractionated heparin (UFH). The pharmacodynamic and pharmacokinetic profiles of the different commercial preparations vary. LMWHs can be delivered subcutaneously. Unlike UFHs, they usually do not require laboratory monitoring of activity. Contraindications to any heparin include a history of heparin-induced thrombotic thrombocytopenia. Contraindications to treatment with LMWH include known sensitivity to pork, and caution should be used in extremes of weight or severe renal dysfunction.

Low molecular weight heparins versus unfractionated heparin

Although the American College of Cardiology/American Heart Association (ACC/AHA) guidelines recommend that LMWH is preferable to UFH in patients who develop UA/NSTEMI, both agents exhibit comparable efficacy and safety. A recent meta-analysis compared enoxaparin with UFH in six trials involving 21,946 patients who develop UA/NSTEMI [20]. Although enoxaparin reportedly showed a NNT of 110 to reduce death or MI with no increase in NNH, one of the six trials accounted for most of the positive effect. In this trial, thrombolysis in myocardial infarction (TIMI)-11b, patients were randomized to UFH for an average of 3 days and compared with enoxaparin treatment for 6 weeks [21]. Given the difference in duration of these treatments, which was structured into the study design, direct comparison of outcomes for these regimens is questionable. If this study is removed from the analysis, no statistically significant difference exists in outcomes in the remaining 18,775 patients. Analysis of UFH compared with two other LMWHs, dalteparin [22] and nadroparin [23], showed no statistically significant benefit over UFH.

American College of Cardiology/American Heart Association recommendations

Class 1:

- Anticoagulation with subcutaneous LMWH or IV UFH should be added to antiplatelet therapy with ASA or clopidogrel.

Class 2a:

- Enoxaparin is preferable to UFH as an anticoagulant in patients who develop UA/STEMI in the absence of renal failure and unless CABG is planned within 24 hours.

Heparin dosing in acute coronary syndrome

Intravenous unfractionated heparins

- 60–70 U/kg IV bolus (max 5000 U) and 12–15 U/kg/h infusion (max 1000 U/h)
- Maintain partial thromboplastin time (PTT) 60–80 seconds based on nomogram

Low molecular weight heparins approved for use in unstable angina/non-ST elevation myocardial infarction

- Enoxaparin 1 mg/kg subcutaneously twice a day
- Dalteparin 120 IU/kg subcutaneously twice a day

Adenosine diphosphate receptor antagonists

Ticlopidine and clopidogrel are thienopyridines, which are noncompetitive antagonists of platelet adenosine diphosphate receptor. They irreversibly inhibit platelet activation but require several days to take complete effect. For secondary prevention, both have been shown to reduce adverse events in patients who develop atherosclerotic vascular disease. Clopidogrel is the preferred agent, demonstrating fewer adverse effects than ticlopidine (thrombotic thrombocytopenia purpura and neutropenia) [24].

In the acute setting, clopidogrel has been studied in UA/NSTEMI and seems to have some benefit in combination with ASA. In the CURE trial, patients who presented with UA/NSTEMI received usual care and were randomized to clopidogrel versus placebo [25]. The NNT was 50 to prevent cardiovascular death, stroke, or MI. The NNH with major bleeding was 100. Of note, the Clopidogrel in Unstable angina to prevent Recurrent Events trial only found benefit in patients who exhibited ST depression or positive cardiac markers (the definite UA/NSTEMI group). The initial study protocol, which included high-risk patients without these findings, was modified after the first 3000 patients because of lack of benefit.

In patients who underwent coronary artery bypass graft surgery (CABG) after angiography, patients treated with clopidogrel showed a significantly increased rate of major perioperative bleeding—9% versus 6% [25]. For this reason, it is recommended that, clopidogrel should be withheld for 5 to 7 days before CABG. In the acute setting, any patient going to angiography may prove to be a CABG candidate; therefore, patients who have suspected ACS and are selected for angiography should be treated only with clopidogrel after the need for CABG has been precluded.

American College of Cardiology/American Heart Association recommendations
Class 1:

- Give clopidogrel to all patients who have ACS that are ASA allergic.
- Give clopidogrel to patients who have ischemic ST depression or elevated cardiac markers.
- Initiate treatment as early as possible.
- Withhold clopidogrel treatment in patients undergoing angiography until the need for emergent CABG has been excluded.

Dosing in ACS:

- Clopidogrel: 300–600 mg by mouth initially, then 75 mg by mouth each day
- Ticlopidine: 500 mg loading dose, then 250 mg by mouth twice a day

Glycoprotein IIb/IIa receptor antagonists

Thrombus formation occurs when activated platelets form clot by initial adhesion to the endothelium and then aggregation with each other. Platelets aggregate when activated fibrin links platelets together by binding to the glycoprotein (GP) 2b3a receptor on each. By blocking this receptor, GP 2b3a antagonists block thrombus formation. Of the three agents approved for use in the United States (Box 2), two of these, tirofiban and eptifibatide, are approved for use in medical management of ACS. The efficacy of GP 2b3a antagonists in decreasing adverse outcomes in ACS patients receiving percutaneous coronary intervention (PCI) have been documented in numerous trials. In pooled data of trials from 4952 patients who experience UA/NSTEMI and received PCI treated with GP 2b3a antagonists compared with placebo, the NNT was 17 to prevent death or MI [2].

Although the ACC/AHA guidelines recommend use of these agents in certain UA/NSTEMI patients who are managed medically, definitive evidence of benefit in this setting is lacking [26]. Only one trial has been designed specifically to study this question. Seven thousand eight hundred patients who present with ST-segment depression or elevated cardiac markers who were not undergoing early revascularization were randomized to usual care in addition to placebo compared with two dosage regimens for abciximab [27]. No difference existed in the individual or combined endpoints of death or MI. Boersma and colleagues [28] performed a meta-analysis reviewing all large, randomized placebo-controlled trials of patients who experience UA/NSTEMI receiving GP 2b3a antagonists. The NNT to prevent death or MI was 100 in 31,402 treated patients; however, analysis of the 19,416 medically managed patients who did not undergo coronary revascularization revealed no reduction in death or MI [28]. NNH with major bleeding was 100.

Box 2. GP 2b3a receptor antagonists approved in the United States

Abciximab
- Murine Fab fragment
- Approved only for PCI
- 0.25 mg/kg bolus, then 0.125 μg/kg/min infusion (max-10 μg/min) for 12–24 hours

Tirofiban
- Synthetic non peptide
- Approved for PCI or medical management of ACS
- 0.4 μg/kg/min for 30 minutes (equals 0.2 μg/kg bolus), then 0.1 μg/kg/min infusion for 48–96 hours

Eptifibatide
- Synthetic cyclic heptapeptide
- Approved for PCI or medical management of ACS
- 180 μg/kg bolus then 2.0 μg/kg/min infusion for 72–96 hours

Why, then, is there controversy about whether GP 2b3a antagonists are of benefit in medically managed patients who experience UA/NSTEMI? Possibly, in patients who are randomized to treatment, those that undergo PCI account for all the benefit demonstrated in the treatment group. Based on this evidence, the strength of recommendation for the use of GP 2b3a antagonists in medically managed patients who develop UA/NSTEMI patients was downgraded from class 1 to class 2a in the 2002 ACC/AHA guidelines. Although treatment with GP 2b3a antagonists is still deemed acceptable in patients who experience continuing ischemia, an elevated troponin, or "other high-risk features," these should be given only to patients who are believed to have UA/NSTEMI (ie, elevated cardiac markers or clearly ischemic ECG changes). It is controversial whether the evidence at this time supports the use of these agents in any patient with UA/NSTEMI not undergoing PCI.

American College of Cardiology/American Heart Association recommendations

Class 1:

- Administer a platelet GP 2b3a antagonist to patients in whom catheterization and PCI are planned. They may be administered just before PCI. From an ED standpoint, deferring administration of GP 2b3a antagonists until the catheterization determines the coronary anatomy is acceptable.

Class 2a:

- Eptifibatide or tirofiban should be administered to patients who experience continuing ischemia, an elevated troponin, or high-risk features when PCI is not planned.
- Treatment with ASA, heparin, and clopidogrel should proceed as recommended whether or not GP 2b3a antagonist treatment is indicated.

Direct thrombin inhibitors

Direct thrombin inhibitors (DTI) are anticoagulants that specifically bind to thrombin, theoretically providing more predictable effects than anticoagulants, such as heparin, which require a cofactor, such as antithrombin, for thrombin inactivation. The first agent in this class, hirudin, was extracted from the medicinal leech. The agents approved in the United States are lepirudin and desirudin (recombinant forms of hirudin), bivalirudin (a synthetitic hirudin analog previously known as hirulog), and argatroban (a synthetic molecule unrelated to hirudin) [29]. Of these, only bivalirudin is approved for patients who have ACS and only for patients who experience UA undergoing PCI.

Some benefit may exist from the use of DTIs in patients who experience UA/NSTEMI, although the only currently approved uses in these patients are for PCI or for anticoagulation of patients who have a history of heparin-induced thrombocytopenic purpura. The GUSTO-IIb trial randomized patients who presented with suspected MI to 72 hours of IV recombinant hirudin versus UFH [30]. In the 8011 patients who presented without ST elevation, no statistically significant benefit existed in death or MI at 30 days. OASIS 2 [31] compared higher doses of recombinant hirudin (0.4 mg/kg bolus and 0.15 mg/kg/h infusion compared with 0.1 mg/kg bolus and 0.1 mg/kg/h infusion) to UFH in 10,141 patients who presented with UA/NSTEMI. Again, no statistically significant difference existed in death or MI at 7 days, although the NNT was 110 to prevent the combined endpoint of death, MI, or refractory ischemia. Number needed to harm was 200 to cause major bleeding. When these two trials were combined with nine smaller trials in a recent meta-analysis, DTI treatment compared with heparin resulted in a NNT of 110 to prevent death or MI in 20,570 patients who presented with UA/NSTEMI [32]. No difference existed in intracranial bleeding, and major bleeding was decreased by 0.4% overall. DTIs were shown to be of equivalent efficacy to GP 2b3a antagonists in patients undergoing PCI [33].

Percutaneous coronary intervention—conservative versus early invasive strategies

Emergent PCI was shown to have significant benefit in patients experiencing STEMI. The results are less clear in patients who present with UA/NSTEMI. In an early conservative strategy, patients who present with UA/NSTEMI are selected for cardiac catheterization using echocardiography, stress testing, and recurrent symptoms to identify persistent ischemia or decreased left ventricular function. In an early invasive approach, routine cardiac catheterization is performed either emergently or, more commonly, within 48 hours after admission. Use of the conservative strategy typically results in cardiac catheterization of one third to one half of the patients. Initial studies suggested that a conservative strategy was equivalent to or better than routine catheterization for all patients presenting with UA/NSTEMI [34–36].

More recent studies, however, have shown benefit from an early invasive strategy for patients who develop definite UA/NSTEMI (elevated cardiac markers or ST depression). This benefit may be caused by improved outcomes in PCI with the use of GP 2b3a antagonists and coronary stents. In TACTICS-TIMI-18, 2220 patients who presented with UA/NSTEMI were randomized to an early invasive versus conservative strategy [37]. The NNT was 45 to prevent death or MI at 6 months with the early invasive approach. In FRISC-2, the two approaches were compared in 2457 patients who presented with UA/NSTEMI [38]. Criteria for catheterization in the conservative arm were more stringent than other studies, and only 10% of patients received cardiac catheterization. The NNT was 37 to prevent one death or MI at 6 months using the early invasive approach. Currently, either strategy is considered acceptable.

American College of Cardiology/American Heart Association recommendations for early cardiac catheterization
Class 1

- Recurrent angina/ischemia with low-level activities despite intensive anti-ischemic therapy
- Troponin elevation
- Ischemic ST depression
- Ischemia with shock, heart failure, or depressed systolic function
- High risk findings on noninvasive stress testing
- Sustained ventricular tachycardia
- PCI within 6 months or prior CABG
- In the absence of above-mentioned findings, either an early conservative or early invasive strategy may be offered if no contraindications for revascularization.

Summary

ED management of patients who present with UA/NSTEMI is unique because these patients often present with suspected rather than proven disease. Because the impact of treatment varies depending on severity of illness and certainty of diagnosis, treatment selection in patients who present with UA/NSTEMI should be tailored to these factors. In general, patients with ECG changes, such as ischemic ST depression or elevation of cardiac markers, can be classified as definite UA/NSTEMI. Although all patients who have suspected or definite disease should be given ASA, and most patients should receive beta-blockers, medications such as heparin and clopidogrel have been shown to be of clearest benefit in patients who have definite disease. GP 2b3a antagonists have been shown to be of clearest benefit in patients receiving PCI. Other treatments are of benefit in select situations.

References

[1] Second International Study of Infarct Survival Collaborative Group (ISIS-2). Randomised trial of intravenous streptokinase, oral aspirin, both, or neither among 17,187 cases of suspected acute myocardial infarction: ISIS-2. Lancet 1988;2(8607):349–60.

[2] Braunwald E, Antman EM, Beasley JW, et al. ACC/AHA guideline update for the management of patients with unstable angina and non-ST-segment elevation myocardial infarction—summary article: a report of the American College of Cardiology/American Heart Association task force on practice guidelines (Committee on the Management of Patients with Unstable Angina). J Am Coll Cardiol 2002;40(7):1366–74.

[3] The RISC Group. Risk of myocardial infarction and death during treatment with low dose aspirin and intravenous heparin in men with unstable coronary artery disease. Lancet 1990; 336(8719):827–30.

[4] Cairns JA, Gent M, Singer J, et al. Aspirin, sulfinpyrazone, or both in unstable angina: results of a Canadian multicenter trial. N Engl J Med 1985;313(22):1369–75.

[5] Lewis HD Jr, Davis JW, Archibald DG, et al. Protective effects of aspirin against acute myocardial infarction and death in men with unstable angina. Results of a Veterans Administration Cooperative Study. N Engl J Med 1983;309(7):396–403.

[6] Theroux P, Ouimet H, McCans J, et al. Aspirin, heparin, or both to treat acute unstable angina. N Engl J Med 1988;319(17):1105–11.

[7] The MIAMI Trial Research Group. Metoprolol in acute myocardial infarction (MIAMI): a randomised placebo-controlled international trial. Eur Heart J 1985;6(3):199–226.

[8] First International Study of Infarct Survival Collaborative Group (ISIS-1). Randomised trial of intravenous atenolol among 16,027 cases of suspected acute myocardial infarction: ISIS-1. Lancet 1986;2(8498):57–66.

[9] Gruppo Italiano per lo Studio della Sopravvivenza nell'infarto Miocardico (GISSI-3). Effects of lisinopril and transdermal glyceryl trinitrate singly and together on 6-week mortality and ventricular function after acute myocardial infarction. Lancet 1994;343(8906): 1115–22.

[10] Fourth International Study of Infarct Survival Collaborative Group (ISIS-4). A randomised factorial trial assessing early oral captopril, oral mononitrate, and intravenous magnesium sulphate in 58,050 patients with suspected acute myocardial infarction. Lancet 1995; 345(8951):669–85.

[11] Gorman MW, Sparks HV Jr. Nitroglycerin causes vasodilatation within ischaemic myocardium. Cardiovasc Res 1980;14(9):515–21.

[12] Kinch JW, Ryan TJ. Right ventricular infarction. N Engl J Med 1994;330(17):1211–7.

[13] Antman EM, Anbe DT, Armstrong PW, et al. ACC/AHA guidelines for the management of patients with ST-elevation myocardial infarction: a report of the American College of Cardiology/American Heart Association task force on practice guidelines (Committee to Revise the 1999 Guidelines for the Management of Patients with Acute Myocardial Infarction). Circulation 2004;110(9):e82–292.

[14] ACE Inhibitor Myocardial Infarction Collaborative Group. Indications for ACE inhibitors in the early treatment of acute myocardial infarction: systematic overview of individual data from 100,000 patients in randomized trials. Circulation 1998;97(22):2202–12.

[15] Lubsen J, Tijssen JG. Efficacy of nifedipine and metoprolol in the early treatment of unstable angina in the coronary care unit: findings from the Holland Interuniversity Nifedipine/metoprolol Trial (HINT). Am J Cardiol 1987;60(2):18A–25A.

[16] Furberg CD, Psaty BM, Meyer JV. Nifedipine. Dose-related increase in mortality in patients with coronary heart disease. Circulation 1995;92(5):1326–31.

[17] Pepine CJ, Faich G, Makuch R. Verapamil use in patients with cardiovascular disease: an overview of randomized trials. Clin Cardiol 1998;21(9):633–41.

[18] Gibson RS, Boden WE, Theroux P, et al. Diltiazem and reinfarction in patients with non-Q-wave myocardial infarction. Results of a double-blind, randomized, multicenter trial. N Engl J Med 1986;315(7):423–9.

[19] Oler A, Whooley MA, Oler J, et al. Adding heparin to aspirin reduces the incidence of myocardial infarction and death in patients with unstable angina. A meta-analysis. JAMA 1996;276(10):811–5.

[20] Petersen JL, Mahaffey KW, Hasselblad V, et al. Efficacy and bleeding complications among patients randomized to enoxaparin or unfractionated heparin for antithrombin therapy in non-ST-segment elevation acute coronary syndromes: a systematic overview. JAMA 2004;292(1):89–96.

[21] Antman EM, McCabe CH, Gurfinkel EP, et al. Enoxaparin prevents death and cardiac ischemic events in unstable angina/non-Q-wave myocardial infarction. Results of the thrombolysis in myocardial infarction (TIMI) 11B trial. Circulation 1999;100(15):1593–601.

[22] Klein W, Buchwald A, Hillis SE, et al. Comparison of low-molecular-weight heparin with unfractionated heparin acutely and with placebo for 6 weeks in the management of unstable coronary artery disease. Fragmin in unstable coronary artery disease study (FRIC). Circulation 1997;96(1):61–8.

[23] FRAXIS study group. Comparison of two treatment durations (6 days and 14 days) of a low molecular weight heparin with a 6-day treatment of unfractionated heparin in the initial management of unstable angina or non-Q wave myocardial infarction: FRAXIS (Fraxiparine in Ischaemic Syndrome). Eur Heart J 1999;20(21):1553–62.

[24] Tran H, Anand SS. Oral antiplatelet therapy in cerebrovascular disease, coronary artery disease, and peripheral arterial disease. JAMA 2004;292(15):1867–74.

[25] Yusuf S, Zhao F, Mehta SR, et al. Effects of clopidogrel in addition to aspirin in patients with acute coronary syndromes without ST-segment elevation. N Engl J Med 2001;345(7):494–502.

[26] Schriger DL, Herbert ME. Platelet glycoprotein inhibitors in patients with medically managed acute coronary syndrome: does the enthusiasm exceed the science? Ann Emerg Med 2001;38(3):249–55.

[27] Simoons ML. Effect of glycoprotein IIb/IIIa receptor blocker abciximab on outcome in patients with acute coronary syndromes without early coronary revascularisation: the GUSTO IV-ACS randomised trial. Lancet 2001;357(9272):1915–24.

[28] Boersma E, Harrington RA, Moliterno DJ, et al. Platelet glycoprotein IIb/IIIa inhibitors in acute coronary syndromes: a meta-analysis of all major randomised clinical trials. Lancet 2002;359(9302):189–98.

[29] Lincoff AM. Direct thrombin inhibitors for non-ST-segment elevation acute coronary syndromes: what, when, and where? Am Heart J 2003;146(Suppl 4):S23–30.

[30] The Global Use of Strategies to Open Occluded Coronary Arteries (GUSTO) IIb Investigators. A comparison of recombinant hirudin with heparin for the treatment of acute coronary syndromes. N Engl J Med 1996;335(11):775–82.

[31] Organisation to Assess Strategies for Ischemic Syndromes(OASIS-2) Investigators. Effects of recombinant hirudin (lepirudin) compared with heparin on death, myocardial infarction,

refractory angina, and revascularisation procedures in patients with acute myocardial ischaemia without ST elevation: a randomised trial. Lancet 1999;353(9151):429–38.
[32] Direct Thrombin Trialists' Collaborative Group. Direct thrombin inhibitors in acute coronary syndromes: principal results of a meta-analysis based on individual patients' data. Lancet 2002;359(9303):294–302.
[33] Lincoff AM, Kleiman NS, Kereiakes DJ, et al. Long-term efficacy of bivalirudin and provisional glycoprotein IIb/IIIa blockade vs heparin and planned glycoprotein IIb/IIIa blockade during percutaneous coronary revascularization: REPLACE-2 randomized trial. JAMA 2004;292(6):696–703.
[34] Boden WE, O'Rourke RA, Crawford MH, et al. Veterans Affairs Non-Q-Wave Infarction Strategies in Hospital (VANQWISH) Trial Investigators. Outcomes in patients with acute non-Q-wave myocardial infarction randomly assigned to an invasive as compared with a conservative management strategy. N Engl J Med 1998;338(25):1785–92.
[35] McCullough PA, O'Neill WW, Graham M, et al. A prospective randomized trial of triage angiography in acute coronary syndromes ineligible for thrombolytic therapy. Results of the medicine versus angiography in thrombolytic exclusion (MATE) trial. J Am Coll Cardiol 1998;32(3):596–605.
[36] Effects of tissue plasminogen activator and a comparison of early invasive and conservative strategies in unstable angina and non-Q-wave myocardial infarction. Results of the TIMI IIIB Trial. Thrombolysis in Myocardial Ischemia. Circulation 1994;89(4):1545–56.
[37] Cannon CP, Weintraub WS, Demopoulos LA, et al. Comparison of early invasive and conservative strategies in patients with unstable coronary syndromes treated with the glycoprotein IIb/IIIa inhibitor tirofiban. N Engl J Med 2001;344(25):1879–87.
[38] Fragmin and Fast Revascularisation during Instability in Coronary Artery Disease Investigators. Invasive compared with non-invasive treatment in unstable coronary-artery disease: FRISC II prospective randomised multicentre study. Lancet 1999;354(9180): 708–15.

ELSEVIER
SAUNDERS

Emerg Med Clin N Am
23 (2005) 1043–1063

EMERGENCY
MEDICINE
CLINICS OF
NORTH AMERICA

Acute Reperfusion Therapy in Acute Myocardial Infarction

Chris A. Ghaemmaghami, MD[a,b,*],
David R. Burt, MD[c]

[a]*Department of Emergency Medicine, University of Virginia Health System, PO Box 800699, Charlottesville, VA 22908-0699, USA*
[b]*Chest Pain Center, University of Virginia Health System, PO Box 800699, Charlottesville, VA 22908-0699, USA*
[c]*Emergency and Cardiovascular Medicine, Spectrum Health System, Grand Rapids, MI 49503, USA*

The electrocardiographic classification of acute myocardial infarctions (AMI) has had a profound influence on the treatment of patients with AMI. Deciding whether a patient has ST-segment elevations, a new left bundle branch block (LBBB), or neither of these findings on ECG launches the treating physician down two different treatment pathways: (a) patients with ST-elevation MI (STEMI) need to be assessed for immediate reperfusion therapy; whereas (b) patients with non-ST-elevation MI (NSTEMI) are best treated with aggressive medical management without acute reperfusion.

The pathophysiologic reasoning behind these different approaches is based on the fact that the presence of ST-segment elevation or new LBBB patterns on ECG in the appropriate clinical scenario has a high specificity for both the diagnosis of AMI and for that MI to be caused by an acute thrombosis in one of the major epicardial coronary arteries. DeWood and colleagues [1] have demonstrated that nearly 90% of patients who undergo angiography for transmural AMI have total coronary occlusions within 4 hours of the symptom onset. By contrast, NSTEMI patients have a wide variety of nonocclusive lesions, small vessel disease, and infarctions related to high metabolic demands of the myocardium. These conditions are best treated through measures to restore and preserve microvascular flow and reduce oxygen demand. A STEMI, on the other hand, requires treatment

* Corresponding author.
E-mail address: cg3n@virginia.edu (C.A. Ghaemmaghami).

doi:10.1016/j.emc.2005.07.014
emed.theclinics.com

focused on the immediate relief of the coronary obstruction and restoration of forward flow through the coronary arteries.

Within seconds of a coronary arterial occlusion, cellular ATP levels begin to drop, and contractile dysfunction can occur in less than 2 minutes. By 20 to 30 minutes after occlusion, irreversible myocardial cellular necrosis begins. As ATP levels continue to decline, microvascular injury within the myocardium progresses particularly at the subendocardial level [2]. If occlusion is unrelieved, a wavefront of necrosis extends from the initial area of necrosis to cause a transmural infarction (Fig. 1) [3]. The first 2 hours account for the most rapid period of cellular necrosis. From 2 to 6 hours after onset, necrosis continues but the rate begins to decline, and by 6 to 12 hours, the rate of cellular death slows considerably (Fig. 2) [4].

As the area of infarction grows, mechanical and electrical functions of the heart are progressively impaired, and the risk rises for life-threatening dysrhythmias and cardiogenic shock. The goal of reperfusion therapy is to

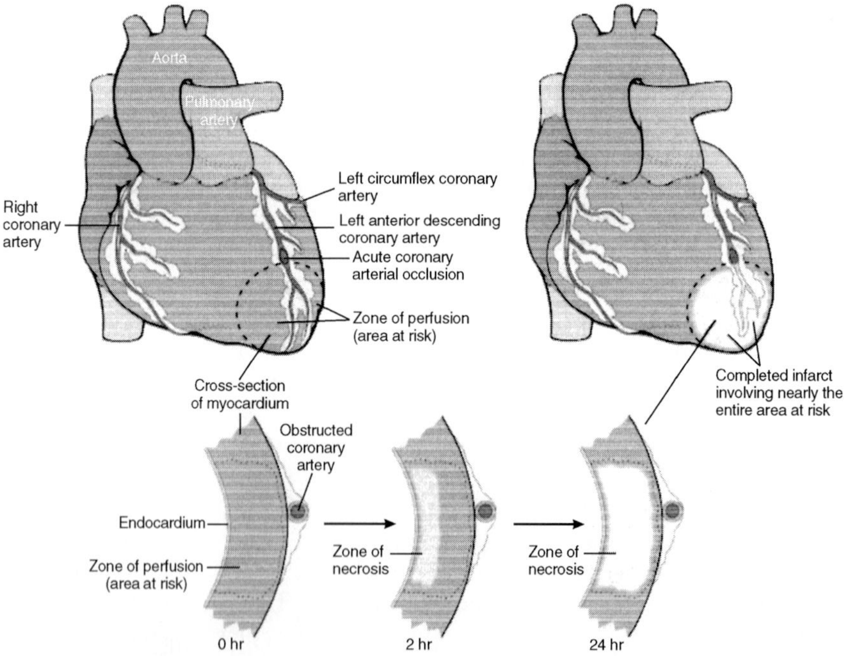

Fig. 1. Progression of myocardial necrosis after coronary artery occlusion. Necrosis begins in a small zone of the myocardium beneath the endocardial surface in the center of the ischemic zone. This entire region of myocardium (*dashed outline*) depends on the occluded vessel for perfusion and is the area at risk. Note that a very narrow zone of myocardium immediately beneath the endocardium is spared from necrosis because it can be oxygenated by diffusion from the ventricle. (*From* Schoen FJ. The heart. In: Cotran RS, Kumar V, Collins T, editors. Pathologic basis of disease. 6th edition. Philadelphia: WB Saunders; 1999. p. 557; with permission.)

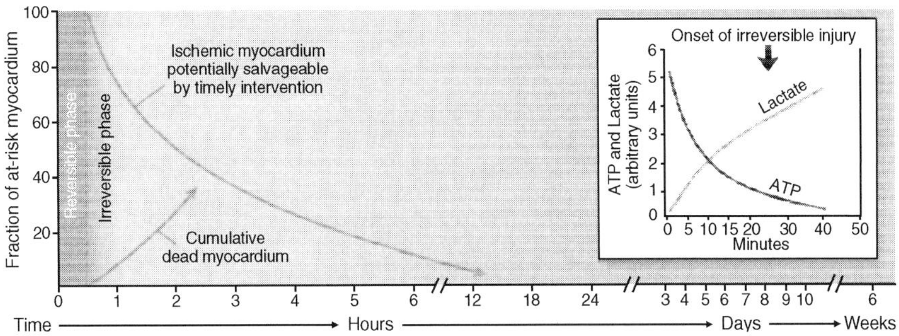

Fig. 2. Temporal sequence of early biochemical, ultrastructural, histochemical, and histologic findings after onset of severe myocardial ischemia. For approximately 30 minutes after the onset of even the most severe ischemia, myocardial injury is potentially reversible. Thereafter, a progressive loss of viability occurs that is complete by 6 to 12 hours. The benefits of reperfusion are greatest when it is achieved early, with progressively smaller benefit occurring as reperfusion is delayed. (*Modified from* Antman E. Acute myocardial infarction. In: Braunwald E, Zipes DP, Libby P, editors. Heart disease: a textbook of cardiovascular medicine. 6th edition. Philadelphia: WB Saunders; 2001. pp. 1114–1231; with permission.)

minimize irreversible myocardial necrosis thus reducing the immediate risk of death and long-term cardiac dysfunction.

Indications and contraindications for reperfusion therapy

Presently, there are two strategies in widespread use for the acute reperfusion of AMI patients, fibrinolytic agents and percutaneous coronary intervention (PCI). The general indications for both strategies are similar, and the basis for the rational selection between the two is discussed below.

In the first 12 hours after symptom onset, immediate reperfusion is indicated for patients who have the following findings on a standard 12-lead ECG.

- An ST elevation $\geq$0.1 mV in at least two contiguous precordial leads or at least two adjacent limb leads
- New or presumably new LBBB
- Findings consistent with a true posterior MI

Acute reperfusion therapy also may be considered in STEMI patients within 12 to 24 hours of symptom onset, who show continued ischemic symptoms and persistent ST-segment elevation of $\geq$0.1 mV in at least two contiguous precordial leads or at least two adjacent limb leads.

Acute surgical reperfusion with coronary artery bypass grafting (CABG) also is an option in patients who have STEMIs, who have refractory ischemia, cardiogenic shock, or life-threatening ventricular dysrhythmias that also have operable left main or multivessel coronary artery disease (CAD) or contraindications to both fibrinolytic therapy and PCI. It is important to recognize that diagnostic coronary angiography is required before the decision to operate. For the emergency physician, therefore, the surgical option can essentially be combined with PCI when deciding between a pharmacologic versus a mechanical reperfusion strategy.

Contraindications to fibrinolysis are listed in Box 1. Major hemorrhage is the most common serious complication from fibrinolytic therapy. The average intracranial hemorrhage (ICH) rate for patients treated in clinical trials with fibrinolytic agents ranges from 0.6% to 1% [5]. An increased risk of ICH in fibrinolytic-treated patients appears to be most closely related to advanced patient age (particularly ages $\geq$75) and the presence of systemic hypertension [6–9]. Other risk factors include low body weight, previous strokes, and excessive anticoagulation. Subsets of patients who have multiple risk factors for ICH can have ICH rates as high as 4% [10]. Other common sites of major hemorrhagic complications may include the gastrointestinal tract and sites of recent surgery or vascular puncture. Ultimately, the decision to use a fibrinolytic agent must be based on an assessment of the net survival benefit while taking into consideration the risk for serious morbidity from hemorrhage.

Contraindications for PCI include serious adverse reactions to intravenous contrast dyes, poor arterial access for catheters, and a known history of CAD with lesions precluding percutaneous intervention. Relative contraindications include chronic renal failure short of the need for hemodialysis.

Because it is now well documented that restoration of forward flow through the culprit vessel is one of the primary factors influencing the short- and long-term outcomes in the patient having a STEMI, the conservative management option without reperfusion therapy should be chosen only in the exceptional case. In the rare patient for whom conservative treatment is justifiable, care should be taken to document the circumstances and reasoning in the medical record.

Impact of time to treatment from symptom onset

Clinical studies of AMI patients undergoing early reperfusion therapy show a strong correlation between time-related myocardial necrosis and reperfusion therapy, with respect to the resultant left ventricular function and patient survival. The efficacy of fibrinolytic agents in lysing thrombus diminishes with time, and the survival benefit begins to decline [11]. In an analysis of all major fibrinolytic AMI trials before 1994, the number of lives saved per thousand treated declined from 35 when treated within the first hour of symptom onset to 25 when treated between the second and third hours after symptom onset. Fibrinolytic therapy administered within the first hour can occasionally abort even an evolving MI [12]. The rate of decline in the survival benefit decelerates sharply between the sixth and

Box 1. Contraindications and cautions for fibrinolysis in ST elevation myocardial infarction

Absolute contraindications
Any prior ICH
Known structural cerebral vascular lesion (eg, arteriovenous malformation)
Known malignant intracranial neoplasm (primary or metastatic)
Ischemic stroke within 3 months *except* acute ischemic stroke within 3 hours
Suspected aortic dissection
Active bleeding or bleeding diathesis (excluding menses)
Significant closed-head or facial trauma within 3 months

Relative contraindications
History of chronic, severe, or poorly controlled hypertension
Severe uncontrolled hypertension on presentation (systolic blood pressure ≥180 mmHg or diastolic blood pressure ≥110 mmHg)
History of ischemic stroke greater than 3 months, dementia, or known intracranial pathology not covered in contraindications
Traumatic or prolonged (greater than 10 minutes) cardiopulmonary resuscitation
Major surgery (within less than 3 weeks)
Recent (within 2–4 weeks) internal bleeding
Noncompressible vascular punctures
For streptokinase/anistreplase: previous exposure (more than 5 days ago) or previous allergic reaction to these agents
Pregnancy
Active peptic ulcer
Current use of anticoagulants: the higher the international normalized ratio (INR), the higher the risk of bleeding

Adapted from ACC/AHA guidelines for the management of patients with ST-elevation myocardial infarction: executive summary: a report of the American College of Cardiology/American Heart Association Task Force on Practice Guidelines (Writing Committee to Revise the 1999 Guideline on Acute Myocardial Infarction). Circulation. 2004;110(5):588–636.

twelfth hours [9]. In the National Registry of Myocardial Infarction (NRMI) 2 and 3, a comparison of time to fibrinolytic agents to survival has revealed a significant trend: compared with door-to-therapy times under 30 minutes, the adjusted odds of death increased by 11% and 23% for patients who had door-to-therapy times between 61 and 90 minutes and greater than

90 minutes, respectively. Similarly, an increase in the risk of significant left ventricular (LV) functional impairment also increased at each 30-minute interval [12–14]. Furthermore, an analysis of NRMI 2 registry data shows that in PCI-treated patients, a door-to-balloon time greater than 2 hours is associated with an increased relative risk of mortality compared with individuals managed with PCI that is initiated earlier in the hospital course (odds ratio 1.41) [12]. According to current American College of Cardiology (ACC)/American Heart Association (AHA) guidelines, the initiation of fibrinolytic therapy (eg, door-to-needle time) is recommended within 30 minutes of arrival at the emergency department (ED). In the case of a PCI-based strategy, the target is a maximum time of 90 minutes from ED presentation to the time of the first intracoronary balloon inflation (eg, door-to-balloon time) [15].

Fibrinolytic therapy

Pharmacologic reperfusion therapy for the treatment of acute myocardial infarction has been used on thousands of patients over the past 20 years and has been examined critically in multiple major trials. More than 150,000 patients have been randomized in trials of fibrinolysis [9,16–18]. The International Study of Infarct Survival (ISIS)-2 trial [16] has established the efficacy of streptokinase—and the fibrinolytic concept—by demonstrating a 25% relative reduction in 35-day mortality in comparison with placebo when used in conjunction with aspirin. The subsequent Global Utilization of Streptokinase and Tissue Plasminogen Activator for Occluded Coronary Arteries (GUSTO) trial [19] has shown a slight superiority of tPA over streptokinase in respect to 30-day survival and no significant difference in major bleeding complications. Further investigations of the newer agents reteplase (rPA) and tenecteplase (TNK-tPA) in comparisons with alteplase (tissue-type plasminogen activator [tPA]) have been shown to have equivalent survival benefits and comparable risks of major hemorrhage [20–22].

Prompt fibrinolysis inarguably has been shown to increase immediate survival and salvage myocardium and to reduce long-term morbidity and mortality [16,23–25]. The Fibrinolytic Therapy Trialists' Collaborative Group [9] has demonstrated an 18% relative reduction in subject mortality compared with control patients. The survival benefits were particularly impressive in subsets of patient with left bundle branch blocks and ST-segment elevations on ECG, in which 49 and 37 lives per 1000 patients, respectively, were saved with treatment. Multivariate analysis revealed that patients who do not reperfuse after receiving fibrinolytic therapy have significantly higher rates of left ventricular dysfunction than those who have the restoration of nearly normal coronary flow [26].

Currently, there are four commonly used US Food and Drug Administration-approved fibrinolytic agents for the treatment of AMI:

streptokinase, alteplase (tPA), reteplase (rPA), and tenecteplase (TNK-tPA) (Table 1; also see Box 1). Streptokinase is considered to be the first generation of fibrinolytic agents. Streptokinase is a natural product that binds plasminogen and converts it into a plasmin-like agent. This agent in turn converts both circulating and fibrin-bound plasminogen into circulating plasmin. The ensuing systemic lytic state depletes fibrinogen, plasminogen, and factors V and VIII [5]. Because of the associated anticoagulation seen with streptokinase, concomitant heparin administration may be of little benefit and can increase the risk of major hemorrhage. Patients can develop antistreptococcal antibodies after the administration of streptokinase. This sensitization can cause a serious hypersensitivity reaction, especially on a re-exposure. Hypotension on administration may rarely be encountered and may be treated by temporarily halting the infusion, elevating the feet of the patient, or administering fluid.

With recombinant tissue plasminogen activator (tPA), the second generation of fibrinolytic agents was introduced. tPA has more specificity for action against fibrin located in clots but can cause a mild general fibrinogen depletion that is less severe than that seen with streptokinase. tPA has a relatively short half-life of 3 to 8 minutes, so it is administered as an infusion rather than a bolus. The so-called accelerated or "front-loaded" method for administering tPA refers to the 90-minute protocol used in the GUSTO trial (Table 2). The third generation of fibrinolytic agents consists of variants of tPA that have been identified as spontaneous human mutations (eg, reteplase) or specifically engineered to have certain beneficial properties (eg, tenecteplase). Both reteplase and tenecteplase are recombinant products and are nonantigenic. These agents appear to provide greater earlier patency rates of infarct vessels over streptokinase or tPA [22]. Notably, reteplase causes greater fibrinogen depletion than tPA but less than streptokinase. By contrast, tenecteplase has more fibrin specificity and an increased resistance to plasminogen activator inhibitor-1 [27]. Both tenecteplase and reteplase have longer half-lives than tPA, allowing for single- and double-bolus administration, respectively.

Table 1
Fibrinolytic agents

Chemical name	Streptokinase	tPA	rPA	TNK-tPA
Generic name	N/A	Alteplase	Reteplase	Tenecteplase
Trade name	N/A	Activase	Retevase	TNKase
Plasminogen activation	Indirect	Direct	Direct	Direct
Patency at 90 mins				
TIMI grade 3	29%–32%	45%–63%	60%	66%
TIMI grade 2 or 3	54%–60%	73%–82%	83%	88%
Cost	~$300	$2200	$2200	$2200
Antigenic properties	Yes	No	No	No

Table 2
Fibrinolytic and heparin dosing guidelines

Fibrinolytic agent	Dosage		Heparin
Streptokinase	1.5 million units IV, over 60 min		UFH: 12500 units SC every 12 hours
tPA (alteplase)	Bolus: 15 mg IV		UFH: 60 units/kg bolus (max 4000 units) then 12 units/kg/h (max 1000 units/h); maintain APTT 50–70 s
	Infuse: 0.75 mg/kg IV over 30 min (max 50 mg) then 0.50 mg/kg IV over 60 min (max 35 mg)		
rPA (reteplase)	Double bolus: 10 U IV bolus followed by a second 10 U IV bolus in 30 min		UFH: 60 units/kg bolus (max 4000 units) then 12 units/kg/h (max 1000 units/h); maintain APTT 50–70 s
TNK-tPA (tenecteplase)	Weight-based single IV bolus		Enoxaparin: 30 mg IV then 1 mg/kg SC every 12 h
	≤ 60 kg	30 mg	<OR>
	60–69 kg	35 mg	UFH: 60 unit/kg bolus (max 4000 units) then 12 units/kg/h (max 1000 units/h) maintain APTT 50–70 s
	70–79 kg	40 mg	
	80–89 kg	45 mg	
	≥ 90 kg	50 mg	

Abbreviations: APTT, activated partial thromboplastin time; IV, intravenous; SC, subcutaneous; UFH, unfractionated heparin.

Despite the higher cost of tPA over streptokinase, the absolute survival benefit of 1.1% was justified in a formalized cost-effectiveness analysis based on outcomes from the GUSTO trial, revealing a cost per year of life saved of $32,678 [28]. Because the pricing of all second and third generation fibrinolytics is equivalent, the findings related to tPA should be generalizable to the entire class of new agents.

Multiple combinations of a fibrinolytic agent with anticoagulants, thrombin inhibitors, or platelet aggregation inhibitor have been studied in randomized controlled trials [29]. The Assessment of the Safety and Efficacy of a New Thrombolytic (ASSENT)-3 study group [29] has reported the superiority of a combined treatment regimen of tenecteplase plus enoxaparin or reduced-dose tenecteplase plus abciximab over tenecteplase plus unfractionated heparin in terms of efficacy and safety at 30 days (Table 3). A bolus administration significantly reduces the potential for medication errors and greatly simplifies its use, thereby decreasing times to therapy initiation. Considering the excellent clinical outcomes, the ease of administration (bolus therapy for both agents), and lower comparative cost, the tenecteplase/enoxaprin regimen appears to be the most attractive fibrinolytic option at this time (see Table 2 for heparin dosing guidelines).

Ultimately, the selection of fibrinolytic agent is less important than the prompt decision to administer one. The benefits of early administration of a fibrinolytic agent outweigh the differences in survival benefit between any

Table 3
ASSENT-3 results: combination regimens using tenecteplase for treatment of STEMI

Endpoints	TNK-tPA + enoxaparin (%) (n = 2040)	TNK-tPA + abciximab (%) (n = 2017)	TNK-tPA + UFH (%) (n = 2038)	*P* value
Death at 30 days	5.4	6.6	6.0	.25
In-hospital reinfarction	2.7	2.2	4.2	.0009
Refractory ischemia	4.6	3.2	6.5	<.0001
Intracranial hemorrhage	0.9	0.9	0.9	.98
Major bleeding (not ICH)	3.0	4.3	2.2	.0005
Combined endpoints				
Efficacy (death, reinfarct, ischemia)	11.4	11.1	15.4	.0001
Efficacy and safety (death, reinfarct, ischemia, ICH, major bleeding)	13.8	14.2	17.0	.0081

Abbreviation: UFH, unfractionated heparin.

Adapted from Assessment of the safety and efficacy of a new thrombolytic regimen (ASSENT)-3 Investigators. Efficacy and safety of tenecteplase in combination with enoxaparin, abciximab, or unfractionated heparin: the ASSENT-3 randomised trial in acute myocardial infarction. Lancet 2001;358:605; with permission.

of the individual agents, and the selection of agents depends primarily on availability.

Clinical assessment of reperfusion after fibrinolysis

After pharmacologic reperfusion therapy has been performed, the treating physician must continue monitoring the patient closely to ensure that reperfusion occurs. Reperfusion may occur very early after anticoagulation, but 60 to 90 minutes may pass before reperfusion is achieved. The resolution of symptoms, a reduction of at least 50% of peak ST-segment elevation, and the occurrence of accelerated idioventricular rhythms are signs that fibrinolysis has been successful. By contrast, persistent ischemic symptoms, hemodynamic instability, the persistence of ST-segment elevation, and the occurrence of ventricular tachyarrhythmias strongly suggest that fibrinolysis has failed [30]. Referral for "rescue PCI" is indicated in patients who fail pharmacologic reperfusion.

Percutaneous coronary intervention

Primary PCI has been shown repeatedly to be an ideal reperfusion strategy in the treatment of acute STEMI. Multiple studies have shown its superiority to pharmacologic reperfusion, provided the patient receives early treatment. For patients who present later than 3 hours from symptom onset and have high-risk features or present in cardiogenic shock, PCI is the preferred strategy. PCI has a lower rate of ICH and can be performed in most patients in whom fibrinolytic therapy is contraindicated. PCI has the advantage of higher initial reperfusion rates and lower subsequent rates of adverse events such as stroke, death, and reinfarction [31–34]. Multiple small clinical trials have been conducted comparing primary PCI with fibrinolysis for STEMI [35]. In a quantitative review of 10 trials comparing primary PCI with fibrinolytic therapy conducted before 1996, Weaver and colleagues [35] describe lower rates of 30-day mortality, reinfarction, total stroke rate, and hemorrhagic stroke rate in patients undergoing PCI. These trials were conducted before the advent of routine intracoronary stenting and the adjunctive use of Glycoprotein IIb/IIIa receptor inhibitor (GPI) [36–39]. Subsequent trials comparing PCI combined with stents or GPI with PCI alone showed incremental benefits to the combined approach [40,41].

Presently, primary PCI is regarded widely as the preferred therapeutic option for treatment of those STEMI patients in whom PCI can be performed within 90 minutes of first medical contact. However, primary PCI requires an experienced team, and only hospitals with an established interventional cardiology program should use primary PCI as their preferred strategy for STEMI patients. Strict performance criteria must be developed and monitored consistently and accurately to ensure that door-to-balloon time remains acceptable. This requires a great degree of co-operation and interaction among the emergency medical services (EMS), emergency medicine, and cardiology.

As with the administration of fibrinolytics, it has been shown that early revascularization is preferable, and the door-to-treatment times should be minimized. Studies have reported increasing mortality rates with increasing door-to-balloon times [42,43]. Decreases in infarct size, improved LV function, and improved long-term outcomes also are apparent in patients treated earlier.

Patients with acute MI presenting with signs of cardiogenic shock warrant special consideration. Cardiogenic shock occurs in 7% to 10% of patients who have acute MI, and these patients have a high mortality rate ($\geq$10%). Fibrinolytic therapy has not been shown to benefit these patients, regardless of the time of administration. Primary PCI, however, was demonstrated in the Should We Emergently Revascularize Occluded Coronaries for Cardiogenic Shock (SHOCK) trial [44] to reduce 30-day absolute mortality rates by 9% compared with immediate medical stabilization. Improvements in functional outcomes and survival extended past 6 months and continued improving from baseline, indicating the benefit in these patients is real and sustained. Thus, in patients who have cardiogenic shock, added emphasis should be placed on transporting them to facilities with primary PCI capabilities.

With the evolution of cardiac stents, primary stenting has been compared with primary angioplasty alone in multiple studies. Mortality and reinfarction rates were unchanged, but major cardiac event rates declined because of a significant reduction in the need for subsequent target vessel revascularization [45–47].

Currently, there has been considerable interest in the use of drug-eluting stents in the treatment of STEMI patients [48]. Vessel patency rates and short-term adverse event rates appear to be unaffected, but the 30-day combined event rate of revascularization, reinfarction, and death decreased from 10.4% to 7.5% in the group receiving drug-eluting stents.

Rescue percutaneous coronary intervention after failed fibrinolysis

At best, 90-minute patency after fibrinolysis for STEMI occurs at a rate of 85% [49]. Referral for PCI after fibrinolysis, or "rescue PCI," is indicated when lytic agents fail to result in adequate reperfusion. If rescue PCI can be performed within the first 3 to 6 hours after symptom onset, significant myocardium may be salvaged. Rescue PCI can establish antegrade coronary flow in 90% of patients. Relative reductions in mortality when rescue PCI is performed within 90 minutes after fibrinolytic treatment can approach 50% versus conservative management and result in better long-term left ventricular function [50].

Evolving concepts

Advanced prehospital protocols

Despite increasing awareness of the importance of expediently administered reperfusion therapy and attempts to reduce presentation to treatment times, the barrier imposed by long prehospital transport times continues to impede progress toward ideal reperfusion times. Increasing attention has been placed on the role of prehospital care and the possibilities for the EMS provider to initiate reperfusion therapy in the field. Improved paramedic training, the ability to transmit 12-lead ECGs for physician review, and bolus fibrinolytics make feasible the possibility of pre-hospital administration of fibrinolytics for STEMI. Based on our knowledge of the pathophysiology of acute MI, it would be expected that prehospital fibrinolysis would reduce the time to treatment and improve outcomes. It has been difficult to confirm these expectations in clinical trials.

The Comparison of Angioplasty and Prehospital Thrombolysis in Acute Myocardial infarction (CAPTIM) trial [51] was designed to compare prehospital thrombolysis to primary PCI. Results were inconclusive but suggested that prehospital thrombolysis may be preferable to primary PCI for patients treated within the first 2 hours after symptom onset. The ASSENT-3 PLUS trial shows that prehospital reperfusion therapy with tenecteplase and enoxaparin or unfractionated heparin (UFH) allowed treatment within 2 hours of symptom onset in 50% of patients who have STEMI, with an average reduction in treatment time of 47 minutes. It also showed a slightly greater risk of ICH and bleeding in patients who were older than age 75 and who were treated with enoxaparin as opposed to UFH [52]. In a meta-analysis of six trials enrolling 6434 patients, an average of

58 minutes was saved by performing fibrinolysis in the prehospital setting, and a survival benefit with an odds ratio of 0.83 (95% CI, 0.70-0.95) favored prehospital fibrinolysis [53]. Additional studies are pending, but at this time, prehospital thrombolytics are not used in most areas of the United States.

An additional possibility is the use of prehospital 12-lead EKG to assist in the triage of identified STEMI patients to appropriate facilities. Assessing the STEMI patient for contraindications to thrombolytics, cardiogenic shock, and time since symptom onset would be used to determine the destination of the patient, either to a non-PCI facility for thrombolysis or to a PCI center for mechanical intervention [54]. In large urban areas with a close proximity of PCI, the best model may develop of an integrated system to quickly identify STEMI patients prehospital and transport them to the nearest known available PCI center, similar to the concept of a trauma center. This has been done successfully in several areas, including Boston [55]. However, this model may not be applicable in many areas of the country with lower densities of people and PCI centers. An assessment of each individual system is important to develop strategies and protocols appropriate to each region.

Facilitated percutaneous coronary intervention

Although pharmacologic fibrinolysis and primary PCI are proven effective therapies for acute MI, both have limitations. A plateau has likely been reached in the effectiveness of fibrinolysis. ICH, a serious complication of fibrinolysis, still occurs in up to 1% of patients. PCI, although showing generally superior results to lytics if given in the same time interval, has limited availability and potentially long transit times, which may negate some or all benefit. Many portions of the United States remain relatively distant from high-quality PCI centers. These conditions are not likely to change quickly, given the geography of our country, the status of EMS coverage, and factors affecting patient delay in presentation.

"Facilitated PCI," a process for combining the best aspects of both fibrinolytics and PCI in an effort to optimize outcomes is being studied currently in several large trials worldwide. The concept is simple: on presentation to an outlying facility without PCI capability, the STEMI patient is treated with a combination of fibrinolytic or antithrombotic agents to enhance early reperfusion and antegrade flow while limiting infarct size. Generally, the patient receives a fibrinolytic agent (often at half dose to minimize bleeding risks) along with a glycoprotein IIb/IIIa receptor inhibitor. The patient is then quickly transported to a PCI center for post-treatment PCI and stenting if merited. The hypothesis is that early fibrinolytics may provide adequate reperfusion early in the course of the STEMI to minimize damage and that "follow-up" PCI (even outside the 90–120-minute preferred window) subsequently provides benefit by improving Thrombolysis in Myocardial Infarction (TIMI)-grade flow with balloon angioplasty or stenting. The early opportunity to evaluate cardiac artery anatomy and access to quality cardiac care at an interventional facility also may prove beneficial.

Intuitively, the concept is sensible and has generated considerable enthusiasm. Several studies are in progress to more fully investigate this concept; however, results have been inconclusive at this point [56–58]. In one recent study, results of patients receiving half-dose reteplase and abciximab before transit to the cardiac catheterization lab were compared with patients receiving abciximab alone. Although coronary artery patency rates were higher in those receiving the reteplase, this did not improve clinical outcomes [59]. In addition, patients who received combination therapy had a slightly increased rate of bleeding complications. Other investigations have shown conflicting results. Currently, several well-designed studies are underway to provide more information on this concept [60].

At this time then, the benefits of facilitated PCI remain unproven, and this strategy cannot be recommended routinely. However, in the relatively uncomplicated patient with minimal risk factors for bleeding, it may be an option, particularly if long delays to reperfusion are unavoidable.

Selection of reperfusion strategy

It is clear from multiple studies that fibrinolytic therapy and primary PCI are both effective strategies for the treatment of acute MI. Equally clear is that the time from symptom onset to definitive treatment also is critically important, particularly when fibrinolytic therapy is used. This focus on time is appropriate because early aggressive evaluation and treatment clearly reduces morbidity and mortality.

More controversial is the selection of a treatment strategy. PCI is superior to fibrinolytic therapy as a reperfusion strategy in STEMI when performed quickly and competently at high-volume PCI centers. For patients presenting to PCI centers, the choice of treatment, rapid PCI, is clear. However, fewer than 25% of United States hospitals offer PCI programs. Thus, physicians at these hospitals have two treatment options: on-site fibrinolytic therapy or rapid patient transfer to a primary PCI site. Interfacility transport is feasible, but careful consideration for the ultimate benefit for the patient must be considered.

The PRAGUE-2 study [61] has examined the issue of transportation of patients for primary PCI. This study shows that thrombolysis is substantially less effective in patients who have greater than 3 hours of symptoms, suggesting a transfer for these patients if PCI availability was reasonably timely. It did not show a benefit of transfer for patients with symptom duration less than 3 hours. The Danish Multicenter Randomized Study on Fibrinolytic Therapy versus Acute Coronary Angioplasty in Acute Myocardial Infarction (DANAMI-2) [62] also compared the issue of patient transfer for primary angioplasty versus the use of on-site fibrinolysis. The authors' conclusions suggest that PCI is superior if transport times do not exceed 2 hours. The majority of benefit, however, was in the rate of reinfarction.

These two and other studies also suggest that the transport of acute MI patients is reasonably safe yet not without risk. In the PRAGUE-2 study [61] 4 of 425 patients were not transported because of hemodynamic deterioration. Of the 421 transported patients, three patients lapsed into successfully treated ventricular fibrillation and two died, a rate of 1.2%. It also should be noted that in the DANAMI-2 trial [62], the median interhospital transfer time was 32 minutes. In the PRAGUE-2 trial, the time between randomization and catheter inflation was 97 minutes.

Clearly, there is a disparity between what is achievable in tightly controlled studies in largely metropolitan areas and what is reported in generalized practice. The diverse nature of United States geography and patient densities, as well as considerable variation in the level of skill, availability, and transport equipment of EMS providers make generalizing difficult. This situation is not likely to change in the near future. The PRAGUE-2 AND DANAMI-2 reports contrast markedly with the recent NRMI-4 data that revealed a median door-to-balloon time of less than 90 minutes in only 4.2% of transferred patients in the United States. The median total presentation-to-balloon time for transfer patients in the United States undergoing primary PCI was 180 minutes, double that of the current ACC/AHA guidelines [63]. Patients presenting with atypical symptoms during nonbusiness hours and to rural teaching hospitals also had longer delays to treatment.

Data from the CAPTIM trial [51] show that the early treatment of STEMI with fibrinolytics is preferable to primary PCI for most patients treated within the first 2 hours after symptom onset but that the benefit over PCI declines rapidly thereafter. Similarly, a meta-analysis by Nallamothu and colleagues [64] suggests that benefits associated with primary PCI may be lost if transport time exceeds 1 hour (Fig. 3).

In view of these and similar findings, the 2004 ACC/AHA [65] guidelines for the treatment of STEMI contain the following principal:

"PCI is the generally preferred strategy if a skilled PCI lab is available and door-to-balloon time is reasonably expected to be less than 90 minutes including transport time. Patients in cardiogenic shock and those at higher risk of ICH or other contraindications to fibrinolysis should also be considered for primary PCI, even outside the 90 minute window. In addition, late presenters (symptom onset greater than three hours ago) are preferentially recommended for PCI, if it can be done in an expedient fashion...PCI is the preferred strategy if the diagnosis of STEMI is in doubt."

Fibrinolytics are preferred for those patients who present with less than 3 hours of symptoms but who will have a delay to an invasive strategy that places them over the 90 minute door-to-balloon threshold for PCI (from the

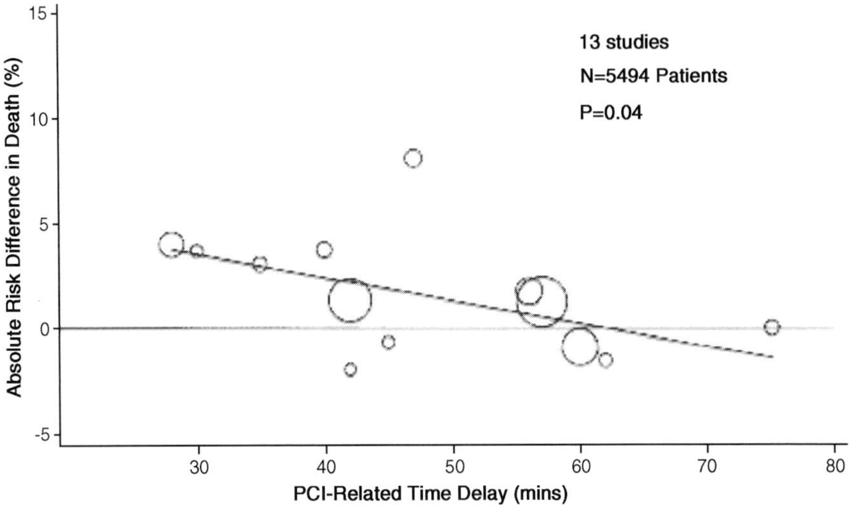

Fig. 3. Absolute risk reduction in short-term mortality rates with primary PCI as a function of PCI-related time delay in 13 studies involving recombinant (r)tPA. The size of the circles reflect the sample sizes of the patient studies. Solid line, weighted meta-regression analysis. Values ≥ 0 represent benefit with PCI, and values ≤ 0 represent harm. (*From* Nallamothu BK, Antman EM, Bates ER. Primary percutaneous coronary intervention versus fibrinolytic therapy in acute myocardial infarction: does the choice of fibrinolytic agent impact on the importance of time-to-treatment. Am J Cardiol 2004;94(6):772–4; with permission.)

time of first medical presentation). These conditions include prolonged transport time in excess of 1 hour or a situation in which an appropriate PCI lab will not reasonably be available in time to meet the door-to-balloon goal of 90 minutes. If transport can be accomplished within 1 hour, a patient can be expected statistically to benefit from PCI even if he or she could have received fibrinolytics more quickly. In addition, patients better suited for PCI (eg, at high risk for ICH, presence of cardiogenic shock, and other factors) should be transferred to a PCI facility with less consideration given to transport time.

Transfer protocols

Rather than engaging in the ongoing "either/or" strategy debate, the treatment of the acute MI patient is best served by adopting reasonable treatment guidelines such as those espoused by the AHA/ACC, coupled with the concentrated effort to improve the efficiency of the entire system.

For those STEMI patients who are being considered for interfacility transfer, a reasonable yet quick assessment must be made of the transfer situation (Box 2). First, a realistic (not optimistic) estimate of transfer time must be made. Generous allowances must be made for patient preparation time, notification delays, and other delays. Currently, in most situations in

Box 2. Suggested evaluation course for STEMI patients at non-PCI facilities

Step 1. *Confirm through 12-lead ECG that a STEMI is occurring*
Step 2. *Initiate early activation of transportation system, unless transport clearly will not be indicated*
Step 3. *Determine time of symptom onset*
Step 4. *Determine strategy selection*

A. If symptoms began less than 2 to 3 hours ago, consider fibrinolytics as first option *unless*
   - Patient has absolute contraindications to fibrinolytics (eg, recent bleeding or head trauma)
   - Patient appears to be in cardiogenic shock.
   - Transport time to a PCI capable facility is reasonably ≤1 hour
   - Individual patient factors (eg, previous CABG) indicate that the primary PCI will most likely be more beneficial
   - Diagnosis of STEMI is in doubt

B. If symptoms began more than 3 hours but less than 12 ago, consider transport for primary PCI *unless*
   - The catheterization lab is not available or is not a reasonable option
   - Patient has extended transport time, in which case fibrinolytics may still be the preferred option (should be discussed with a cardiologist)
   - If primary PCI is not a viable option for patients presenting between 3 and 12 hours of symptom onset, fibrinolytics should still be strongly considered.

C. If symptoms began more that 12 hours ago, acute reperfusion is not indicated, unless there are continuing ischemic symptoms or under special circumstances; consider transfer to cardiac care unit for further treatment.

the United States, the EMS must be called in for transport, a source of delay that is often overlooked. If a patient is being considered for transport, the EMS must be summoned without hesitation, and preparation of the patient for transfer must continue, even if the decision is still uncertain.

Second, information on the absolute length of transport, the options available to shorten transport (eg, flight transport), and possible delaying factors (eg, weather or traffic conditions) must be available. This is especially important in areas with high traffic volumes or during times of inclement weather.

Third, an assessment must be made of the "downstream care" that the patient will receive. The ability and training of transport personnel to deal with complications must be assessed; and most important, contact must be made with the receiving facility to ensure that primary PCI will be available without delay on the patient's arrival.

Once the above information has been obtained and evaluated, a final realistic assessment of the transfer should be made by the transferring physician. Unless a patient is in cardiogenic shock or presents later than 3 hours after symptom onset or has a firm contraindication to fibrinolysis, the transferring physician should consider erring on the side of caution and administering a fibrinolytic. This decision will be supported by the knowledge that early treatment is superior to later treatment and that transport and processing times usually are underestimated in real-world situations. It is in this final assessment that the competence of overall judgment of the physician is most critical.

A system designed to incorporate EMS, the referring emergency departments, and the receiving cardiology teams has the best chance for successfully meeting reperfusion time goals and ensuring optimal patient outcomes. Each community should endeavor to develop such an integrated approach to the care of their STEMI patients.

References

[1] DeWood MA, Spores J, Notske R, et al. Prevalence of total coronary occlusion during the early hours of transmural myocardial infarction. N Engl J Med 1980;303(16):897–902.

[2] Schoen FJ. The heart. In: Cotran RS, Kumar V, Collins T, editors. Pathologic basis of disease. 6th edition. Philadelphia: WB Saunders; 1999. p. 557.

[3] Reimer KA, Lowe JE, Rasmussen MM, et al. The wavefront phenomenon of ischemic cell death: 1: myocardial infarct size vs duration of coronary occlusion in dogs. Circulation 1977; 56(5):786–94.

[4] Antman E. Acute myocardial infarction. In: Braunwald E, Zipes DP, Libby P, editors. Heart disease: a textbook of cardiovascular medicine. 6th edition. Philadelphia: WB Saunders; 2001. p. 1114–231.

[5] Ohman EM, Harrington RA, Cannon CP, et al. Intravenous thrombolysis in acute myocardial infarction. Chest 2001;119:253–77.

[6] Simoons ML, Maggioni AP, Knaterud G, et al. Individual risk assessment for intracranial hemorrhage during thrombolytic therapy. Lancet 1993;342:1523.

[7] Angeja BG, Rundle AC, Gurwitz JH, et al. Death or nonfatal stroke in patients with acute myocardial infarction treated with tissue plasminogen activator. Am J Cardiol 2001;87:627.

[8] Barron HV, Rundle AC, Gore JM, et al. Intracranial hemorrhage rates and effect of immediate beta-blocker use in patients with acute myocardial infarction treated with tissue plasminogen activator. Am J Cardiol 2000;85:294.

[9] Fibrinolytic Therapy Trialists' (FTT) Collaborative Group. Indications for fibrinolytic therapy in suspected acute myocardial infarction: collaborative overview of early mortality and major morbidity results from all randomised trials of more than 1000 patients. Lancet 1994;343:311–22.

[10] Brass LM, Lichtman JH, Wang Y, et al. Intracranial hemorrhage associated with thrombolytic therapy for elderly patients with acute myocardial infarction: results from the Cooperative Cardiovascular Project. Stroke 2000;31:1802–11.

[11] Zeymer U, Tebbe U, Essen R, et al for the ALKK-Study Group. Influence of time to treatment on early infarct-related artery patency after different thrombolytic regimens. Am Heart J 1999;137:34–8.

[12] Cannon CP, Gibson CM, Lambrew CT, et al. Relationship of symptom-onset-to-balloon time and door-to-balloon time with mortality in patients undergoing angioplasty. JAMA 2000;283:2941.
[13] Peterson LR, Chandra NC, French WJ, et al. Reperfusion therapy in patients with acute myocardial infarction and prior coronary artery bypass surgery (National Registry of Myocardial Infarction-2). Am J Cardiol 1999;84:1287.
[14] Cannon CP, Gibson CM, Lambrew CT, et al. Longer thrombolysis door-to-needle times are associated with increased mortality in acute myocardial infarction: an analysis of 85,589 patients in the National Registry of Myocardial Infarction 2 and 3. J Am Coll Cardiol 2000; 35(Suppl A):376A.
[15] Ryan TJ, Antman EM, Brooks NH, et al. 1999 update: ACC/AHA guidelines for the management of patients with acute myocardial infarction. J Am Coll Cardiol 1999;34:890.
[16] Second International Study of Infarct Survival Collaborative Group. Randomised trial of intravenous streptokinase, oral aspirin, both, or neither among 17,187 cases of suspected acute myocardial infarction: ISIS-2. Lancet 1988;2:349–60.
[17] Third International Study of Infarct Survival Collaborative Group. ISIS-3: a randomised comparison of streptokinase vs tissue plasminogen activator vs anistreplase and of aspirin plus heparin vs aspirin alone among 41,299 cases of suspected acute myocardial infarction. Lancet 1992;339:753–70.
[18] The International Study Group. In-hospital mortality and clinical course of 20,891 patients with suspected acute myocardial infarction randomised between alteplase and streptokinase with or without heparin. Lancet 1990;336:71–5.
[19] GUSTO Investigators. An international randomized trial comparing four thrombolytic strategies for acute myocardial infarction. N Engl J Med 1993;329:673.
[20] GUSTO III Investigators. A comparison of reteplase with alteplase for acute myocardial infarction. N Engl J Med 1997;337:1118.
[21] Assessment of the Safety and Efficacy of a New Thrombolytic Investigators (ASSENT-2). Single-bolus tenecteplase compared with frontloaded alteplase in acute myocardial infarction: the ASSENT-2 double blind randomized trial. Lancet 1999;354:716.
[22] Bode C, Smalling RW, Berg G, et al. Randomized comparison of coronary thrombolysis achieved with double-bolus reteplase and front-loaded, accelerated alteplase in patients with acute myocardial infarction. Circulation 1996;94:891.
[23] Gruppo Italiano per lo Studio della Streptochinasi nell'Infarto Miocardico (GISSI). Effectiveness of intravenous thrombolytic treatment in acute myocardial infarction. Lancet 1986;1:397–402.
[24] Wilcox RG, von der Lippe G, Olsson CG, et al. Trial of tissue plasminogen activator for mortality reduction in acute myocardial infarction: Anglo-Scandinavian Study of Early Thrombolysis (ASSET). Lancet 1988;2:525–30.
[25] AIMS Trial Study Group. Long-term effects of intravenous anistreplase in acute myocardial infarction: final report of the AIMS study. Lancet 1990;335:427–31.
[26] Ross AM, Coyne KS, Moreyra E, et al, for the Global Utilization of Streptokinase and Tissue Plasminogen Activator for Occluded Coronary Arteries Trial (GUSTO-I) Angiographic Investigators. Extended mortality benefit of early postinfarction reperfusion. Circulation 1998;97:1549–56.
[27] Keyt BA, Paoni NF, Refino CJ, et al. A faster acting and more potent form of tissue plasminogen activator. Proc Natl Acad Sci USA 1994;91:3670.
[28] Mark DB, Hlatky MA, Califf RM, et al. Cost effectiveness of thrombolytic therapy with tissue plasminogen activator as compared with streptokinase for acute myocardial infarction. N Engl J Med 1995;332:1418.
[29] Assessment of the Safety and Efficacy of a New Thrombolytic Regimen (ASSENT)-3 Investigators. Efficacy and safety of tenecteplase in combination with enoxaparin, abciximab, or unfractionated heparin: the ASSENT-3 randomised trial in acute myocardial infarction. Lancet 2001;358:605.

[30] Zimetbaum PJ, Josephson ME. Use of the electrocardiogram in acute myocardial infarction. N Engl J Med 2003;348:933–40.

[31] Zijlstra F, Hoorntje JC, de Boer MJ, et al. Long-term benefit of primary angioplasty as compared with thrombolytic therapy for acute myocardial infarction. N Engl J Med 1999; 341:1413–9.

[32] Global Use of Strategies to Open Occluded Coronary Arteries in Acute Coronary Syndromes (GUSTO IIb) Angioplasty Substudy Investigators. A clinical trial comparing primary coronary angioplasty with tissue plasminogen activator for acute myocardial infarction. N Engl J Med 1997;336:1621–8.

[33] Weaver WD, Simes RJ, Betriu A, et al. Comparison of primary coronary angioplasty and intravenous thrombolytic therapy for acute myocardial infarction: a quantitative review. JAMA 1997;278:2093–8.

[34] Andersen HR, Neilsen TT, Rasmussen K, et al. A comparison of coronary angioplasty with fibrinolytic therapy in acute myocardial infarction. N Engl J Med 2003;349:733–42.

[35] Weaver WD, Simes RJ, Betriiu A, et al. Comparison of primary angioplasty and intravenous thrombolytic therapy for acute myocardial infarction: a quantitative review [abstract]. JAMA 1997;278:2093–8.

[36] Grines CL, Browne KF, Marco J, et al. A comparison of immediate angioplasty with thrombolytic therapy for acute myocardial infarction. N Engl J Med 1993;328:673.

[37] Ziljstra F, de Boer MJ, Hoorntje J, et al. A comparison of immediate coronary angioplasty with intravenous streptokinase in acute myocardial infarction. N Engl J Med 1993;328:680.

[38] Gibbons RJ, Holmes DR, Reeder GS, et al. Immediate angioplasty compared with the administration of a thrombolytic agent followed by conservative treatment for myocardial infarction. N Engl J Med 1993;328:685.

[39] de Boer MJ, Hoorntje J, Ottervanger JP, et al. Immediate coronary angioplasty versus intravenous streptokinase in acute myocardial infarction: left ventricular ejection fraction, hospital mortality and reinfarction. J Am Coll Cardiol 1994;23:1004.

[40] Zorman S, Zorman D, Noc M. Effects of abciximab pretreatment in patients with acute myocardial infarction undergoing primary angioplasty. Am J Cardiol 2002;90:533.

[41] Suryapranata H, van't Hof A, Hoorntje J, et al. Randomized comparison of coronary stenting with balloon angioplasty in selected patients with acute myocardial infarction. Circulation 1998;97:2502.

[42] Berger PB, Ellis SG, Holmes DR, et al. Relationship between delay in performing direct coronary angioplasty and early clinical outcome in patients with acute myocardial infarction: results from the Global Use of Strategies To Open Occluded Arteries in Acute Coronary Syndromes (GUSTO-IIb) trial. Circulation 1999;100:14.

[43] Cannon CP, Gibson CM, Lambrew CT, et al. Relationship of symptom-onset-to-balloon time and door-to-balloon time with mortality in patients undergoing angioplasty for acute myocardial infarction. JAMA 2000;283:2941–7.

[44] Hochman JS, Sleeper LA, Webb JG, et al, for the Should We Emergently Revascularize Occluded Coronaries for Cardiogenic Shock (SHOCK) Investigators. Early revascularization in acute myocardial infarction complicated by cardiogenic shock. N Engl J Med 1999; 341:625–34.

[45] Maillard L, Hamon M, Khalife K, et al, for the STENTIM-2 Investigators. A comparison of systematic stenting and conventional balloon angioplasty during primary percutaneous transluminal coronary angioplasty for acute myocardial infarction. J Am Coll Cardiol 2000; 35:1729–36.

[46] Scheller B, Hennen B, Severin-Kneib S, et al. Long-term follow-up of a randomized study of primary stenting versus angioplasty in acute myocardial infarction. Am J Med 2001;110: 1–6.

[47] Zhu MM, Feit A, Chadow H, et al. Primary stent implantation compared with primary balloon angioplasty for acute myocardial infarction: a meta-analysis of randomized clinical trials. Am J Cardiol 2001;88:297–301.

[48] Lemos PA, Saia F, Hofma SH, et al. Short- and long-term clinical benefit of sirolimus-eluting stents compared to conventional bare stents for patients with acute myocardial infarction. J Am Coll Cardiol 2004;43:704–8.
[49] Granger CB, White HD, Bates ER, et al. A pooled analysis of coronary arterial patency and left ventricular function after intravenous thrombolysis for acute myocardial infarction. Am J Cardiol 1994;74:1220–8.
[50] Ellis SG, da Silva ER, Heyndrickx G, et al. Randomized comparison of rescue angioplasty with conservative management of patients with early failure of thrombolysis for acute anterior myocardial infarction. Circulation 1994;90:2280–4.
[51] Steg PG, Bonnefoy E, Chabaud S, et al, for the Comparison of Angioplasty and Prehospital Thrombolysis In acute Myocardial infarction (CAPTIM) Investigators. Impact of time to treatment on mortality after prehospital fibrinolysis or primary angioplasty: data from the CAPTIM randomized clinical trial. Circulation 2003;108:2851–6.
[52] Wallentin L, Goldstein P, Armstrong PW, et al. Efficacy and safety of tenecteplase in combination with the low-molecular-weight heparin enoxaparin or unfractionated heparin in the prehospital setting: the Assessment of the Safety and Efficacy of a New Thrombolytic Regimen (ASSENT)-3 PLUS randomized trial in acute myocardial infarction. Circulation 2003;108:135–42.
[53] Morrison LJ, Verbeek PR, McDonald AC, et al. Mortality and prehospital thrombolysis for acute myocardial infarction: a meta-analysis. JAMA 2000;283:2686–92.
[54] Jacobs AK. Primary angioplasty for acute myocardial infarction: is it worth the wait? N Engl J Med 2003;349:798–800.
[55] Moyer P, Feldman J, Levine J, et al. Implications of the mechanical (PCI) vs thrombolytic controversy for ST segment elevation myocardial infarction on the organization of emergency medical services: the Boston EMS experience. Critical Pathways in Cardiology 2004;3:53–61.
[56] Cannon CP. Bridging the gap with new strategies in acute ST elevation myocardial infarction: bolus thrombolysis, glycoprotein IIb/IIIa inhibitors, combination therapy, percutaneous coronary intervention, and "facilitated" PCI. J Thromb Thrombolysis 2000; 9:235–41.
[57] Herrmann HC, Moliterno DJ, Ohman EM, et al. Facilitation of early percutaneous coronary intervention after reteplase with or without abciximab in acute myocardial infarction: results from the SPEED (GUSTO-4 Pilot). Trial. J Am Coll Cardiol 2000;36: 1489–96.
[58] Ross AM, Coyne KS, Reiner JS, et al, for the Plasminogen-activator Angioplasty Compatibility Trial (PACT) investigators. A randomized trial comparing primary angioplasty with a strategy of short-acting thrombolysis and immediate planned rescue angioplasty in acute myocardial infarction: the PACT trial. J Am Coll Cardiol 1999;34: 1954–62.
[59] Kastrati A, Mehilli J, Schlotterbeck K, et al, for the Bavarian Reperfusion Alternatives Evaluation (BRAVE) Study Investigators. Early administration of reteplase plus abciximab vs abciximab alone in patients with acute myocardial infarction referred for percutaneous coronary intervention: a randomized controlled trial. JAMA 2004;291:947–54.
[60] Ellis SG, Armstrong P, Betriu A, et al, for the FINESSE Investigators. Facilitated percutaneous coronary intervention versus primary percutaneous coronary intervention: design and rationale of the Facilitated Intervention with Enhanced Reperfusion Speed to Stop Events (FINESSE) trial. Am Heart J 2004;147:E16.
[61] Widimsky P, Budesinsky T, Vorac D, et al, for the PRAGUE Study Group Investigators. Long distance transport for primary angioplasty vs immediate thrombolysis in acute myocardial infarction: final results of the randomized national multicentre trial: PRAGUE-2. Eur Heart J 2003;24:94–104.
[62] Andersen HR, Nielsen TT, Rasmussen K, et al. A comparison of coronary angioplasty with fibrinolytic therapy in acute myocardial infarction. N Engl J Med 2003;349:733.

[63] Nallamothu BK, Bates ER, Herrin J, et al, for the NRMI Investigators. times to treatment in transfer patients undergoing primary percutaneous coronary intervention in the United States: National Registry of Myocardial Infarction (NRMI)-3/4 analysis. Circulation 2005; 111:761–7.

[64] Nallamothu BK, Antman EM, Bates ER. Primary percutaneous coronary intervention versus fibrinolytic therapy in acute myocardial infarction: does the choice of fibrinolytic agent impact on the importance of time-to-treatment. Am J Cardiol 2004;94(6):772–4.

[65] American College of Cardiology, American Heart Association. ACC/AHA guidelines for the management of patients with ST-elevation myocardial infarction: executive summary: a report of the American College of Cardiology/American Heart Association Task Force on Practice Guidelines (Writing Committee to Revise the 1999 Guideline on Acute Myocardial Infarction). Circulation 2004;110(5):588–636.

ELSEVIER
SAUNDERS

Emerg Med Clin N Am
23 (2005) 1065–1082

EMERGENCY
MEDICINE
CLINICS OF
NORTH AMERICA

Arrhythmic Complications of Acute Coronary Syndromes

Andrew D. Perron, MD*, Timothy Sweeney, MD

Department of Emergency Medicine, 22 Bramhall Street, Maine Medical Center, Portland, ME 04102, USA

Cardiac arrhythmias routinely manifest during or following an acute coronary syndrome (ACS). Although the incidence of arrhythmia is directly related to the type of ACS the patient is experiencing (higher with ST-elevation myocardial infarction [STEMI] and lower with non–ST-elevation myocardial infarction [NSTEMI] and unstable angina pectoris [UAP]), the clinician needs to be cautious with all patients in these categories. For example, nearly 90% of patients who experience acute myocardial infarction (AMI) develop some cardiac rhythm abnormality and 25% have a cardiac conduction disturbance within 24 hours of infarct onset [1–5]. In this patient population, the incidence of serious arrhythmias, such as ventricular fibrillation (4.5%), is greatest in the first hour of an AMI and declines rapidly thereafter [2–6].

ACS patients, particularly those with STEMI, demand a rapid and multifaceted approach. Decisions regarding reperfusion strategy (eg, angioplasty versus thrombolysis), adjunctive medical therapy (eg, aspirin, heparin, beta-adrenergic blockade, nitrates, and other medicines), and management of complicating factors (eg, congestive heart failure [CHF]) all compete for the clinician's attention. Concomitantly, the clinician has to be prepared to recognize arrhythmias and treat those that require intervention because they can exacerbate ischemia and lead to clinical instability. Further, with emergency department (ED) administration of thrombolytics, the clinician should be aware of common "reperfusion" arrhythmias and their potential significance.

This article addresses the identification and treatment of arrhythmias and conduction disturbances that complicate the course of patients who have

* Corresponding author.
E-mail address: perroa@mmc.org (A.D. Perron).

doi:10.1016/j.emc.2005.07.002
emed.theclinics.com

ACS, particularly AMI and thrombolysis. Emphasis is placed on mechanisms and therapeutic strategies.

Basic mechanisms for arrhythmias and conduction disturbances

In the setting of AMI, several factors contribute to the development of cardiac arrhythmias. Alterations in ion currents, hypoxia, and electrolyte imbalances provide a milieu for cardiac arrhythmia [1,7,8]. Furthermore, enhanced automaticity of the myocardium and Purkinje system is precipitated by autonomic dysfunction of the heart in the face of generalized autonomic imbalance [9,10]. Enhanced efferent sympathetic activity, increased concentrations of circulating catecholamines, and local release of catecholamines from nerve endings within the heart muscle itself have been implicated. Furthermore, transmural infarction can interrupt afferent and efferent limbs of the sympathetic nervous system innervating myocardium distal to the area of infarction [11]. The net result of this autonomic imbalance is the promotion of arrhythmia development [11,12].

Other postulated mechanisms include the presence of elevated free fatty acid levels and oxygen-derived free radicals that may contribute to the development of arrhythmias in ACS [1]. Additionally, electrolyte abnormalities, such as hypokalemia, hypomagnesemia, and acidosis, have received increased attention as potentially important (and treatable) causes of serious rhythm disturbances [1,12,13]. The severity of all these potential abnormalities, combined with infarct size and residual flow in the infarct-related artery, determines the patient's risk for arrhythmia, and careful attention to correcting potential contributors is prudent [1,12,13]. Treatment of coexisting conditions is essential (eg, gastrointestinal bleed), which can potentially result in sinus tachycardia, supraventricular tachyarrhythmias, increased myocardial oxygen demand, and hypoxemia. Although many peri-infarct arrhythmias are benign and self-limited, arrhythmias, in general, require aggressive treatment when they result in (1) hypotension; (2) increased myocardial oxygen requirements; or (3) predisposition to further malignant ventricular arrhythmias [1].

Supraventricular tachyarrhythmias

Sinus Tachycardia

Sinus tachycardia is defined as a heart rate of more than 100 beats per minute with consistent association of the P wave with each QRS complex [14]. Although sinus tachycardia is a normal physiologic response to stress, persistent sinus tachycardia following AMI carries an unfavorable prognosis with an increased mortality risk [15]. Sinus tachycardia is associated with enhanced sympathetic activity and can result in transient hypertension or hypotension. The elevated heart rate increases myocardial oxygen demand, whereas decreased time spent in diastole compromises coronary flow, worsening myocardial ischemia. Persistent sinus tachycardia may be caused by heart failure, hypovolemia, ongoing pain, anxiety, hypoxemia, anemia, pericarditis, pulmonary embolism, or the previous administration of drugs, such as atropine, epinephrine, or dopamine.

Persistent sinus tachycardia in the patient who has ACS demands workup and appropriate therapy, such as adequate pain medication for ongoing discomfort, diuretics for heart failure, oxygen, intravascular volume replacement for hypovolemia, anti-inflammatory agents for fever or pericarditis, and beta-blockers or nitroglycerine for ischemia. For example, administration of a beta-blocker (eg, metoprolol, 5 mg intravenous [IV], repeated every 5 minutes to a total dose of 15 mg) has been shown to be helpful in reducing myocardial oxygen demand and heart rate in ACS. However, beta-blockers are generally contraindicated in patients who experience hypovolemia or pump failure. Thus, a thorough investigation of the cause of sinus tachycardia is first required. If the cause cannot be determined to a high degree of confidence, an ultra–short-acting beta-blocker, such as esmolol (25–200 mg/kg/min) may be considered to ascertain the patient's response to slowing of the heart rate [16].

Premature atrial contractions

Premature atrial contractions often occur before the development of paroxysmal supraventricular tachycardia, atrial flutter, or atrial fibrillation [17]. They may be caused by atrial distention from increased left ventricular diastolic pressure, by inflammation associated with pericarditis, and, less frequently, by atrial ischemia or infarction [18–20]. No specific therapy is indicated; however, attention should be given to identifying the underlying disease process, particularly occult CHF.

Paroxysmal supraventricular tachycardia

Paroxysmal supraventricular tachycardia occurs in less than 10% of patients who experience AMI but requires rapid and aggressive management to reduce additional ischemia caused by the rapid ventricular rate [21]. Vagal maneuvers, such as Valsalva or carotid sinus massage (following careful assessment for carotid bruits), may occasionally restore sinus rhythm and are of low risk. The drug of choice for paroxysmal supraventricular tachycardia in non-AMI patients is adenosine (6–12 mg rapid IV push for more than 1–3 seconds) [21]. Although little data exist to guide therapy with adenosine in the AMI patient, many experts believe it can be used safely provided that hypotension (systolic blood pressure $<$ 100 mm Hg) is not present [1]. In patients without significant left ventricular failure, IV diltiazem (15–20 mg), metoprolol (5–15 mg), or verapamil (5–10 mg) are acceptable alternatives. IV beta-blockers combined with IV verapamil should be avoided because their combined administration may cause severe hypotension or high grade atrioventricular (AV) nodal block [22]. In patients who develop severe CHF or hypotension, synchronized cardioversion with an initial dose of 50 J (or biphasic equivalent) is indicated. Although digitalis has been shown to be useful in converting paroxysmal supraventricular tachycardia, it has fallen out of favor because of its delayed onset of action, adverse drug profile, and the presence of more desirable medications discussed earlier that can be used [1,14].

Atrial flutter

Atrial flutter is the least common sustained atrial arrhythmia associated with AMI and occurs in fewer than 5% of patients [23]. Atrial flutter is usually transient and in AMI results from sympathetic overstimulation of the atria. In patients who experience CHF or pulmonary emboli, atrial flutter often occurs and intensifies hemodynamic deterioration [24]. Treatment strategies for persistent atrial flutter mirror those for atrial fibrillation and are described in later discussion.

Atrial fibrillation

Atrial fibrillation is much more common than atrial flutter, with an incidence of 10% to 15% in patients who experience AMI [17]. The onset of atrial fibrillation in the first hours of AMI is usually caused by left atrial ischemia [25]. Pericarditis, and all conditions leading to elevated left atrial pressure can lead to atrial fibrillation in association with ACS [17,26]. Presence of atrial fibrillation during AMI is associated with increased mortality and stroke, particularly in patients who experience anterior-wall myocardial infarctions (MIs) [1,27]. The poor prognosis seen with atrial fibrillation may be caused by its appearance in patients who experience greater tissue damage, larger infarct size, and cardiac failure [17,27].

As with sinus tachycardia, atrial fibrillation with rapid ventricular response increases myocardial oxygen demand, worsening ischemia, and left ventricular function. A critical first step in choosing the appropriate treatment is the assessment of the rate of ventricular response, whether ischemia is being precipitated or worsened, or cardiac output is being seriously compromised. If the patient is experiencing new or worsening ischemic pain, hypotension, or both, immediate electrical cardioversion should be performed. Electrical cardioversion begins with 25 to 50 J (or biphasic equivalent) for atrial flutter and 50 to 100 J (or biphasic equivalent) for atrial fibrillation, with gradual increase if the initial shock is unsuccessful [22].

If the patient is not seriously compromised, initial attention should be focused on slowing the ventricular response [14]. For patients who do not develop hypotension, a beta-blocker (eg, metoprolol in 5-mg IV boluses every 5–10 minutes to a total dose of 15 mg, followed by 25–50 mg by mouth every 6 hours) should be used to reduce the combined effects of ischemia and increased sympathetic tone. If there is concern about the patient's ability to tolerate beta-blockade, IV esmolol may again be used [1]. Because of its short half-life, adverse effects dissipate quickly after the infusion is terminated. IV diltiazem (0.25 mg/kg IV) or verapamil are effective alternatives that promptly slow the ventricular rate, although they should be used with caution (if at all) in patients who experience CHF [1]. Because of increased risk for thromboembolism in atrial fibrillation, IV anticoagulation with heparin should be administered unless contraindicated. For patients who experience atrial flutter refractory to medical therapy, overdrive atrial pacing is available as an important therapeutic option [17].

Accelerated junctional rhythm

An uncommon rhythm in AMI is accelerated junctional rhythm, or nonparoxysmal junctional tachycardia. This rhythm occurs when there is increased automaticity of the junctional tissue that assumes the role of pacemaker appearing at a rate of 70 to 130 beats per minute. An important diagnostic feature in this arrhythmia is that sinus beats are *not* slowed, as with junctional escape rhythms; instead, the ventricular rate usurps control. As with all the tachyarrhythmias, the increased heart rate has potential for increasing myocardial ischemia [28]. This dysrhythmia is more common in patients who develop inferior compared with anterior MI and also may be seen in patients who develop digitalis intoxication [1]. Treatment is aimed at resolving the underlying conditions, such as ischemia or digitalis intoxication [17].

Bradyarrhythmias

Sinus bradycardia

Sinus bradycardia is defined as a sinus rate less than 60 beats per minute with normal association of P waves and the QRS complex and is a common arrhythmia in patients who have ACS [29,30], particularly those with inferior and posterior AMI [29]. In the initial 1 to 2 hours after inferior infarction onset, bradycardia is present in approximately 40% of patients, but by 4 hours the incidence decreases to approximately 20% [17,29,30]. The postulated mechanism is stimulation of cardiac vagal afferent receptors, which are more common in the inferoposterior portion of the left ventricle. This mechanism results in efferent cholinergic stimulation of the heart, leading to bradycardia and hypotension [1] and is a manifestation of the Bezold-Jarisch reflex. The Bezold-Jarisch reflex is mediated by the vagus nerves [31] and can also be seen during reperfusion, especially of the right coronary artery [32]. The vasovagal response is also commonly responsible for sinus bradycardia, which can be intensified by severe pain and also by morphine administration [33]. In the early phases of AMI, the resultant sinus bradycardia may actually be protective, reducing myocardial oxygen demands [29]. Profound sinus bradycardia that produces cerebral and cardiac hypoperfusion, low cardiac output, and hypotension, however, may increase the likelihood of repetitive ventricular arrhythmias and should be aggressively treated [17].

In the absence of adverse signs or symptoms (eg, chest pain, shortness of breath, decreased level of consciousness, hypotension, shock, pulmonary congestion, or CHF), therapy for bradyarrythmia is not required. If emergent therapy is indicated, atropine sulfate may be given at a dose of 0.5 to 1.0 mg every 3 to 5 minutes (up to a total of 0.03–0.04 mg/kg [2–3 mg total]) [17,34]. Occasionally, a low dose of atropine may further aggravate sinus node slowing, whereas a high dose may produce sinus tachycardia, resulting in increased ischemia [35]. The inability to reverse hypotension with atropine in patients who develop sinus bradycardia and inferior MI suggests volume depletion, right ventricular infarction, or both. When atropine is ineffective and the patient is symptomatic or hypotensive, transcutaneous or transvenous pacing is indicated. Denervated, transplanted hearts do not respond to atropine and require cardiac pacing as the initial intervention [22]. If these interventions fail, additional pharmacologic intervention includes dopamine (5–20 μg/kg/min IV), epinephrine (2–10 μg/min), and, potentially, isoproterenol [22]. The latter, however, should be used with extreme caution and at low doses if at all because it can potentiate cardiac ischemia [22].

Junctional bradycardia

An atrioventricular junctional escape rhythm at a rate of 35 to 60 beats per minute in patients who develop inferior MI is not uncommon [17,20]. Importantly this arrhythmia is usually a benign (protective) escape rhythm without hemodynamic compromise, and therapy, therefore, is usually not required. When there is hemodynamic impairment, transcutaneous or transvenous pacing may be necessary to maintain adequate perfusion [1].

Atrioventricular block

First-degree AV block

First-degree AV block is defined as prolongation of the PR interval greater than 0.20 seconds and occurs in approximately 15% of patients who develop AMI, most commonly inferior infarction [17]. Almost all patients who develop first-degree AV block have conduction disturbances located above the bundle of His. This distinction is important, because progression to complete heart block or ventricular asystole occurs almost exclusively in patients who experience first-degree AV block in whom the conduction disturbance is *below* the bundle of His [1]. For this reason, the clinical significance of first-degree AV block is usually minimal, and no specific therapy is indicated.

Concomitant therapy with digoxin, beta-blockers, or calcium channel blockers, such as diltiazem or verapamil may be partially responsible for first-degree AV block; however, discontinuation of these drugs may potentially increase ischemia. Only if hemodynamic impairment or higher degree block occurs should these agents be stopped. If first-degree AV block is associated with sinus bradycardia and hypotension, administration of atropine is indicated. Continued ECG monitoring is required for early detection of the possibility of progression to higher degrees of block [1,17,36].

Second-degree AV block

Second-degree AV block manifests as intermittent failure of atrial impulses to conduct to the ventricles and exists in two forms: (1) Mobitz type I or Wenckebach AV block and (2) Mobitz type II block.

Mobitz type I or Wenckebach AV block

Mobitz type I block occurs in approximately 10% of patients who experience AMI and accounts for 90% of all patients who experience AMI and second-degree AV block [1,37]. Mobitz type I block is defined as a failure of the atrial impulse to conduct to the ventricles, with a nonconducted beat usually following a progressive lengthening of the PR interval and shortened RP intervals (PR-RP reciprocity). The following features characterize Mobitz type I block: (1) it occurs as the result of ischemia of the AV node; (2) it is common (10%) in AMI; (3) it is associated with a narrow QRS complex; (4) it is most commonly associated with inferior MI; (5) it is usually transient, may be intermittent, and rarely progresses to complete AV block; and (6) it does not affect prognosis [1,14,17].

Mobitz type I block does not necessarily require treatment unless the ventricular rate is unable to sustain perfusion or there is coexisting cardiac failure or bundle branch block. If the heart rate is inadequate for perfusion or the coexisting conditions are present, immediate treatment with atropine (0.5–1.0 mg IV) is indicated. Transcutaneous or temporary transvenous pacing is rarely required.

Mobitz type II AV block

Mobitz type II AV block is uncommon, representing only 10% of all cases with second-degree AV block (overall incidence less than 1%) [38] and is defined as an intermittent failure of atrial impulses to conduct to the ventricles, characterized by a uniform PR interval before the nonconducted atrial beat. In contrast to Mobitz type I block, Mobitz type II block is characterized by the following features: (1) the conduction abnormality is located below the bundle of His; (2) it is associated with impaired conduction distal to the bundle of His, reflecting trifascicular block and usually leading to a wide QRS complex; (3) it is almost always associated with anterior infarction; (4) it often progresses suddenly to complete heart block; and (5) it is associated with a poor prognosis (mortality rate associated with a progression of Mobitz type II block to complete heart block is approximately 80%) [1,14,17].

Mobitz type II second-degree AV block should be immediately treated with transcutaneous pacing or atropine (0.5–1.0 mg IV), with the latter showing improvement in only one half of cases and occasionally even worsening the block [22]. Ultimately, a temporary transvenous demand pacemaker needw to be established [1].

Third-degree AV block

Third-degree AV block, or complete heart block, occurs in 5% to 15% of patients who experience AMI [39]. The cardiac conduction system has a dual blood supply, from the AV branch of the right coronary artery and the septal perforating branch of the left anterior descending coronary artery [1,40]. Prognosis with this condition depends on the location of the block in the conduction system and the size of MI [41]. In patients who develop inferior MI, the block occurs at or above the bundle of His in 70% of cases [17,41]. The block usually develops gradually, progressing from first-degree or type I second-degree block. The escape rhythm is usually stable, with a narrow QRS complex and a rate exceeding 40 beats per minute [1]. In 30% of cases, the block is below the bundle of His, resulting in an escape rhythm with a rate slower than 40 beats per minute and a wide QRS complex. Complete heart block in patients who develop inferior MI is usually responsive to pharmacologic intervention and resolves in most patients within a few days [37]. The mortality rate for inferior MI patients who develop complete heart block is approximately 15% unless there is coexisting right ventricular infarction, in which case the mortality rate is doubled [42].

With inferior MI and high-degree AV block, the possibility of volume depletion as a cause for hypotension must be eliminated, especially if there is coexisting right ventricular infarction whereby preload becomes more important relative to RV output in driving blood through the pulmonary vasculature. Volume challenge, therefore, is a reasonable clinical strategy before implementing pharmacologic intervention or temporary pacing [17,37]. Immediate treatment with atropine (0.5–1.0 mg IV) is indicated with the same caveats as with Mobitz II: it may not help and potentially worsen the block [22]. Temporary transcutaneous or transvenous pacing should be implemented in symptomatic patients who are unresponsive to atropine. Patients with inferior MI who develop persistent symptomatic bradycardia or conduction abnormalities should be considered for permanent pacing.

In patients who develop anterior MI, third-degree AV block usually is preceded by intraventricular block or Mobitz type II AV block (not first-degree or Mobitz type I) and occurs suddenly. The block is located below the bundle of His, resulting in escape rhythms with wide QRS complexes and rates less than 40 beats per minute. This rhythm may progress suddenly to asystole and is associated with a mortality rate of 80% [1,43].

Immediate treatment with atropine (0.5–1.0 mg IV repeated every 3–5 minutes for a total dose of 2–3 mg) or transcutaneous pacing is indicated, followed by temporary transvenous pacing. Patients with anterior MI who develop third-degree AV block and survive to hospitalization often receive a permanent pacemaker.

Intraventricular block

Electrical conduction from the bundle of His is relayed through three fascicles (the anterior and posterior divisions of the left bundle and the right bundle). Approximately 15% of patients who experience AMI develop disturbances in one or more of these fascicles [17]. Isolated left anterior fascicular block occurs in 3% to 5% of patients who experience AMI and is unlikely to progress to complete AV block [44]. Isolated left posterior fascicular block occurs in only 1% to 2% of patients who experience AMI but this fascicle has a larger blood supply than the anterior fascicle and anterior fascicular block is therefore associated with a larger infarct and higher mortality [44]. The right bundle-branch, like the posterior fascicle, has a redundant blood supply. The presence of a new Right bundle branch block (RBBB), seen in approximately 2% of AMI cases, suggests a large infarct territory, typically in an anteroseptal distribution. Not surprisingly, progression to complete heart block is frequent [1,45]. In patients who develop anterior MI and new right bundle branch block, there is substantial risk for death caused by cardiogenic shock reflecting the extensive size of the myocardial infarct [45].

The combination of right bundle branch block with a left anterior or posterior fascicular block or the combination of left anterior and posterior fascicular blocks (left bundle branch block) is known as bifascicular block. If a new block occurs in two of the three conduction fascicles, the risk for developing complete AV block is high [1,45]. Mortality is also high because of the extensive myocardial necrosis required to produce the bifascicular block [1,46]. Bifascicular block in the presence of first-degree AV block (prolongation of the PR interval) is termed trifascicular block. Nearly 40% of such patients progress to complete heart block [44].

Whether a bundle branch block is new or old is often unclear and difficult to determine in the emergency department setting. Irrespective, the presence of a new or old bundle branch block with coexisting AMI identifies a patient who is more likely to develop high-degree AV block, CHF, ventricular fibrillation (VF), and death [44]. Old or indeterminate bundle branch block associated with AMI generally does not require temporary or permanent pacing.

New right or left bundle branch block, bifascicular blocks, and all forms of trifascicular block are more commonly associated with anterior infarction. They are therefore associated with larger infarcts in older patients who have a higher incidence of arrhythmias, CHF, and higher mortality rates when compared with AMI patients who do not develop bundle branch block [1,7].

Asystole

The incidence of asystole following MI varies widely depending on the definition. Approximately 1% of patients who experience AMI experience transient episodes of asystole caused by abnormalities in the AV conduction system. In these instances, immediate transcutaneous pacing followed by establishment of a transvenous pacemaker is indicated [48]. Patients who develop asystole as a terminal complication from AMI have a mortality rate that approaches 100% [1,14,17].

Indications for temporary and permanent pacing

Temporary pacing

Indications for temporary pacing in patients who experience AMI include asystole, complete heart block, persistent Mobitz type II second-degree AV block especially with a wide QRS complex/BBB, symptomatic bradycardia, sinus pauses lasting 3.5 seconds or more, and transient asystole unresponsive to atropine [49]. In addition, any bradycardia unresponsive to atropine that is associated with hypotension or signs and symptoms of ischemia may require temporary pacing [17,49].

Permanent pacing

AMI patients require permanent pacing if they have persistent high-degree block (Mobitz type II or third-degree heart block) with a wide QRS complex or have transient advanced AV block associated with bundle branch block [17,50]. Persistent symptomatic bradycardias or conduction defects also warrant consideration for permanent pacing [17,50].

Ventricular arrhythmias

Premature ventricular contractions

In the past, there was believed to be an association between "warning arrhythmias" (eg, >5 premature ventricular contractions [PVCs]/min, PVCs with multiform configuration, R-on-T phenomenon, and repetitive patterns in the form of couplets or salvos) and the risk for VF [14,51]. It is now clear, however, that such warning arrhythmias occur with the same frequency in patients who do and do not subsequently develop VF [52]. In fact, several studies have demonstrated that primary VF occurs without any antecedent warning arrhythmias in many patients and can develop despite pharmacologic suppression of warning arrhythmias [1,53,54]. Further, these "warning arrhythmias" frequently are observed in patients who experience AMI who never develop VF [53,55]. For these reasons, the prior practice of prophylactic suppression of PVCs with antiarrhythmic drugs, such as lidocaine, is no longer indicated. Prophylaxis has been shown to be associated with increased risk for fatal bradycardia or asystole, as a result of suppression of escape pacemakers [56–59].

Based on this evidence, most clinicians pursue a conservative course at the time PVCs are observed in an ACS patient and do not routinely administer prophylactic antiarrythmics [1]. Instead, attention should be directed toward resolving any electrolyte or metabolic abnormalities and identifying and treating recurrent ischemia [1,14]. If PVCs are encountered in the presence of sinus tachycardia early in the process of an evolving MI, the use of IV beta-blockers may reduce the incidence of subsequent VF [60]. Available antiarrhythmic agents should be used only to suppress symptomatic, immediately life-threatening arrhythmias [14].

Accelerated idioventricular rhythm

Accelerated idioventricular rhythm is seen in up to 20% of patients who experience AMI [1] and is defined as a ventricular rhythm (characterized by a wide QRS complex) with a variable rate between 60 and 125 beats per minute [1,14]. Most episodes are of short duration and terminate spontaneously. This rhythm has two postulated, possibly coexisting causes. First, the SA or AV node may suffer structural damage with depression of nodal automaticity potentiated by enhanced vagal tone. Second, an abnormal ectopic focus within the ventricle may assume the role of dominant pacemaker. The presence of accelerated idioventricular rhythm does not affect prognosis, and there is no definitive evidence that, if left untreated, the incidence of VF or death is increased [61]. This rhythm occurs somewhat more frequently in patients who develop early reperfusion, although it is neither sensitive nor specific enough to merit consideration as a marker of reperfusion [14]. Temporary pacing is not indicated unless the rhythm is sustained and results in hypotension or ischemic symptoms. Suppression of the rhythm with antiarrhythmic therapy is also nonbeneficial and may cause hemodynamic compromise [14]. Accelerated idioventricular rhythm is the result of failure of the proximal pacemakers and represents an appropriate escape rhythm. If an antiarrythmic, such as lidocaine, is given, suppression of this escape rhythm can result in profound bradycardia or even asystole [54,58,59].

Ventricular tachycardia

Nonsustained ventricular tachycardia

Nonsustained ventricular tachycardia is defined as three or more consecutive ventricular ectopic beats at a rate of greater than 100 beats per minute and lasting less than 30 seconds [1]. As the spectrum of clinical significance moves from isolated premature beats toward nonsustained ventricular tachycardia, the issue of risk and benefit of antiarrhythmic agents becomes more complicated [14]. In patients who experience multiple runs of nonsustained ventricular tachycardia, the risk for sudden hemodynamic collapse may be substantial. Nonetheless, nonsustained ventricular tachycardia in the immediate peri-infarction period does not appear to be associated with an increased mortality risk, and there is no demonstration that effective antiarrhythmic treatment results in a morbidity or mortality benefit [62]. In stark contrast, nonsustained ventricular tachycardia occurring more than 48 hours after infarction in patients who experience depressed left ventricular function (left ventricular ejection fraction $< 40\%$) is a marker for increased risk for sudden cardiac death. In this subgroup, electrophysiologic testing and therapy are appropriate [63].

Multiple episodes of nonsustained ventricular tachycardia demands intensified monitoring and attention to electrolyte imbalances [14]. Serum potassium levels should be maintained above 4.5 mEq/L and serum magnesium above 2 mEq/L [64]. Ongoing ischemia should be aggressively searched for and corrected if found.

Sustained ventricular tachycardia

Sustained ventricular tachycardiais defined as three or more consecutive ventricular ectopic beats at a rate greater than 100 beats per minute and lasting longer than 30 seconds or causing hemodynamic compromise that requires intervention [1]. Monomorphic ventricular tachycardia is more likely to be caused by a myocardial scar and require aggressive strategies to prevent its recurrence, whereas polymorphic ventricular tachycardia may be more responsive to measures directed against ischemia [24,47,56]. Sustained polymorphic ventricular tachycardia following AMI is associated with a hospital mortality of 20% [62].

Emergency treatment of sustained ventricular tachycardia is mandatory because of its hemodynamic effects and because it frequently deteriorates into VF. Rapid (greater than 150 beats per minute) polymorphic ventricular tachycardia associated with hemodynamic instability should be treated with immediate direct-current unsynchronized cardioversion of 200 J (or biphasic energy equivalent), whereas monomorphic ventricular tachycardia should be treated with a synchronized discharge of 100 J (or bipasic energy equivalent) [22]. If sustained ventricular tachycardia is well tolerated, the following antiarrhythmic therapies (rather than initial direct-current cardioversion) may be attempted first [22]:

1. Lidocaine (initial bolus of 1.0–1.5 mg/kg followed by additional boluses of 0.5–0.75 mg/kg every 5–10 minutes as needed to a maximum of 3 mg/kg. A maintenance of infusion of 1–4 mg per minute should then be initiated).

2. Procainamide (loading dose of 12–17 mg/kg over 20–30 minutes, followed by a maintenance infusion of 1–4 mg/min).
3. Amiodarone (loading dose of 150 mg followed by a constant infusion of 1.0 mg/min for up to 6 hours and then a maintenance infusion of 0.5 mg per minute).

After conversion to sinus rhythm, every effort should be made to identify and correct precipitating causes, such as electrolyte abnormalities, acid-base disturbances, hypoxia, or medication effects. For persistent ventricular tachycardia despite the above interventions, overdrive pacing may be effective in electrically converting the patient to sinus rhythm.

Ventricular fibrillation

The incidence of primary VF (4.5%) is greatest in the first hour following infarct onset and thereafter rapidly declines [6,65]. Approximately 60% of episodes occur within 4 hours and 80% within 12 hours [66]. Secondary or "late" VF occurs more than 48 hours following MI and is usually associated with terminal pump failure and clinical cardiogenic shock [52]. Risk of secondary VF increases with larger infarct size, intraventricular conduction delay, anteroseptal AMI, persistent sinus tachycardia, atrial flutter, or atrial fibrillation early in the clinical course [1]. Secondary VF in association with cardiogenic shock has a poor prognosis with an in-hospital mortality rate of 40% to 60% [67]. Primary VF in hospitalized AMI patients has uncertain prognostic implications [68–71].

Treatment for VF is unsynchronized electrical countershock with at least 200 to 300 J (or biphasic energy equivalent) implemented as rapidly as possible [22]. The likelihood for survival decreases 10% for each minute of time after the onset of uncorrected VF [22]. Successful conversion of VF and prevention of refractory recurrent episodes is facilitated by administration of amiodarone, 300-mg bolus followed by infusion; procainamide, 30 mg/min infusion with a maximal total dose of 17 mg/kg; or lidocaine, 1- to 1.5-mg/kg bolus. Following conversion of VF, antiarrhythmic therapy is generally continued by constant IV infusion for 12 to 24 hours [14,22].

As outlined previously, prophylactic lidocaine has been shown to reduce the incidence of VF but is not used because it seems to have an excess mortality risk owing to bradycardic and asystolic events [72]. In contradistinction, early use of beta-blockers in patients who experience AMI has been shown not only to reduce the incidence of VF but also mortality [6,73,74]. These data support the contention that IV beta-blockers should be administered early in the course of all appropriate AMI patient candidates.

Reperfusion arrhythmias

The sudden onset of rhythm disturbances in AMI patients following treatment with thrombolytic therapy has traditionally been believed to be a marker of successful coronary reperfusion [75]. A high incidence of identical rhythm disturbances exists in AMI patients who do not experience successful coronary reperfusion [76–78]; therefore, the sensitivity or specificity of reperfusion arrhythmias for detecting successful reperfusion are too low to be clinically useful [68]. In addition, clinical features, such as relief of chest pain are poor markers of successful reperfusion [76]. It is unfortunate that no single clinical finding or constellation of findings has been shown to be reliably predictive of angiographically demonstrated coronary artery patency [1,76,79].

In a meta-analysis of many thrombolytic therapy trials, Solomon and colleagues reported no increase in the risk for ventricular tachycardia or VF in patients receiving thrombolytic therapy [80]. The incidence of these arrhythmias, then, seems to be similar in patients not receiving thrombolytic therapy. These arrhythmias may be a consequence of spontaneous coronary artery reperfusion or related to the infarct process itself. For these reasons, arrhythmias associated with AMI following treatment with thrombolytic therapy cannot be relied on to determine reperfusion status and should be treated as discussed earlier [1,75,76,80].

References

[1] Antman EM. Acute myocardial infarction. In: Braunwald E, editor. Heart disease: a textbook of cardiovascular medicine. 5th edition. Philadelphia: WB Saunders; 1997. p. 1245–53.

[2] Mangrum MJ. Diagnosis and treatment of acute myocardial infarction. Emerg Med Clin North Am 2001;19(2):385–95.

[3] Al-Khatib SM, Granger CB, Huang Y, et al. Sustained ventricular arrhythmias among patients with acute coronary syndromes with no ST-segment elevation: incidence, predictors, and outcomes. Circulation 2002;106:309–12.

[4] Guidry UC, Evans JC, Larson MG, et al. Temporal trends in event rates after Q-wave myocardial infarction: The Framingham Heart Study. Circulation 1999;100:2054.

[5] Furman MI, Dauerman HL, Goldberg RJ, et al. Twenty-two year (1975 to 1997) trends in the incidence, in-hospital and long-term case fatality rates from initial Q-wave and non-Q-wave myocardial infarction: A multi-hospital, community-wide perspective. J Am Coll Cardiol 2001;37:1571–80.

[6] O'Doherty M, Tayler DI, Quinn E, et al. Five hundred patients with myocardial infarction monitored within one hour of symptoms. BMJ 1983;286:1405–8.

[7] Janse MJ, Wit AL. Electrophysiological mechanisms of ventricular arrhythmias resulting from myocardial ischaemia and infarction. Physiol Rev 1989;69:1049–169.

[8] Figueras J, Segura R, Bermejo B. Repeated 15-minute coronary occlusions in pigs increase occlusion arrhythmias but decrease reperfusion arrhythmias that are associated with extracellular hypokalemia. J Am Coll Cardiol 1996;28:1589–97.

[9] Hartikainen J, Kuikka J, Mantysaari M, et al. Sympathetic reinnervation after acute myocardial infarction. Am J Cardiol 1996;77:5–9.

[10] Arnar DO, Bullinga JR, Martins JB. Role of the Purkinje system in spontaneous ventricular tachycardia during acute ischemia in a canine model. Circulation 1997;96:2421–9.

[11] Barber MJ, Mueller TM, Davies BG, et al. Interruption of sympathetic and vagal-mediated afferent responses by transmural myocardial infarction. Circulation 1985;72:623–31.

[12] Shusterman V, Aysin B, Gottipaty V, et al. Autonomic nervous system activity and the spontaneous initiation of ventricular tachycardia. J Am Coll Cardiol 1998;32:1891–9.
[13] Tansey MJ, Opie LH. Relation between plasma free fatty acids and arrhythmias within the first twelve hours of acute myocardial infarction. Lancet 1983;2:419–22.
[14] Califf RM. Acute myocardial infarction. In: Antman EM, editor. Cardiovascular therapeutics: a companion to braunwald's heart disease. Philadelphia: WB Saunders; 1996. p. 153–4.
[15] Crimm A, Severance HW Jr, Coffey K, et al. Prognostic significance of isolated sinus tachycardia during first three days of acute myocardial infarction. Am J Med 1984;76:983–8.
[16] Kirshenbaum JM, Kloner RF, McGowan N, et al. Use of an ultrashort-acting beta receptor blocker (esmolol) in patients with acute myocardial ischemia and relative contraindications to beta-blockade therapy. J Am Coll Cardiol 1988;12:773–80.
[17] Roberts R, Morris D, Pratt CM, et al. Pathophysiology, recognition, and treatment of acute myocardial infarction and its complications. In: Schlant RC, Alexander RW, et al, editors. Hurst's the heart: arteries and veins. 8th edition. New York: McGraw-Hill; 1994. p. 1139–44.
[18] Gordon S, Finck DR, Perera RD, et al. Atrial infarction complicating an acute inferior myocardial infarction. Arch Intern Med 1984;144:193.
[19] Nielsen FE, Andersen HH, Gram-Hansen P, et al. The relationship between ECG signs of atrial infarction and the development of supraventricular arrhythmias in patients with acute myocardial infarction. Am Heart J 1992;123:69–72.
[20] Heidbuchel H, Tack J, Vanneste L, et al. Significance of arrhythmias during the first 24 hours of acute myocardial infarction treated with alteplase and effect of early administration of a β-blocker or a bradycardic agent on their incidence. Circulation 1994;89:1051–9.
[21] Ganz LI, Friedman PL. Supraventricular tachycardia. N Engl J Med 1995;332:162–73.
[22] The American Heart Association in collaboration with the International Liaison Committee on Resuscitation. Guidelines 2000 for cardiopulmonary resuscitation and emergency cardiovascular care: part 6: advanced cardiovascular life support; section 7: algorithm approach to ACLS emergencies; section 7A: principles and practice of ACLS. Circulation 2000;102:136–9.
[23] Berisso MZ, Carratino L, Ferroni A, et al. Frequency, characteristics, and significance of supraventricular tachyarrhythmias detected by 24-hour electrocardiographic recording in the late hospital phase of acute myocardial infarction. Am J Cardiol 1990;65:1064–70.
[24] DeSanctis RW, Block P, Hutter AM. Tachyarrhythmias in myocardial infarction. Circulation 1972;45:681–702.
[25] Hod H, Lew AS, Keltai M, et al. Early atrial fibrillation during evolving myocardial infarction: a consequence of impaired left atrial perfusion. Circulation 1987;75:146–50.
[26] Sugiura T, Owasaka T, Takahashi N, et al. Factors associated with atrial fibrillation in Q wave anterior myocardial infarction. Am Heart J 1991;121:1409–12.
[27] Goldberg RJ, Seeley D, Becker RC, et al. Impact of atrial fibrillation on the in-hospital and long-term survival of patients with acute myocardial infarction: a community-wide perspective. Am Heart J 1990;119:996–1001.
[28] Konecke LL, Knoebel SB. Nonparoxysmal junctional tachycardia complicating acute myocardial infarction. Circulation 1972;45:367–74.
[29] Grauer LE, Gershen BJ, Orlando MM, et al. Bradycardia and its complications in the prehospital phase of acute myocardial infarction. Am J Cardiol 1973;32:607–11.
[30] Pantridge JF, Webb SW, Adgey AAJ. Arrhythmias in the first hours of acute myocardial infarction. Prog Cardiovasc Dis 1981;23:265–78.
[31] Mark AL. The Bezold-Jarisch reflex revisited: clinical implications of inhibitory reflexes originating in the heart. J Am Coll Cardiol 1983;1:90–102.
[32] Wei JY, Markis JE, Malagold M, et al. Cardiovascular reflexes stimulated by reperfusion of ischemic myocardium in acute myocardial infarction. Circulation 1983;67:796–801.
[33] Come PC, Pitt B. Nitroglycerin-induced severe hypotension and bradycardia in patients with acute myocardial infarction. Circulation 1976;54:624–8.

[34] Swart G, Brady WJ, DeBehnke DJ, et al. Acute myocardial infarction complicated by hemodynamically unstable bradyarrythmia: prehospital and ED treatment with atropine. Am J Emerg Med 1999;17(7):647–52.
[35] Chadda KD, Lichstein E, Gupta PK, et al. Effects of atropine in patients with bradyarrhythmias complicating myocardial infarction. Am J Med 1977;63:503–10.
[36] Norris RM, Mercer CJ. Significance of idioventricular rhythms in acute myocardial infarction. Prog Cardiovasc Dis 1974;16:455–68.
[37] Clemmensen P, Bates ER, Califf RM, et al. Complete atrioventricular block complicating inferior wall acute myocardial infarction treated with reperfusion therapy: TAMI Study Group. Am J Cardiol 1991;67:225–30.
[38] Bhandari AK, Sager PT. Management of peri-infarctional ventricular arrhythmias and conduction disturbances. In: Naccarelli GV, editor. Cardiac arrhythmias: a practical approach. New York: Futura Publishing; 1991. p. 283.
[39] Berger PB, Ruocco NA Jr, Ryan TJ, et al. Incidence and prognostic implications of heart block complicating inferior myocardial infarction treated with thrombolytic therapy: results from TIMI II. J Am Coll Cardiol 1992;20:533–40.
[40] Fisch JR, Zipes DP, Fisch C. Bundle branch block in sudden death. Prog Cardiovasc Dis 1980;23:187–92.
[41] Goldberg RJ, Zevallos JC, Yarzebski J, et al. Prognosis of acute myocardial infarction complicated by complete heart block (the Worcester Heart Attack Study). Am J Cardiol 1992;69:1135–41.
[42] Mavric Z, Zaputovic L, Matana A, et al. Prognostic significance of complete atrioventricular block in patients with acute inferior myocardial infarction with and without right ventricular involvement. Am Heart J 1990;119:823–8.
[43] Kostuk WJ, Beanlands DS. Complete heart block associated with acute myocardial infarction. Am J Cardiol 1970;26:380–4.
[44] Hindman MC, Wagner GS, Jaro M, et al. The clinical significance of bundle branch block complicating acute myocardial infarction: II. Indications for temporary and permanent pacemaker insertion. Circulation 1978;58:689–99.
[45] Klein RC, Vera Z, Mason DT. Intraventricular conduction defects in acute myocardial infarction: Incidence, prognosis, and therapy. Am Heart J 1984;108:1007–13.
[46] Lamas GA, Mueller JE, Turi AG, et al. A simplified method of predicting occurrence of complete heart block during acute myocardial infarction. Am J Cardiol 1986;57:1213–4.
[47] Dubois C, Pierard LA, Smeets JP, et al. Short- and long-term prognostic importance of complete bundle-branch complicating acute myocardial infarction. Clin Cardiol 1988;11:292–6.
[48] Zoll PM, Zoll RH, Falk RH, et al. External noninvasive temporary cardiac pacing: clinical trials. Circulation 1985;71:937–44.
[49] American College of Cardiology/American Heart Association Task Force. Guidelines for the early management of patients with acute myocardial infarction. Circulation 1990;82:664–707.
[50] Dreifus LS, Fisch C, Griffin JC, et al. Guidelines for implantation of cardiac pacemakers and antiarrhythmic devices: a report of the American College of Cardiology/American Heart Association Task Force on assessment of diagnostic and therapeutic cardiovascular procedures. Circulation 1991;84:455–67.
[51] Lown B, Calvert AF, Armington R, et al. Monitoring for serious arrhythmias and high risk of sudden death. Circulation 1975;52:189–98.
[52] Campbell RWF. Arrhythmias. In: Julian D, Braunwald E, editors. Management of acute myocardial infarction. Philadelphia: WB Saunders; 1994. p. 223.
[53] El-Sherif N, Myerburg RJ, Scherlag BJ, et al. Electrocardiographic antecedents of primary ventricular fibrillation: value of the R-on-T phenomenon in myocardial infarction. Br Heart J 1976;38:415–22.

[54] Weinberg B, Zipes D. Strategies to manage the post-MI patient with ventricular arrhythmias. Clin Cardiol 1989;12:86–90.
[55] Lee KJ, Wellens HJJ, Dorsnar E, et al. Observations on patients with primary ventricular fibrillation complicating acute myocardial infarction. Circulation 1975;52:755–9.
[56] Antman EM, Berlin JA. Declining incidence of ventricular fibrillation in myocardial infarction: implications for the use of lidocaine. Circulation 1992;84:764–73.
[57] Hine LK, Laird N, Hewitt P, et al. Meta-analytic evidence against prophylactic use of lidocaine in acute myocardial infarction. Arch Intern Med 1989;149:2694–8.
[58] Sadowski ZP, Alexander JH, Skrabucha B, et al. Multicenter randomized trial and a systematic overview of lidocaine in acute myocardial infarction. Am Heart J 1999;137:792–8.
[59] Alexander JH, Granger CB, Sadowski Z, et al, for the GUSTO-I and GUSTO-IIb Investigators. Prophylactic lidocaine use in acute myocardial infarction: incidence and outcomes from two international trials. Am Heart J 1999;137:799–805.
[60] Norris RM, Barnaby PF, Brown MA, et al. Prevention of ventricular fibrillation during acute myocardial infarction by intravenous propranolol. Lancet 1984;2:883–6.
[61] Bigger JR Jr, Dresdale RJ, Heissenbuttel RH, et al. Ventricular arrhythmias in ischemic heart disease: mechanism, prevalence, significance, and management. Prog Cardiovasc Dis 1977;19:255–300.
[62] Eldar M, Sievner Z, Goldbourt U, et al. Primary ventricular tachycardia in acute myocardial infarction: clinical characteristics and mortality. The SPRINT Study Group. Ann Intern Med 1992;117:31–6.
[63] Volpi A, Cavalli A, Turato R, et al. Incidence and short-term prognosis of late sustained ventricular tachycardia after myocardial infarction: results of the Gruppo Italiano per lo Studio della Sopravvivenza nell'Infarto Miocardico (GISSI-3) Data Base. Am Heart J 2001;142:87–92.
[64] Antman EM. General hospital management. In: Julian DG, Braunwald E, editors. Management of acute myocardial infarction. Philadelphia: WB Saunders; 1994. p. 29.
[65] Wyse DG. Management of early and late arrhythmias in acute myocardial infarction. In: Anderson JL, editor. Modern management of acute myocardial infarction in the community hospital. New York: Marcel Dekker; 1991. p. 343.
[66] Campbell RWF, Murray A, Julian DG. Ventricular arrhythmias in first 12 hours of acute myocardial infarction: natural history study. Br Heart J 1981;46:351–7.
[67] Behar S, Reicher Ress H, Schechter M, et al. Frequency and prognostic significance of secondary ventricular fibrillation complicating acute myocardial infarction. Am J Cardiol 1993;71:152–6.
[68] Chiriboga D, Yarzebski J, Goldberg RJ, et al. Temporal trends (1975 through 1990) in the incidence and case-fatality rate of primary fibrillation complicating acute myocardial infarction: a community-wide perspective. Circulation 1994;89:998–1003.
[69] Volpi A, Cavalli A, Franzosi MG, et al. One-year prognosis of primary ventricular fibrillation complicating acute myocardial infarction. Am J Cardiol 1989;63:1174–8.
[70] Volpi A, Maggioni A, Franzosi MG, et al. In-hospital prognosis of patients with acute myocardial infarction complicated by primary ventricular fibrillation. N Engl J Med 1987;317:257–61.
[71] Thompson CA, Yarzebski J, Goldberg RJ, et al. Changes over time in the incidence and case-fatality rates of primary ventricular fibrillation complicating acute myocardial infarction: perspectives from the Worcester heart attack study. Am Heart J 2000;139:1014–21.
[72] MacMahon S, Collins R, Peto R, et al. Effects of prophylactic lidocaine in suspected acute myocardial infarction: an overview of results from the randomized, controlled trials. JAMA 1988;260:1910–6.
[73] ISIS-1 (First International Study of Infarct Survival) Collaborative Group. Randomized trial of intravenous atenolol among 16,027 cases of suspected acute myocardial infarction. Lancet 1986;2:57–66.

[74] Freemantle N, Cleland J, Young P, et al. Beta blockade after myocardial infarction: systematic review and meta regression analysis. BMJ 1999;318:1730–7.

[75] Goldberg S, Greenspon AJ, Urban PL, et al. Reperfusion of arrhythmia: a marker of restoration of antegrade flow during intracoronary thrombolysis for acute myocardial infarction. Am Heart J 1983;105:26–32.

[76] Califf RM, O'Neill W, Stack RS, et al. Failure of simple clinical characteristics to predict perfusion status after intravenous thrombolysis. Ann Intern Med 1988;108:658–62.

[77] Newby KH, Thompson T, Stebbins A, et al, for the GUSTO Investigators. Sustained ventricular arrhythmias in patients receiving thrombolytic therapy: incidence and outcomes. Circulation 1998;98:2567–73.

[78] Gorgels APM, Vos MA, Letsch IS, et al. Usefulness of the accelerated idioventricular rhythm as a marker for myocardial necrosis and reperfusion during thrombolytic therapy in acute myocardial infarction. Am J Cardiol 1988;61:231–5.

[79] DiMarco JP, Lerman BB, Kron IL, et al. Sustained ventricular tachyarrhythmias within 2 months of acute myocardial infarction: results of medical and surgical therapy in patients resuscitated from the initial episode. J Am Coll Cardiol 1985;6:759–68.

[80] Solomon SD, Ridker PM, Antman EM. Ventricular arrhythmias in trials of thrombolytic therapy for acute myocardial infarction: a meta-analysis. Circulation 1993;88:2575–81.

ELSEVIER
SAUNDERS

Emerg Med Clin N Am
23 (2005) 1083–1103

EMERGENCY
MEDICINE
CLINICS OF
NORTH AMERICA

Cocaine-Associated Chest Pain

Joel T. Levis, MD, PhD[a,b,c,*], Gus M. Garmel, MD[a,b,c]

[a]*Kaiser Santa Clara Medical Center, Department of Emergency Medicine, 900 Kiely Boulevard, Santa Clara, CA 95051, USA*

[b]*Division of Emergency Medicine, Stanford University School of Medicine, 701C Welch Road, Stanford, CA 94304, USA*

[c]*Stanford/Kaiser Emergency Medicine Residency Program, 701C Welch Road, Stanford, CA 94304, USA*

History and epidemiology

Cocaine is a large alkaloid extracted from the leaves of the *Erythroxylum coca* plant found primarily in South America [1]. The practice of chewing the coca leaves dates back at least 5000 years, based on archaeological findings in Ecuador [2]. This practice was continued by Incans, who recognized coca's ability to boost energy, relieve fatigue, and lessen hunger [3]. The German chemist Friedrich Gaedcke was the first person to isolate alkaloidal cocaine from the coca leaf in 1855, while Albert Niemann is credited with chemically characterizing the substance in 1859 [2]. Cocaine use became popular in the United States in the 1880s and 1890s. During this time, cocaine could be found in many patented medicines, including Cocaine Toothache Drops, Vin Mariani (coca-based wine), and Coca Cola [4,5]. Sigmund Freud proposed using cocaine as a treatment for patients' depression, cachexia, asthma, and morphine addiction [6,7]. During this same period, cocaine was also used as a local anesthetic based partly on research conducted by William Halsted, who later developed an addiction to cocaine [7].

Cocaine use was legal in the United States until the passage of the Food and Drug Act of 1906 and the Harrison Narcotic Act of 1914, which banned the importation of coca and cocaine except for pharmaceutical purposes [7,8]. The Controlled Substances Act of 1970 further prohibited the manufacture, distribution, and possession of cocaine, except for limited medicinal use [7,8]. Cocaine is currently classified as a Schedule II drug. This

* Corresponding author. Kaiser Santa Clara Medical Center, Department of Emergency Medicine, 900 Kiely Boulevard, Santa Clara, CA 95051.

E-mail address: joel.levis@kp.org (J.T. Levis).

0733-8627/05/$ - see front matter
doi:10.1016/j.emc.2005.07.009

indicates its high potential for abuse in addition to its high incidence of psychologic and physical dependence, while recognizing that it possesses some medicinal value [9].

During the year 2000, 2.8 million chronic cocaine users were estimated in the United States [10]. Users spent $35 billion on cocaine that year, a decrease from $70 billion spent in 1990. This reduction in money spent on cocaine can be attributed to a reduction in cocaine's price, an increase in the consumer price index, and a decrease in cocaine consumption throughout the 1990s [10]. Americans consumed 259 metric tons of cocaine in 2000, a decrease from the 447 metric tons consumed in 1990. According to the US Department of Health and Human Services' *Results from the 2002 National Survey on Drug Use and Health: National Findings*, more than 33 million people age 12 and older (14.4%) reported using cocaine at least once in their lifetime [11]. This report also identified more than 8 million Americans age 12 and older (3.6%) having tried crack cocaine at least once in their lifetime. Elderly patients also use cocaine; one study from an urban emergency department (ED) found 2% of its patients over 60 years old tested positive for cocaine [12]. According to ED data collected by the Drug Abuse Warning Network (DAWN), there were 199,198 reported mentions of cocaine in 2002 [13]. A drug mention refers to a substance that was recorded ("mentioned") during a drug-related ED episode.

ED visits for cocaine-related problems include but are not limited to psychiatric, neurologic, cardiopulmonary, trauma, and addiction-related symptoms and complaints [14,15]. Cardiopulmonary complaints related to cocaine use are common, with chest pain being the most common symptom (20%–40%) among cocaine users presenting to two urban EDs [16,17]. Although the differential diagnosis for chest pain resulting from cocaine use includes mechanical, traumatic and infectious causes, the most concerning and extensively studied is myocardial ischemia. In 1995, cocaine-related chest pain led to the evaluation of an estimated 64,000 patients for myocardial ischemia [18]. These patients had an admission rate of 57%, with an annual cost of more than $83 million. Since that time, the evaluation and management of patients with cocaine-associated chest pain has evolved significantly as a result of tremendous research on this topic. This article reviews cocaine's pharmacology, its role in the pathogenesis of chest pain with specific emphasis on its role in inducing myocardial ischemia, and current diagnostic and management strategies for cocaine-associated chest pain encountered in the ED.

Pharmacology

Cocaine (benzoylmethylecgonine) can be isolated as water-soluble crystalline salt, cocaine hydrochloride, or as free cocaine base in powder or pellet ("crack") form. Cocaine hydrochloride is 89% cocaine by weight, melts at 195°C, and decomposes on heating [19,20]. The cocaine alkaloid ("free base") is soluble in acetone and alcohol, melts at 98°C, and vaporizes at higher temperatures without decomposing, thereby allowing it to be smoked. Crack cocaine is formed by evaporating the free base's solvent, leaving pure cocaine crystals. The name "crack" is derived from the popping sound it makes when it is heated [20].

Cocaine hydrochloride is well-absorbed through mucous membranes. Thus, users may achieve a high blood concentration from intranasal, sublingual, intravaginal, or rectal administration [21]. The mucosal administration of cocaine results in a slower onset of action (1–3 minutes) secondary to local vasoconstriction, a later peak effect (20–30 minutes), and a longer duration of action (60–90 minutes) compared with intravenous (IV) injection of the drug [7,21]. Smoking crack cocaine delivers drug to the circulation within seconds to minutes, with pharmacokinetics approaching those of the IV route [22]. The euphoria obtained when crack cocaine is smoked occurs within seconds and is short-lived. Because of the rapid and intense "high" obtained when crack cocaine is smoked, this form of cocaine is considered the most potent and addictive form.

Cocaine's primary effect on the nervous system is the alteration of nerve transmission. After local administration, cocaine's anesthetic properties are derived by the drug's ability to inhibit membrane permeability to sodium during depolarization, thereby blocking the initiation and transmission of electrical signals [21,23–25]. Following systemic administration, cocaine blocks the presynaptic reuptake of norepinephrine, dopamine, epinephrine, and serotonin, producing an excess of these neurotransmitters at the site of the postsynaptic receptor. In essence, cocaine is a potent sympathomimetic agent, acting as a central nervous system stimulant. In addition to the general feeling of well-being, euphoria, and dysphoria that ensues with its use, cocaine also produces hypertension and tachycardia by stimulating the vasomotor center [23]. Cocaine's elevation of heart rate is also partly a result of increased peripheral catecholamine levels resulting from the drug's ability to block the presynaptic reuptake of norepinephrine. These catecholamines further stimulate alpha- and beta-adrenergic receptors, resulting in the systemic effects of hypertension, tachycardia, diaphoresis, tremor, mydriasis, and localized vasoconstriction [1,7].

The serum half-life of cocaine is less than 1 hour; less than 5% of cocaine appears unchanged in the urine [1,4,16,24]. Rapid metabolism of cocaine occurs by serum cholinesterase, although cocaine is also metabolized by the liver. Two major metabolites (benzoylecgonine and ecgonine methyl ester) account for more than 80% of cocaine's known metabolites [4]. Benzoylecgonine does not have significant clinical effects when administered parenterally in animals [26,27]. However, benzoylecgonine is a sensitive and specific marker for recent cocaine use because urinary elimination of this metabolite has been detected 2 to 3 days after use, even longer in chronic users [16,28]. Aside from a mild vasodilatory effect, most animal studies suggest that ecgonine methyl ester is pharmacologically inactive [26].

Individuals with pseudocholinesterase deficiency may be more sensitive to cocaine's metabolites; one study demonstrated an association with more serious toxicity in subjects who had lower plasma cholinesterase levels [29].

Cocaethylene, a pharmacologically active metabolite formed after co-ingestion of cocaine and alcohol, is similar to cocaine with respect to several neurochemical and pharmacologic properties. One study demonstrated that despite the similarity between cocaine and cocaethylene's psychotropic and cardiovascular effects, the pharmacokinetics of the two compounds differed significantly in bioavailability, clearance, and volume of distribution [30]. Cocaethylene's clearance is slower than cocaine, with its average elimination $T_{1/2}$ 24% longer. In another study, ED patients who tested positive for alcohol and cocaine were more likely to be involved in violent trauma and were more often admitted to the intensive care/intermediate care units with a longer mean length of hospital stay [31]. Because 62% to 90% of cocaine abusers concurrently abuse ethanol [32], cocaethylene has important clinical implications in patients simultaneously using cocaine and alcohol.

Pathophysiology of cocaine-induced myocardial ischemia

Current research indicates that multiple factors contribute to cocaine-induced myocardial ischemia and infarction. Several mechanisms have been proposed for the manner in which cocaine causes cardiac ischemia and infarction in individuals who use or abuse this drug. These mechanisms include coronary vasoconstriction, increased platelet aggregation, thrombus formation leading to myocardial infarction (MI), myocardial toxicity, and an increased cardiac demand for oxygen resulting from adrenergic stimulation [8,33–36]. The exact extent to which these mechanisms interact is unknown. Persons who chronically abuse cocaine may also be susceptible to accelerated atherosclerosis [37].

Cocaine use can result in coronary artery vasoconstriction by alpha-adrenergic stimulation. Lange and colleagues [38,39] demonstrated that coronary vascular resistance increased, whereas coronary artery diameter decreased following low doses of intranasal administration of cocaine in human subjects undergoing cardiac catheterization for the evaluation of chest pain. These effects were reversed with phentolamine, an alpha-adrenergic blocker. Lange and colleagues [40] have also shown that the vasoconstrictive effects of cocaine were potentiated following intracoronary administration of propranolol, a beta-adrenergic blocker, further decreasing coronary blood flow in subjects pretreated with intranasal cocaine. Cocaine-mediated coronary vasoconstriction seems to be significantly enhanced at sites of significant coronary artery stenosis, as demonstrated by Flores and colleagues [41]. Diseased arterial segments with more endothelial dysfunction have greatly impaired (or absent) production of endothelium-derived relaxing factor, resulting in marked vasoconstriction of these arterial segments in the setting of intense alpha-adrenergic stimulation seen with cocaine use [41]. Finally, verapamil has also been shown to alleviate cocaine-induced coronary vasoconstriction in human subjects following administration of intranasal cocaine, lending further support to cocaine's vasoconstrictive role in promoting myocardial ischemia [39,42].

Although most cardiac risk factors are generally absent in patients who experience cocaine-associated myocardial ischemia, cigarette smoking among this group is common. Rates of tobacco use in these individuals range from 80% to 90% [43–45]. Analysis of 51 patients who had used cocaine and tobacco revealed that the interval between cocaine and tobacco use was often related to the onset of chest pain; as the time between tobacco and cocaine use shortened, the development of chest pain occurred more rapidly [46]. Nicotine, like cocaine, is known to induce coronary vasoconstriction. The co-administration of these drugs was studied in human subjects to assess this degree of coronary vasoconstriction [47]. In this study, these drugs administered together resulted in significantly greater decreases in the diameter of diseased coronary arterial segments seen angiographically compared with either drug alone.

Cocaine's role in promoting thrombosis, platelet aggregation and accelerated atherosclerosis may contribute to the incidence of myocardial ischemia and infarction in patients using this drug. Cocaine has been shown to increase human platelet aggregation in vitro in response to adenosine diphosphate [48] and arachidonic acid [49], in addition to increasing thromboxane production and release following pretreatment of platelets with cocaine in vitro [49]. Bement and colleagues [50] demonstrated that repeated arterial injury can serve as a nidus for platelet aggregation and fibrin deposition in a rabbit model of cocaine-induced arterial injury. Cocaine administration in a pig model has also been shown to increase the reactivity of platelets exposed to subendothelium, lending further support to the concept that cocaine administration has a prothrombotic effect by facilitating the interaction of platelets with damaged arteries [51]. In healthy human subjects, intranasal administration of cocaine resulted in platelet activation, platelet-containing microaggregate formation, and decreased bleeding times [52]. The findings of coronary thrombi in patients who have recently used cocaine without significant known coronary artery disease (CAD) further supports cocaine's role in promoting coronary thrombogenesis [33].

Cocaine may globally affect the cardiac muscle through elevations of norepinephrine levels. Autopsies of 30 individuals who experienced cocaine-related deaths revealed a 93% incidence of myocardial contraction band necrosis [53]. The severity of the band necrosis correlated with serum and urine cocaine concentrations. Similar contraction band necrosis has also been seen in autopsies of hearts from patients with high circulating levels of catecholamines from pheochromocytomas. These contraction bands may serve as substrate for potentially lethal dysrhythmias associated with cocaine use [53].

The tachycardia and hypertension caused by cocaine results in increased myocardial oxygen demand [33,36,38–40]. Myocardial ischemia occurs when the myocardial oxygen demand exceeds oxygen supply. Although it is not believed that cocaine's sympathomimetic effects on heart rate and blood pressure alone cause myocardial ischemia and infarction in cocaine users, these effects may act synergistically with other factors, such as accelerated atherogenesis, thrombus formation, or platelet aggregation leading to myocardial ischemia and infarction [33].

Chronic cocaine users may be prone to premature atherosclerosis of the coronary arteries [7,16,18,21]. Coronary atherosclerosis is found with increasing frequency in autopsies of young cocaine users when compared with age-matched controls [54–57]. Of 21 patients presenting with cocaine-associated chest pain and MI, 67% had clinical evidence of reperfusion after thrombolytic therapy, indicating significant CAD in this group [58]. Similarly, coronary angiography has demonstrated significant CAD in young persons who abuse cocaine [33,59–63]. The mechanisms by which cocaine contributes to accelerated CAD in young people is unclear, but seems to be multifactorial. Repeated episodes of coronary vasoconstriction, increased endothelial damage, increased platelet aggregation, and adrenergically-stimulated increases in heart rate and blood pressure are each likely to contribute [62].

Patients withdrawing from cocaine addiction demonstrate evidence of myocardial ischemia after cessation of cocaine use. Nademanee and colleagues [64] followed 21 patients admitted for inpatient detoxification with ambulatory (Holter) ECG monitoring. Eight of these 21 patients with cocaine addiction had frequent episodes of ST-segment elevation during Holter monitoring, with most episodes occurring during the first 2 weeks of withdrawal. Eighty-seven percent of these episodes were silent (without symptoms). Exercise treadmill testing was performed on 20 of these 21 patients, with only one test positive for ischemia. These results show that chronic cocaine users continue to have risk for myocardial ischemia even during the first weeks following drug cessation [64].

Differential diagnosis

Patients presenting to the ED with chest pain after cocaine use must be evaluated for intrathoracic processes that could cause their pain, including but not limited to myocardial ischemia and infarction. Barotrauma resulting in pneumothorax, pneumomediastinum, and pneumopericardium have each been reported in patients smoking crack cocaine [65–70]. Chest pain and dyspnea are the two most common presenting symptoms related to barotrauma. This barotrauma seems to be related to the increase in the intra-alveolar pressure caused by deep inhalation followed by Valsalva maneuver, or from severe cough triggered by the cocaine [71]. This increase in intra-alveolar pressure leads to alveolar rupture, with air dissecting through the peribronchiolar connective tissue into the mediastinum, pericardium, pleural space, or subcutaneous soft tissues.

Aortic dissection, though rare, has been reported after cocaine use [72–77]. It is believed to be a result of a rapid increase in blood pressure and heart rate resulting from the sympathetic stimulation caused by inhibited reuptake of epinephrine and norepinephrine at neuronal synapses [74,78]. These sudden changes increase shear stress in the thoracic aorta, resulting in small intimal tears that can then propagate antegrade along the aorta and retrograde into the coronary vessels and pericardium. Severe, sharp pain in the chest and upper back is the most common presenting symptom, although the clinical presentation of aortic dissection is highly variable. Aortography, transesophageal echocardiography (TEE), and CT scan of the chest help confirm the diagnosis of aortic dissection. Once aortic dissection is suspected, efficient evaluation and management is crucial because in-hospital mortality is approximately 27%, with most deaths occurring shortly after the onset of symptoms [78].

Pulmonary complaints may also cause chest pain or dyspnea in patients who use cocaine. Smoking cocaine has been associated with a number of pulmonary complications, including asthma, interstitial pneumonia or fibrosis, bronchiolitis obliterans organizing pneumonia (BOOP), noncardiogenic pulmonary edema, parenchymal hemorrhage, and pulmonary vascular disease [71,79–82]. An entity known as "crack lung syndrome" has been described including any of a combination of features, such as pulmonary hemorrhage, chest pain, pulmonary edema, and an interstitial lung process [71].

Endocarditis should also be considered in patients using IV cocaine presenting with chest pain and fever. One study demonstrated a strong association of endocarditis in patients who use this drug IV compared with users of IV heroin [83]. This association may be related to cocaine's effect on endothelial tissue, differences in bacterial flora, or the manner in which individuals prepare cocaine for IV use.

Thoracic skeletal muscle injury may result in chest pain in patients who use cocaine. Several studies have demonstrated that patients presenting with cocaine-associated chest pain frequently have elevations of serum creatine kinase levels in the absence of elevated creatine kinase–MB (CK-MB) fractions [84,85] or elevated troponin I levels [85], which generally excludes a cardiac origin for the chest pain. In one study of 217 trauma patients tested for drugs of abuse in an urban ED, 38% tested positive for cocaine metabolites [86]. In light of these findings, cocaine-related traumatic injury to the thorax should be considered in patients with cocaine-associated chest pain.

Evaluation of cocaine-associated chest pain

Cocaine-associated MI was first reported in 1982 [87] and has since become a well-recognized complication of cocaine abuse [15,22,23,44,45,58,60,88,89]. The incidence of AMI in cocaine-associated chest pain is small but significant

[90]. Prospective studies of cocaine-associated chest pain including patients discharged from the ED reveal an incidence of MI ranging from 0.7% to 8.7% [43,91–94]. In a prospective study of 246 patients presenting with cocaine-associated chest pain, Hollander and colleagues [43] reported the rate MI at 6.0%, diagnosed by elevated CK-MB levels. In a 1-year follow-up of patients enrolled in this study, 6 deaths occurred though not as the result of cocaine-related MI [44]. Weber and colleagues [95] also found a 6% incidence of AMI in a cohort of 250 patients presenting to an urban ED with cocaine-associated chest pain. Data from a retrospective study of 29 hospital centers throughout the United States identified patients who presented with cocaine-associated MI as generally young (mean age of 38 years), nonwhite (72%), tobacco smokers (91%), and with cocaine use in the past 24 hours (88%) [45]. In a study to determine the prevalence of cocaine-associated chest pain in suburban and urban EDs, the mean age of patients who experienced chest discomfort and positive assays for cocaine was 36 years; however, the frequency of cocaine use was 18% in patients aged 41 to 50 years and 3% in patients aged 51 to 60 years [88]. These studies point out the importance of inquiring about cocaine use in all patients presenting with chest pain.

Patients who experienced cocaine-associated chest pain may be at highest risk for MI in the first several hours following cocaine use. In a prospective, multicenter evaluation of 246 patients having cocaine-associated chest pain, it began a median of 60 minutes after cocaine use and persisted for a median of 120 minutes [43]. Mittleman and colleagues [96] compared the reported use of cocaine in the hour preceding the onset of MI symptoms with its expected frequency by using self-matched control data based on the case-crossover study design. The risk for MI onset was elevated 23.7 times from baseline in these first 60 minutes.

The ECG is nondiagnostic in 60% of patients who later prove to have cocaine-induced MI, and is abnormal in 56 to 84% of patients with cocaine-associated chest pain [18,21,43,61,97,98]. In a prospective evaluation of cocaine-associated chest pain, the ECG was found to have a sensitivity of 35.7% for predicting MI, with specificity, positive and negative predictive values of 89.9%, 17.9%, and 95.8%, respectively [43]. Normal or nonspecific initial ECG findings do not rule out the possibility of MI in cocaine users [18,43,99]. Normal variations, such as J point and ST segment elevations, account for many of the abnormal ECGs observed in young patients who experience cocaine-associated chest pain [100]. As a result, the identification of ischemia on ECG analysis is more difficult in this patient population.

In patients experiencing chest pain without associated cocaine use, serum biochemical markers (creatine kinase, CK-MB, troponins, and myoglobin) are most useful to detect cardiac injury in the evaluation of myocardial ischemia and infarction. Because cocaine produces increased motor activity, hyperthermia, skeletal muscle injury, and rhabdomyolysis, creatine kinase and CK-MB may not be as useful in detecting cardiac injury and MI in this patient population [18,101]. Counselman and colleagues [102] studied 40 patients presenting to an urban ED with any complaint related to cocaine use within the preceding 24 hours (excluding seizures) to determine the incidence of creatine kinase elevations. Twenty-one of the 40 patients (53%) had elevated creatine kinase levels, with mean creatine kinase levels for these patients of 1071 IU/L. No statistically significant difference existed between the patient's initial complaint (musculoskeletal, psychiatric, or cardiovascular) and the incidence of creatine kinase elevation, indicating that some degree of skeletal muscle injury and creatine kinase elevation appear to be common in patients using cocaine. In addition, Hollander and colleagues [43] demonstrated that as many as 50% of patients presenting to EDs with cocaine-associated chest pain have elevated levels of creatine kinase without evidence of MI. Finally, Tokarski and colleagues demonstrated that initial CPK and CK-MB level elevations, which rapidly decline on serial determinations, less commonly indicate infarction than a pattern of continuously rising enzyme concentrations in patients admitted with cocaine-associated chest pain and normal or nondiagnostic ECGs [18,99].

Cardiac troponins appear to be equivalent if not superior to detecting myocardial injury in patients who experience cocaine-associated chest pain when compared with CK-MB [103–105]. In a prospective evaluation of 19 patients presenting with cocaine-associated chest pain who were hospitalized to rule out AMI, total creatine kinase and CK-MB fractions were elevated during the hospital course in 17 of 19 patients, whereas cardiac troponin I and T levels were within normal limits in all patients tested [103]. No patient in this study was diagnosed with AMI. Similarly, Hollander and colleagues [104] evaluated whether recent cocaine use alters the specificity of CK-MB, myoglobin, and cardiac troponin I for AMI in patients seen in the ED for chest pain. Ninety-seven patients were enrolled in this study, 19 (20%) of whom had recently used cocaine. The specificity of cardiac markers in patients who used cocaine and those who did not were as follows: cardiac troponin I, 94% versus 94%; CK-MB, 75% versus 88%; and myoglobin, 50% versus 83%, respectively. Not only do these results demonstrate that cardiac troponin I was the most specific cardiac marker in this study, but they suggest that the specificity of cardiac troponin I was not affected by recent cocaine use. Finally, Kontos and colleagues [105] compared the outcomes of MI by CK-MB elevation, significant disease on coronary angiography, or cardiac death based on troponin I elevations in patients admitted for possible MI after cocaine use. Of 246 admitted patients, 34 (14%) met CK-MB criteria for MI and 38 (16%) had cardiac troponin I elevations. Most patients with cTnI elevations met CK-MB criteria for MI, and also had a high incidence of underlying significant disease based on angiographic findings. In this study, troponin I seemed to have equivalent diagnostic accuracy as CK-MB for diagnosing myocardial wall necrosis in patients who presented with cocaine-associated chest pain and suspected MI.

Stress testing in patients who presented with cocaine-associated chest pain may be useful in ruling out AMI when the cohort is low risk. Feldman and colleagues [106] used myocardial perfusion imaging with technetium-99m tetrofosmin in 14 patients who presented with cocaine-associated chest pain without ECG evidence of acute cardiac ischemia. Although their cohort was small, they did not demonstrate reversible ischemia in the majority (12/14, 86%) of these patients. In a larger prospective study from 1999, Kontos and colleagues [91] looked at the use of myocardial perfusion imaging with technetium-99m sestamibi in patients presenting to the ED with cocaine-associated chest pain. Of 216 patients with cocaine-associated chest pain who underwent perfusion imaging, 5 had positive studies, including 2 with MI. Only 6 of 67 patients undergoing follow-up stress perfusion imaging had reversible defects. At 30 day follow up, no untoward cardiac events occurred in patients who produced negative results after rest perfusion imaging. The researchers concluded that (1) AMI is infrequent in patients presenting with cocaine-associated chest pain; (2) positive results after rest perfusion imaging are uncommon, suggesting that myocardial ischemia is infrequently the cause of cocaine-associated chest pain; and (3) early perfusion imaging may offer an effective alternative to routine admission to the cardiac care unit of patients presenting with cocaine-related cardiac symptoms.

The safety of dobutamine stress echocardiography (DSE) for the ED evaluation of cocaine-associated chest pain has been evaluated in a pilot study by Dribben and colleagues [107]. Of 19 patients completing DSE and reaching their target heart rates, none experienced signs of exaggerated adrenergic response from dobutamine. In addition, 13 of 20 patients (65%) required supplemental atropine to reach their target heart rates, further suggesting the lack of exaggerated adrenergic response. Given that a DSE test may be completed within 6 hours, it might serve as a useful adjunct to more rapidly rule out MI in patients presenting with cocaine-associated chest pain.

Stress testing, such as exercise ECG, myocardial perfusion scanning, or exercise echocardiography in patients experiencing cocaine-associated chest pain and coincidental traditional cardiac risk factors can, in some cases, lead to false-positive results. This is especially true with above average exercise tolerance. Littman and colleagues [108] identified six cases of cocaine-associated chest pain whereby false-positive stress tests within 2 weeks after the last reported cocaine use led to unnecessary costly and potentially harmful invasive interventions. Cardiac risk factors in patients studied included hypertension in three, tobacco use in three, family history of CAD in three, and diabetes in one patient, with no more than two risk factors present for any one patient. Based on this case series, the investigators recommended postponing invasive coronary evaluation until 2 to 3 weeks of abstinence in clinically stable patients with cocaine-associated chest pain who have risk factors for ischemic heart disease.

Treatment

The initial stabilization and treatment of patients with cocaine-associated chest pain is similar to that of patients with typical angina or MI resulting from atherosclerotic CAD. Patients should be placed at rest, given oxygen, and put on a cardiac monitor with frequent cardiac and blood pressure monitoring. Benzodiazepines (diazepam or lorazepam) should be administered, particularly in the agitated patient, as animal models of cocaine toxicity have demonstrated benefit from benzodiazepines [101,109,110]. In patients with hyperdynamic vital signs, which are common with recent cocaine use, this is particularly true. Benzodiazepines have been demonstrated to reduce the heart rate and systemic arterial pressure in cocaine-intoxicated patients [21,111]. Patients whose chest pain may be caused by ischemia should receive aspirin to inhibit platelet aggregation if there are no contraindications, such as known allergy or suspected subarachnoid hemorrhage [7,18,21,101].

Nitroglycerin has been shown to alleviate cocaine-induced vasoconstriction in patients with CAD [112]. In a multicenter observational study by Hollander and colleagues [113], 83 patients with cocaine-associated chest pain were treated with nitroglycerin. Nitroglycerin provided benefit in 41 patients (49%): 37 patients (45%) had relief or reduction in the severity of chest pain and 4 patients (5%) had other beneficial effects. Only one patient in this study sustained an adverse outcome (transient hypotension in the setting of a right ventricular infarct). Therefore, this study provides evidence that nitroglycerin is safe and possibly effective in the treatment of cocaine-associated chest pain.

The early use of lorazepam in combination with nitroglycerin seems to be more efficacious than nitroglycerin alone in relieving chest pain associated with cocaine use. Honderick and colleagues [114] studied 27 patients who presented with cocaine-associated chest pain: 15 patients received only sublingual nitroglycerin every 5 minutes for two doses, the other 12 patients received nitroglycerin plus lorazepam (1 mg IV) every 5 minutes for two doses. Five minutes after the second treatment, patients in the nitroglycerin-plus-lorazepam group reported significantly lower chest pain scores compared with those patients receiving nitroglycerin alone. No adverse effects were reported for either group. However, in a similar study comparing the use of diazepam, nitroglycerin, or both for the treatment of patients who experienced potential cocaine-associated ACS, the combination of diazepam plus nitroglycerin did not offer any advantage over either agent alone [111].

Patients who continue to have chest pain despite the administration of oxygen, benzodiazepines, aspirin, and nitroglycerin may be treated with low-dose IV phentolamine [7,18,21,115]. This nonselective alpha-adrenoreceptor antagonist produces a dose-dependent antagonism of the pressor effect of cocaine in conscious squirrel monkeys [116]. Phentolamine also has been shown to reverse cocaine-induced coronary artery vasoconstriction in humans [38,39]. The administration of phentolamine in a 38 year-old man who presented with cocaine-associated chest pain refractory to oxygen, diazepam, and nitroglycerin resulted in resolution of chest pain and near-normalization of ECG changes consistent with ischemia within 8 minutes of administration [117]. These investigators recommend the use of a low dose (1 mg) of phentolamine in these patients to avoid hypotension while maintaining the anti-ischemic effects of the drug [18,117].

The role of calcium channel blockers in the treatment of cocaine-associated chest pain has not yet been thoroughly evaluated. In rats, nitrendipine has been shown to prevent cardiac toxicity caused by IV cocaine administration [118,119]. In another study in which rats were pretreated with diltiazem, nifedipine, or verapamil and then subjected to high doses of intraperitoneal cocaine, pretreatment with calcium channel blockers resulted in the development of seizures more quickly in pretreated animals than in controls, indicating that calcium channel blockers may actually potentiate cocaine-induced toxicity [120]. Although verapamil has been demonstrated to alleviate cocaine-induced coronary vasoconstriction in patients undergoing cardiac catheterization for the evaluation of chest pain [42], its role in cocaine-related ischemia and infarction remains unclear and requires further investigation. Based on these observations and available data, the use of calcium channel blockers for the treatment of cocaine-associated chest pain is not currently recommended [7,16].

Although patients who present with atherosclerotic heart disease, angina, and MI typically benefit from the use of beta-adrenergic antagonists, beta-blockers are contraindicated in the setting of cocaine-associated myocardial ischemia [7,16,18,36,115,121]. Lange and colleagues [38–40] have demonstrated that cocaine decreases left coronary artery diameter and coronary sinus blood flow while increasing coronary vascular resistance, effects that are exacerbated by beta-adrenergic blockade. These effects presumably occur through unopposed alpha-adrenergic stimulation. Sand and colleagues [122] reported seven cases in which esmolol was used for the treatment of cocaine-associated cardiovascular toxicity, defined as a heart rate greater than 130 beats per minute, a systolic blood pressure greater than 160 mm Hg, or a diastolic blood pressure greater than 120 mm Hg. In this case series, no consistent hemodynamic benefit was identified in patients who received the drug, yet marked exacerbations of hypertension, hypotension, emesis, and lethargy occurred in three patients.

Thrombolytic agents should be used with caution in patients presenting with cocaine-associated AMI. Several cases of complications following the administration of thrombolytic agents in patients who presented with cocaine-associated MI, including intracranial hemorrhage, have been reported in the literature [123–126]; however, no patient died or experienced a major complication in one retrospective cross-sectional survey of 25 patients who received thrombolytic therapy for cocaine-associated MI [58]. The presence or absence of clinical criteria for reperfusion (resolution of

ECG changes, resolution of chest pain, reperfusion dysrhythmias) was noted in the charts of 21 patients who received thrombolytic therapy. Based on these criteria, 14 of these 21 patients (67%) were believed to have undergone reperfusion. Because patients with cocaine-associated chest pain may present with MI without thrombus (ie, injury secondary to diffuse vasospasm), cardiac catheterization, if available, should be considered before thrombolytic agents [7,16,121]. If angiography is unavailable, and contraindications for thrombolytic therapy are not present, these agents should be considered in patients with clinical presentation and ECG changes consistent with AMI [7,16,115,127].

Dysrhythmias

Cocaine can result in ventricular dysrhythmias (idioventricular rhythm, ventricular tachycardia, ventricular fibrillation) and atrial dysrhythmias (supraventricular tachycardia, atrial fibrillation) [4,7,16,128]. Cocaine blocks sodium channels (phase 0 of the action potential) and can produce supraventricular rhythms that are aberrantly conducted during severe intoxication. These wide complex dysrhythmias are similar to those described in tricyclic antidepressant or quinidine poisonings, and have been reported in animals and humans during cocaine toxicity [16,129,130]. In animals, the QRS complex narrows in response to sodium bicarbonate administration, similar to what is seen with tricyclic antidepressants [130]. Therefore, in patients exhibiting signs of acute cocaine intoxication (agitation, hypertension, hyperthermia), sodium bicarbonate is the anti-dysrhythmic agent of choice [7,16,130]. Although lidocaine has been shown to potentiate the toxic effects of cocaine in animals [131], the use of lidocaine was not associated with significant cardiovascular or central nervous system toxicity in a retrospective study of 29 patients who experienced cocaine-associated MI [132]. In a calm patient having cocaine-associated chest pain and normal vital signs, or with evidence of myocardial ischemia or infarction on ECG, a widened QRS-complex rhythm likely represents ventricular tachycardia. Several investigators have proposed lidocaine as the agent of first choice in these patients [7,16,115,132]. When the clinical picture is less clear (eg, an agitated, hypertensive, cocaine-intoxicated patient presenting with chest pain), benzodiazepines and sodium bicarbonate should be given first [7,16].

Disposition

Patients presenting with cocaine-associated chest pain in which a definite cause for the chest pain is not immediately apparent should be evaluated for myocardial ischemia or infarction. In those patients experiencing chest pain who are at low risk for cardiovascular events and who have not recently used cocaine, it has been previously shown that a 12-hour observation period is safe and cost effective [133–135]. Kushman and colleagues [136] performed a retrospective evaluation of patients with cocaine-associated chest pain admitted to a chest pain center (CPC) observation unit. Patients who have a history of CAD, hemodynamic instability, acute ST-segment elevation or depression of greater than 1 mm, or a clinical syndrome consistent with UA, were directly admitted to the hospital and excluded from the study. The CPC protocol entailed continuous ST-segment trend monitoring and serial cardiac troponin I measurements over a 9-hour observation period. Over a 7-year period, 197 patients were enrolled; 171 patients were released from the CPC (86.8%), 22 (11.2%) were admitted for further cardiac evaluation. Four patients left against medical advice during the evaluation period; one of these patients was lost to follow-up. Of 179 patients (90.9%) with reliable 30-day follow-up, one cardiac complication (0.56%) occurred in a patient found to have underlying CAD with multiple cardiac risk factors. The investigators concluded that patients who presented without evidence of myocardial necrosis, ST-segment elevation or ischemia on 12 lead ECG, or hemodynamic instability could be safely and effectively evaluated in a CPC [136].

Recently, a prospective study attempted to validate the use of a 9- to 12-hour observation period in patients who experience cocaine-associated chest pain [94]. In this study, however, high-risk patients presenting with cocaine-associated chest pain were excluded and directly admitted to the hospital (12% of initial study group). The study cohort comprised the remaining 302 patients who reported using, or tested positive for, cocaine. Patients in this study were similar to previous cohorts of patients who experienced cocaine-associated chest pain (young, majority male, cigarette smokers). These patients received protocol-driven care in a CPC. Patients who had normal troponin I levels, no evidence of new ischemic changes on ECG, and no cardiovascular complications (AMI, dysrhythmias, or recurrent symptoms) during the 9- to 12-hour observation period were discharged from the observation unit. During the 30-day follow-up period, none of the patients in this cohort died from a cardiovascular event, and only 4 of the 256 patients with detailed follow-up data available had a MI (1.6%) in this 30-day period. All four nonfatal MIs occurred in patients who continued to use cocaine. These results suggest that an observation period of 9 to 12 hours for low- and moderate-risk patients presenting with cocaine-associated chest pain is likely to be safe, and that continued use of cocaine may result in a small percentage of nonfatal MIs in low- and moderate-risk individuals.

Appropriate disposition strategies for patients with cocaine-associated chest pain have been proposed previously [7,16]. These strategies include admitting all patients with ECGs diagnostic of AMI or having dynamic changes consistent with ischemia, dysrhythmias, or congestive heart failure [16]. All other patients should be evaluated for other possible diagnoses, and treated empirically for ischemic chest pain, with appropriate serum biochemical markers for myocardial injury (creatine kinase, CK-MB, troponin) if noncardiac causes are excluded. Based on recent work by Weber and colleagues [94], patients presenting with cocaine-associated chest pain may be safely discharged from the ED or observation unit after 9 to 12 hours if they are without recurring symptoms, dysrhythmias, or increased serum cardiac markers. Future research may reduce this observation period in patients having low or moderate risk for significant cardiac events.

Summary

Current estimates establish that more than 30 million people in the United States use cocaine. Cardiovascular complaints among patients who present to EDs after cocaine use are common, with chest pain the most common complaint in at least one study [17]. For patients who experience cocaine-associated chest pain, emergency physicians should exclude life-threatening causes of their pain, such as aortic dissection, and other noncardiac etiologies, such as pneumothorax and pneumomediastinum. Although myocardial ischemia and infarction account for only a small percentage of cocaine-associated chest pain complaints, physicians must understand the pathophysiology of cocaine and the diagnostic and treatment strategies necessary to best manage these patients and minimize adverse outcomes. The treatment of individuals who present with cocaine-associated chest pain does not end with patient disposition from the ED. The referral of patients for cocaine detoxification, to abstinence programs and support groups, and for ongoing medical care, including drug-related behavior and cardiac risk factor modification, is essential. The opportunity to impact individuals during their cocaine-related presentations and the initiation of these referrals may, when successful, prevent subsequent medical consequences of future cocaine use.

References

[1] Derlet RW, Horowitz BZ. Advances and updates in cardiovascular emergencies: cardiotoxic drugs. Emerg Med Clin North Am 1995;13(4):771–91.

[2] Van Dyke C, Byck R. Cocaine. Sci Am 1982;246:128–41.

[3] Kennedy J. Coca exotica: the illustrated story of cocaine. Rutherford (NJ): Farleigh Dickinson University Press; 1985.

[4] Warner EA. Cocaine abuse. Ann Intern Med 1993;119(3):226–35.

[5] Karch SB. A brief history of cocaine. Boca Raton (FL): CRC Press; 1998.

[6] Streatfeild D. Cocaine: an unauthorized biography. New York: St. Martin's Press; 2002.

[7] Hahn IH, Hoffman RS. Diagnosis and treatment of acute myocardial infarction: cocaine use and acute myocardial infarction. Emerg Med Clin North Am 2001;19(2):1–18.

[8] Hals G, Richardson W. Drugs of abuse and their complications: emergency department evaluation and management: part I. Emerg Med Rep 2001;22(12):131–46.

[9] US Drug Enforcement Administration. The Controlled Substance Act (CSA). Title II of the Comprehensive Drug Abuse Prevention and Control Act of 1970. Available at: http://www.dea.gov. Accessed August 21, 2005.

[10] Office of National Drug Control Policy What America's Users Spend on Illegal Drugs. 1998–2000; Available at: http://www.whitehousedrugpolicy.gov. Accessed August 21, 2005.
[11] Substance Abuse and Mental Health Statistics (SAMHSA). 2002 National survey on drug use and health: national findings. Available at: http://www.oas.samhsa.gov. Accessed August 21, 2005.
[12] Rivers E, Shirazi E, Aurora T, et al. Brief reports: cocaine use in elder patients presenting to an inner-city emergency department. Acad Emerg Med 2004;11:874–7.
[13] Drug Abuse Warning Network (DAWN). Emergency department trends. Final estimates 1995–2002. Available at: http://www.dawninfo.samhsa.gov. Accessed August 21, 2005.
[14] Rich JA, Singer DE. Cocaine-related symptoms in patients presenting to an urban emergency department. Ann Emerg Med 1991;20(6):616–21.
[15] Cregler LL, Mark H. Special report: medical complications of cocaine abuse. N Engl J Med 1986;315(23):1495–9.
[16] Hoffman RS, Hollander JE. Evaluation of patients with chest pain after cocaine use. Crit Care Clin 1997;13:809–28.
[17] Brody SL, Slovis CM, Wrenn KD. Cocaine-related medical problems: consecutive series of 233 patients. Am J Med 1990;88:325–31.
[18] Hollander JE. Current concepts: the management of cocaine-associated myocardial ischemia. N Engl J Med 1995;333(19):1267–72.
[19] Mueller PD, Benowitz NL, Olson KR. Emergency aspects of drug abuse: cocaine. Emerg Med Clin North Am 1990;8(3):481–93.
[20] Frishman WH, Karpenos A, Molloy TJ. Cocaine-induced coronary artery disease: recognition and treatment. Med Clin North Am 1989;73(2):475–86.
[21] Lange RA, Hillis D. Medical progress: cardiovascular complications of cocaine use. N Engl J Med 2001;345(5):351–8.
[22] Kloner RA, Rezkalla SH. Cocaine and the heart. N Engl J Med 2003;348(6):487–8.
[23] Goldfrank LR, Hoffman RS. The cardiovascular effects of cocaine. Ann Emerg Med 1991; 20(2):165–75.
[24] Burnett LB. Toxicity, cocaine. Emedicine July 2002; p. 1–52.
[25] Erwin MB, Deliargyris EN. Cardiology grand rounds from the University of North Carolina at Chapel Hill: cocaine-associated chest pain. Am J Med Sci 2002;324(1):37–44.
[26] Madden JA, Powers RH. Effects of cocaine and cocaine metabolites on cerebral arteries in vivo. Life Sci 1990;47:1109–14.
[27] Misra AL, Nayak PK, Blouch R, et al. Estimation and disposition of [^{3}H] benzoylecgonine and pharmacological activity of some cocaine metabolites. J Pharm Pharmacol 1975;27: 784–6.
[28] Weiss RD, Gawin FH. Protracted elimination of cocaine metabolites in long-term high-dose cocaine abusers. Am J Med 1988;85:879–80.
[29] Hoffman RS, Henry GC, Howland MA, et al. Association between life-threatening cocaine toxicity and plasma cholinesterase activity. Ann Emerg Med 1992;21:247–53.
[30] McCance EF, Price LH, Kosten TR, et al. Cocaethylene: pharmacology, physiology and behavioral effects in humans. J Pharmacol Exp Ther 1995;274(1):215–23.
[31] Vanek WV, Dickey-White HI, Signs SA, et al. Concurrent use of cocaine and alcohol by patients treated in the emergency department. Ann Emerg Med 1996;28:508–14.
[32] Jatlow P. Cocaethylene: pharmacologic activity and clinical significance. Ther Drug Monit 1993;15:533–6.
[33] Hollander JE, Hoffman RS. Cocaine-induced myocardial infarction: an analysis and review of the literature. J Emerg Med 1992;10:169–77.
[34] Tun A, Khan IA. Myocardial infarction with normal coronary arteries: the pathologic and clinical perspectives. Angiology 2001;52(5):299–304.
[35] Zimmerman FH, Gustafson GM, Kemp HG. Recurrent myocardial infarction associated with cocaine abuse in a young man with normal coronary arteries: evidence for coronary artery spasm culminating in thrombosis. J Am Coll Cardiol 1987;9:964–8.

[36] Frishman WH, Del Vecchio A, Sanal S, et al. Cardiovascular manifestations of substance abuse part 1: cocaine. Heart Dis 2003;5(3):187–201.

[37] Minor RL, Scott BD, Brown DD, et al. Cocaine-induced myocardial infarction in patients with normal coronary arteries. Ann Intern Med 1991;115(10):797–806.

[38] Lange RA, Cigarroa RG, Yancy CW, et al. Cocaine-induced coronary-artery vasoconstriction. N Engl J Med 1989;321(23):1557–62.

[39] Pitts WR, Lange RA, Cigarroa JE, et al. Cocaine-induced myocardial ischemia and infarction: pathophysiology, recognition, and management. Prog Cardiovasc Dis 1997; 40(1):65–76.

[40] Lange RA, Cigarroa RG, Flores ED, et al. Potentiation of cocaine-induced coronary vasoconstriction by beta-adrenergic blockade. Ann Intern Med 1990;112(12):897–903.

[41] Flores ED, Lange RA, Cigarroa RG, et al. Effect of cocaine on coronary artery dimensions in atherosclerotic coronary artery disease: enhanced vasoconstriction at sites of significant stenoses. J Am Coll Cardiol 1990;16:74–9.

[42] Negus BH, Willard JE, Hillis LD, et al. Alleviation of cocaine-induced coronary vasoconstriction with intravenous verapamil. Am J Cardiol 1994;73:510–2.

[43] Hollander JE, Hoffman RS, Gennis P, et al. Prospective multicenter evaluation of cocaine-associated chest pain. Acad Emerg Med 1994;1(4):330–9.

[44] Hollander JE, Hoffman RS, Gennis P, et al. Cocaine-associated chest pain: one-year follow-up. Acad Emerg Med 1995;2:179–84.

[45] Hollander JE, Hoffman RS, Burstein JL, et al. Cocaine-associated myocardial infarction: mortality and complications. Arch Intern Med 1995;155:1081–6.

[46] Hollander JE, Thode HC, Hoffman RS. Chest discomfort, cocaine, and tobacco. Acad Emerg Med 1995;2(3):238.

[47] Moliterno DJ, Willard JE, Lange RA, et al. Coronary-artery vasoconstriction induced by cocaine, cigarette smoking, or both. N Engl J Med 1994;330:454–9.

[48] Rezkalla SH, Mazza JJ, Kloner RA, et al. Effects of cocaine on human platelets in healthy subjects. Am J Cardiol 1993;72:243–6.

[49] Togna G, Tempesta E, Togna AR, et al. Platelet responsiveness and biosynthesis of thromboxane and prostacycline in response to in vitro cocaine treatment. Haemostasis 1985;15(2):100–7.

[50] Bement CL, Cohen L, Nielsen SW, et al. Arterial injury in rabbits following alternate-day injections of cocaine. FASEB J 1989;3:A297.

[51] Zurbano MJ, Heras M, Rigol M, et al. Cocaine administration enhances platelet reactivity to subendothelial components: studies in a pig model. Eur J Clin Invest 1997;27(2): 116–20.

[52] Heesch CM, Wilhelm CR, Ristich J, et al. Cocaine activates platelets and increases the formation of circulating platelet containing microaggregates in humans. Heart 2000;83: 688–95.

[53] Tazelaar HD, Karch SB, Stephens BG, et al. Cocaine and the heart. Hum Pathol 1987;18: 195–9.

[54] Eichhorn EJ, Peacock E, Grayburn PA, et al. Chronic cocaine abuse is associated with accelerated atherosclerosis in human coronary arteries. J Am Coll Cardiol 1992;19(Suppl): 105A [Abstract.].

[55] Mittleman RE, Welti CV. Cocaine and sudden "natural" death. J Forensic Sci 1987;32: 11–9.

[56] Kolodgie FD, Virmani R, Cornhill JF, et al. Increase in atherosclerosis and adventitial mast cells in cocaine abusers: an alternative mechanism of cocaine-associated coronary vasospasm and thrombosis. J Am Coll Cardiol 1991;17(7):1553–60.

[57] Dressler FA, Malekzadeh S, Roberts WC. Quantitative analysis of amounts of coronary arterial narrowing in cocaine addicts. Am J Cardiol 1990;65:303–8.

[58] Hollander JE, Burstein JL, Hoffman RS, et al. Cocaine-associated myocardial infarction: clinical safety of thrombolytic therapy. Chest 1995;107(5):1237–41.

[59] Smith HWB, Liberman HA, Brody SL, et al. Acute myocardial infarction temporally related to cocaine use: clinical, angiographic, and pathophysiologic observations. Ann Intern Med 1987;107:13–8.
[60] Majid PA, Patel B, Kim H-S, et al. An angiographic and histologic study of cocaine-induced chest pain. Am J Cardiol 1990;65:812–4.
[61] Amin M, Gabelman G, Karpel J, et al. Acute myocardial infarction and chest pain syndromes after cocaine use. Am J Cardiol 1990;66:1434–7.
[62] Wilson LD. Rapid progression of coronary artery disease in the setting of chronic cocaine abuse. J Emerg Med 1998;16(4):631–4.
[63] Kontos MC, Jesse RL, Tatum JL, et al. Coronary angiographic findings in patients with cocaine-associated chest pain. J Emerg Med 2003;24(1):9–13.
[64] Nademanee K, Gorelick DA, Josephson MA, et al. Myocardial ischemia during cocaine withdrawal. Ann Intern Med 1989;111:876–80.
[65] Barbera MJA, Vallejo GJ, Velo PM, et al. Spontaneous pneumomediastinum after cocaine inhalation. Respiration (Herrlisheim) 1986;50(3):230–2.
[66] Palat D, Denson M, Sherman M, et al. Pneumomediastinum induced by inhalation of alkaloidal cocaine. N Y State J Med 1988;88(8):438–9.
[67] Hoffman R. New case—summary: adult male with neck discomfort. Int J Med Toxicol 1998;1(4):17.
[68] Maeder M, Ullmer E. Pneomomediastinum and bilateral pneumothorax as a complication of cocaine smoking. Respiration (Herrlisheim) 2003;70(4):407.
[69] Janes SM, Ind PW, Jackson J. Images in thorax: crack inhalation induced pneumo-mediastinum. Thorax 2004;59:360.
[70] Wilson KC, Saukkonen JJ. Acute respiratory failure from abused substances. J Intensive Care Med 2004;19:183–93.
[71] Haim DY, Lippmann ML, Goldberg SK, et al. The pulmonary complications of crack cocaine: a comprehensive review. Chest 1995;107:233–40.
[72] Chang RA, Rossi NF. Intermittent cocaine use associated with recurrent dissection of the thoracic and abdominal aorta. Chest 1995;108(6):1758–62.
[73] Neri E, Toscano T, Massetti M, et al. Cocaine-induced intramural hemotoma of the ascending aorta. Tex Heart Inst J 2001;28(3):218–9.
[74] Nallamothu BK, Saint S, Kolias TJ, et al. Clinical problem-solving: of nicks and time. N Engl J Med 2001;345(5):359–63.
[75] Hsue PY, Salinas CL, Bolger AF, et al. Acute aortic dissection related to crack cocaine. Circulation 2002;105:1592–5.
[76] Perron AD, Gibbs M. Thoracic aortic dissection secondary to crack cocaine ingestion. Am J Emerg Med 1997;15:507–9.
[77] Eagle KA, Isselbacher EM, DeSanctis RW. Cocaine-related aortic dissection in perspective. Circulation 2002;105:1529–30.
[78] Khan IA, Nair CK. Clinical, diagnostic, and management perspectives of aortic dissection. Chest 2002;122:311–28.
[79] Ozkan M, Dweik RA, Ahmad M. Drug-induced lung disease. Cleve Clin J Med 2001;68(9): 782–95.
[80] Osborn HH, Tang M, Bradley K, et al. New-onset bronchospasm or recrudescence of asthma associated with cocaine abuse. Acad Emerg Med 1997;4:689–92.
[81] Tomashefski, JF, Felo JA. The pulmonary pathology of illicit drug and substance abuse. 2004;10(5):413–26.
[82] Hoffman CK, Goodman PC. Pulmonary edema in cocaine smokers. Radiology 1989;172: 463–5.
[83] Chambers HF, Morris DL, Tauber MG, et al. Cocaine use and the risk for endocarditis in intravenous drug users. Ann Intern Med 1987;106(6):833–6.
[84] Rubin RB, Neugarten J. Cocaine-induced rhabdomyolysis masquerading as myocardial ischemia. Am J Med 1989;86(5):551–3.

[85] D'Amore JZ, Gallahue F, Shetty S, et al. Comparison of CPK-MB and troponin I in the evaluation of cocaine chest pain. Acad Emerg Med 2000;7(5):442.
[86] Brookoff D, Campbell EA, Shaw LM. The underreporting of cocaine-related trauma: drug abuse warning network reports vs hospital toxicology tests. Am J Public Health 1993;83(3): 369–71.
[87] Coleman DL, Ross TF, Naughton JL. Myocardial ischemia and infarction related to recreational cocaine use. West J Med 1982;136(5):444–6.
[88] Hollander JE, Todd KH, Green G, et al. Chest pain associated with cocaine: an assessment of prevalence in suburban and urban emergency departments. Ann Emerg Med 1995;26(6): 671–6.
[89] Qureshi AI, Suri MFK, Guterman LR, et al. Cocaine use and the likelihood of nonfatal myocardial infarction and stroke. Circulation 2001;103:502–6.
[90] Carley S, Ali B. Toward evidence based emergency medicine: best BETs from the Manchester Royal 4–175 Infirmary. Acute myocardial infarction in cocaine induced chest pain presenting as an emergency. Emerg Med J 2003;20(2):174–5.
[91] Kontos MC, Schmidt KL, Nicholson CS, et al. Myocardial perfusion imaging with technetium-99m sestamibi in patients with cocaine-associated chest pain. Ann Emerg Med 1999;33(6):639–45.
[92] Feldman JA, Fish SS, Beshansky JR, et al. Acute cardiac ischemia in patients with cocaine-associated complaints: results of a multicenter trial. Ann Emerg Med 2000;36(5):469–76.
[93] Cheng TO. Risk of acute myocardial infarction in cocaine abusers. Circulation 2000;101: e227.
[94] Weber JE, Shofer FS, Larkin L, et al. Validation of a brief observation period for patients with cocaine-associated chest pain. N Engl J Med 2003;348(6):510–7.
[95] Weber JE, Chudnofsky CR, Boczar M, et al. Cocaine-associated chest pain: how common is myocardial infarction? Acad Emerg Med 2000;7:873–7.
[96] Mittleman MA, Mintzer D, Maclure M, et al. Triggering of myocardial infarction by cocaine. Circulation 1999;99(21):2737–41.
[97] Gitter MJ, Goldsmith SR, Dunbar DN, et al. Cocaine and chest pain: clinical features and outcome of patients hospitalized to rule out myocardial infarction. Ann Intern Med 1991; 115:277–82.
[98] Zimmerman JL, Dellinger RP, Majid PA. Cocaine-associated chest pain. Ann Emerg Med 1991;20(6):611–5.
[99] Tokarski GF, Paganussi P, Urbanski R, et al. An evaluation of cocaine-induced chest pain. Ann Emerg Med 1990;19(10):1088–92.
[100] Hollander JE, Lozano M, Fairweather P, et al. "Abnormal" electrocardiograms in patients with cocaine-associated chest pain are due to "normal" variants. J Emerg Med 1994;12(2): 199–205.
[101] Brubacher JR, Hoffman RS. Cocaine toxicity. Top Emerg Med 1997;19(4):1–16.
[102] Counselman FL, McLaughlin EW, Kardon EM, et al. Creatine phosphokinase elevation in patients presenting to the emergency department with cocaine-related complaints. Am J Emerg Med 1997;15:221–3.
[103] McLaurin M, Apple FS, Henry TD, et al. Cardiac troponin I and T concentrations in patients with cocaine-associated chest pain. Ann Clin Biochem 1996;33:183–6.
[104] Hollander JE, Levitt A, Young GP, et al. Effect of recent cocaine use on the specificity of cardiac markers for diagnosis of acute myocardial infarction. Am Heart J 1998;135:245–52.
[105] Kontos MC, Anderson P, Ornato JP, et al. Utility of troponin I in patients with cocaine-associated chest pain. Acad Emerg Med 2002;9(10):1007–13.
[106] Feldman JA, Bui LD, Mitchell PM, et al. The evaluation of cocaine-induced chest pain with acute myocardial perfusion imaging. Acad Emerg Med 1999;6(2):103–9.
[107] Dribben WH, Kirk MA, Trippi JA, et al. A pilot study to assess the safety of dobutamine stress echocardiography in the emergency department evaluation of cocaine-associated chest pain. Ann Emerg Med 2001;38(1):42–8.

[108] Littman L, Miller RF, Monroe MH. Stress testing in patients with cocaine-associated chest pain. J Emerg Med 2004;27(4):417–8.
[109] Guinn MM, Bedford JA, Wilson MC. Antagonism of intravenous cocaine lethality in nonhuman primates. Clin Toxicol 1980;16:499–508.
[110] Catravas JD, Waters IW. Acute cocaine intoxication in the conscious dog: studies on the mechanism of lethality. J Pharmacol Exp Ther 1981;217:350–6.
[111] Baumann BM, Perrone J, Hornig SE, et al. Randomized, double-blind, placebo-controlled trial of diazepam, nitroglycerin, or both for treatment of patients with potential cocaine-associated acute coronary syndromes. Acad Emerg Med 2000;7:878–85.
[112] Brogan WC, Lange RA, Kim AS, et al. Alleviation of cocaine-induced coronary vasoconstriction by nitroglycerin. J Am Coll Cardiol 1991;18(2):581–6.
[113] Hollander JE, Hoffman RS, Gennis P, et al. Nitroglyerin in the treatment of cocaine associated chest pain—clinical safety and efficacy. J Toxicol Clin Toxicol 1994;32(3): 243–56.
[114] Honderick T, Williams D, Seaberg D, et al. A prospective, randomized, controlled trial of benzodiazepines and nitroglycerin or nitroglycerin alone in the treatment of cocaine-associated acute coronary syndromes. Am J Emerg Med 2003;21(1):39–42.
[115] Albertson TE, Dawson A, de Latorre F, et al. Tox-ACLS: toxicologic-oriented advanced cardiac life support. Ann Emerg Med 2001;37(4):S78–90.
[116] Schindler CW, Tella SR, Goldberg SR. Adrenoceptor mechanisms in the cardiovascular effects of cocaine in conscious squirrel monkeys. Life Sci 1992;51(9):653–60.
[117] Hollander JE, Carter WA, Hoffman RS. Use of phentolamine for cocaine-induced myocardial ischemia. N Engl J Med 1992;327(5):361.
[118] Trouve R, Nahas G. Nitrendipine: an antidote to cardiac and lethal toxicity of cocaine. Proc Soc Exp Biol Med 1986;183(3):392–7.
[119] Trouve R, Nahas GG, Manger WM. Catecholamines, cocaine toxicity, and their antidotes in the rat. Proc Soc Exp Biol Med 1991;196(2):184–7.
[120] Derlet RW, Albertson TE. Potentiation of cocaine toxicity with calcium channel blockers. Am J Emerg Med 1989;7(5):464–8.
[121] Keller KB, Lemberg L. The cocaine-abused heart. Am J Crit Care 2003;12(6):562–6.
[122] Sand IC, Brody SL, Wrenn KD, et al. Experience with esmolol for the treatment of cocaine-associated cardiovascular complications. Am J Emerg Med 1991;9(2):161–3.
[123] Bush HS. Cocaine-associated myocardial infarction: a word of caution about thrombolytic therapy. Chest 1988;94(4):878.
[124] LoVecchio F, Nelson L. Intraventricular bleeding after the use of thrombolytics in a cocaine user. Am J Emerg Med 1996;14(7):663–4.
[125] Hollander JE, Wilson LD, Leo PJ, et al. Complications from the use of thrombolytic agents in patients with cocaine associated chest pain. J Emerg Med 1996;14(6):731–6.
[126] Boniface KS, Feldman JA. Thrombolytic therapy and cocaine-associated acute myocardial infarction. Am J Emerg Med 2000;18(5):612–5.
[127] Hoffman RS. Thrombolytic therapy and cocaine-induced myocardial infarction [editorial]. Am J Emerg Med 1996;14(7):693–5.
[128] Chakko S, Myerburg RJ. Cardiac complications of cocaine abuse. Clin Cardiol 1995;18: 67–72.
[129] Beckman KJ, Parker RB, Hariman RJ, et al. Hemodynamic and electrophysiological actions of cocaine. Effects of sodium bicarbonate as an antidote in dogs. Circulation 1991; 83(5):1799–807.
[130] Isner JM, Estes NA, Thompson PD, et al. Acute cardiac events temporally related to cocaine abuse. N Engl J Med 1986;315(23):1438–43.
[131] Derlet RW, Albertson TE, Tharratt RS. Lidocaine potentiation of cocaine toxicity. Ann Emerg Med 1991;20(2):135–8.
[132] Shih RD, Hollander JE, Burstein JL, et al. Clinical safety of lidocaine in patients with cocaine-associated myocardial infarction. Ann Emerg Med 1995;26(6):702–6.

[133] Hoekstra JW, Gibler WB, Levy RC, et al. Emergency-department diagnosis of acute myocardial infarction and ischemia: a cost analysis of two diagnostic protocols. Acad Emerg Med 1994;1(2):103–10.
[134] Gibler WB, Runyon JP, Levy RC, et al. A rapid diagnostic and treatment center for patients with chest pain in the emergency department. Ann Emerg Med 1995;25(1):1–8.
[135] Farkouh ME, Smars PA, Reeder GS, et al. A clinical trial of a chest-pain observation unit for patients with unstable angina. Chest pain evaluation in the emergency room (CHEER) Investigators. N Engl J Med 1998;339(26):1882–8.
[136] Kushman SO, Storrow AB, Liu T, et al. Cocaine-associated chest pai in a chest pain center. Am J Cardiol 2000;85:394–6.

ELSEVIER
SAUNDERS

Emerg Med Clin N Am
23 (2005) 1105–1125

EMERGENCY
MEDICINE
CLINICS OF
NORTH AMERICA

Modern Management of Cardiogenic Pulmonary Edema

Amal Mattu, MD*, Joseph P. Martinez, MD, Brian S. Kelly, MD

Division of Emergency Medicine, University of Maryland School of Medicine, 110 South Paca Street, Sixth Floor, Suite 200, Baltimore, MD 21201, USA

Cardiogenic pulmonary edema (CPE) is a common and potentially deadly condition frequently encountered in emergency medicine. Many conditions exist that directly or indirectly lead to the development of pulmonary edema. Regardless of the underlying cause of CPE, all patients who develop CPE must be diagnosed and managed expeditiously. Patients who have developed CPE can quickly develop respiratory failure if delays occur in recognition or management of the condition. Patients who develop CPE, in fact, have an in-hospital mortality of 15% to 20%, and mortality may be even higher when the condition is associated with acute myocardial infarction (AMI) or acute valvular dysfunction [1–3]. Acute care providers should maintain a high level of vigilance for this condition and initiate management strategies promptly.

Pulmonary edema can be defined as an increase in lung fluid caused by extravasation of fluid from the pulmonary vasculature into the interstitium and alveoli of the lungs [1,2]. The buildup of fluid leads to progressive deterioration of alveolar gas exchange and resulting hypoxia. Pulmonary edema is generally classified as noncardiogenic and cardiogenic. The causes and treatment of non-CPE are beyond the scope of this article. CPE is more common and is discussed in this article. The pathophysiology, etiologies, and emergency department (ED) evaluation is discussed briefly. Modern management strategies are the main focus.

* Corresponding author.
E-mail address: amattu@smail.umaryland.edu (A. Mattu).

doi:10.1016/j.emc.2005.07.005 *emed.theclinics.com*

Pathophysiology

CPE results from leakage of fluid from the pulmonary capillaries and venules into the alveolar space as a result of increased hydrostatic pressure. When the pulmonary capillary hydrostatic pressure exceeds pulmonary interstitial pressure, fluid transudates into the pulmonary alveoli and interstitium [2]. Hydrostatic pressure rises when the left ventricle (LV) is unable to effectively handle its pulmonary venous return [4]. Once fluid begins to build up in the pulmonary interstitium, a vicious self-perpetuating cycle of events follows: alveolar edema leads to impaired gas exchange and hypoxia, leading to increased catecholamine production, leading to increased systemic vascular resistance and blood pressure, leading to increased myocardial wall tension and oxygen demand, leading to myocardial ischemia, leading to LV systolic and diastolic dysfunction, leading to decreased cardiac output and increased end-diastolic pressure, leading to increased pulmonary fluid buildup. During this cycle, activation of the renin-angiotensin-aldosterone system occurs as a result of elevations of end-diastolic pressure and results in increased sympathetic tone. Hypoxia and increased work of breathing result in patient anxiety, which also causes increased catecholamine production and sympathetic tone; therefore, at its most basic level, the end result of this cycle is to have an LV trying in vain to pump against a markedly elevated systemic vascular resistance (increased afterload), resulting in poor cardiac output. Meanwhile, the right-sided filling continues unabated (elevated preload) resulting in even greater pulmonary interstitial fluid. This cycle eventually results in florid pulmonary edema, hypoxia, and respiratory failure unless the cycle is terminated [2].

The goals of management of CPE should focus on breaking this cycle of events by (1) decreasing preload and (2) decreasing afterload. In most cases, accomplishment of these two goals alone results in marked improvement of LV function and significantly increases cardiac output, resolving the pulmonary edema. In some cases, however, further strategies may be needed to (3) improve LV function (inotropic support). In the "Management" section of this article, we discuss optimal strategies to accomplish all three goals.

Etiologies

There are five major causes of CPE in clinical practice (Box 1). The most common cause is an acute exacerbation of chronic LV failure. Chronic LV failure usually is the result of congestive heart failure (CHF) or a cardiomyopathy. An acute exacerbation of chronic LV failure can occur because of medication or dietary noncompliance (eg, discontinuation of diuretic medications, excessive salt intake, and so forth) or from acute cardiac ischemia.

Patients without a prior history of chronic LV failure can develop acute LV dysfunction also. AMI can induce significant deterioration of

Box 1. Major etiologies of cardiogenic pulmonary edema

- Exacerbation of chronic left ventricular failure
- Acute myocardial ischemia/infarction
- Severe systemic hypertension
- Left-sided valvular disorders
- Acute tachydysrhythmias and bradydysrhythmias

myocardial performance and pulmonary edema when infarction occurs in at least 25% of the LV myocardial mass. Acute severe hypertension can also result in LV dysfunction. In this scenario, the heart initially develops impaired ventricular compliance, or relaxation (diastolic dysfunction), which leads to poor ventricular filling and decreased cardiac output. The decrease in cardiac output sets in motion the cascade of events noted in the section "Pathophysiology," eventually resulting in a combination of diastolic and systolic dysfunction leading to pulmonary edema. Additionally, the impaired ventricular compliance produces severely elevated LV pressures, which are then transmitted backward to the pulmonary capillaries, raising hydrostatic pressures and causing fluid transudation.

Patients who experience left-sided valvular (aortic, mitral) disorders can also develop CPE. Patients who experience aortic or mitral regurgitation develop elevated left-sided pressures, similar to patients who develop severe systemic hypertension; this pressure can easily be transmitted backward to the pulmonary circulation and produce interstitial edema. Acute aortic regurgitation, which most often occurs from aortic dissection, infective endocarditis, or blunt trauma; and acute mitral regurgitation, which usually occurs from rupture of the chordae tendinae or papillary muscle dysfunction in association with myocardial infarction (MI), or from infective endocarditis, can easily result in CPE as a result of an abrupt increase in LV pressures. Patients who develop chronic aortic stenosis are also predisposed to the development of CPE. The patients develop noncompliant hypertrophied LVs, which are dependent on high filling pressures to maintain adequate cardiac output [2]. Even slight increases in left-sided pressures in these patients are transmitted backward to the pulmonary capillaries and result in pulmonary edema.

Acute dysrhythmias can also produce CPE. Severe bradydysrhythmias in the face of normal or elevated right-heart filling can induce elevations in pulmonary capillary hydrostatic pressures, leading to CPE. Tachydysrhythmias often lead to CPE caused by poor diastolic filling, which also leads to elevations in pulmonary capillary hydrostatic pressures. Treatment of CPE in either case is simply based on correction of the underlying dysrhythmia using standard Advanced Cardiac Life Support protocols.

Several other conditions can also result in CPE by exacerbating LV function, including sepsis, severe anemia, thyrotoxicosis, myocarditis, and myocardial toxins [1,2]. Additionally, fluid overload in the presence of end-stage renal disease can result in CPE. The general management strategies discussed in "Emergency Department Evaluation" are usually effective for the major etiologies of CPE, although the management should also focus on reversing any of these underlying conditions whenever possible.

Emergency department evaluation

Traditionally, the diagnosis of CPE in the ED has been based on history, physical examination, and chest radiography. Most patients presenting with CPE have a prior history of CHF. Most report the onset of dyspnea on exertion progressing to dyspnea at rest, orthopnea, peripheral edema, and paroxysmal nocturnal dyspnea. The progression of symptoms before ED presentation may take hours to days; however, an episode of acute ischemia or acute valvular dysfunction may cause symptoms to progress much faster. Physical examination findings usually include tachycardia and hypertension from increased catecholamine production, tachypnea, hypoxia, and diaphoresis. Auscultation of the lungs reveals rales or wheezes, and cardiac auscultation may be notable for an S3 heart sound. The remainder of the examination may be notable for jugular venous distension, hepatojugular reflux, and peripheral edema. When CPE is associated with cardiogenic shock, evidence of poor tissue perfusion including skin mottling or pallor may be found. Unfortunately, none of these vital signs or physical examination findings have greater than 70% sensitivity [5]. As many as one third of these patients have chronic obstructive pulmonary disease (COPD) and many also have risk factors for pulmonary embolism and AMI [4,5], any of which can mimic CPE, which further complicates the ability to make an accurate clinical diagnosis.

Chest radiography compliments the history and physical examination in the initial evaluation of patients who experience CPE. The classic radiographic findings of CPE include cardiomegaly (in patients who experience underlying CHF), pulmonary vascular redistribution, thickening of interlobular septa (Kerley B lines), alveolar edema, pleural effusions, and bilateral infiltrates in a "bat wing" pattern [3,6]; however, these classic radiographic findings are not always found at the time of initial presentation. As much as a 12-hour delay may occur between the onset of symptoms and the development of significant radiographic abnormalities when the onset of CPE is abrupt [7,8]. Even the presence of cardiomegaly, which is often considered one of the most reliable radiographic abnormalities associated with systolic dysfunction, often is absent in patients who have developed CPE [9]. Other limitations of chest radiography also exist. Patients who develop chronic lung abnormalities may have scarring that impairs image quality or may mimic vascular redistribution. Image quality is also often impaired in obese patients and patients who develop COPD [10].

The clinical diagnosis of acute heart failure is estimated to be incorrect in more than 50% of cases, with frequent overdiagnosis and underdiagnosis [11–13]. Because of the limitations of clinical assessment and chest radiography in distinguishing acute heart failure and CPE from other causes of acute dyspnea, B-type natriuretic peptide (BNP) testing has emerged as a valuable diagnostic tool in ED practice. BNP is an endogenous cardiac neurohormone that is secreted from the ventricles in response to increased wall tension. BNP counteracts the effects of the renin-angiotensin-aldosterone system by promoting natriuresis, diuresis, and vasodilation. In the setting of acute heart failure and CPE, plasma BNP levels increase. These measurable levels of BNP have been demonstrated to correlate with the severity of LV filling pressures, clinical status, short-term and long-term mortality, and response to in-hospital therapy [10,14–18]. Measurement of BNP levels in patients presenting to the ED with acute dyspnea can be helpful in distinguishing acute heart failure and CPE from other acute or chronic lung diseases [11,19]. A BNP level less than 100 pg/mL makes acute heart failure unlikely and is associated with a negative predictive value of 90%. Conversely, a BNP level greater than 500 pg/mL makes acute heart failure likely and is associated with a positive predictive value of 90%. A BNP level in the range of 100 to 500 pg/mL can be caused by acute heart failure but can also be caused by other conditions that induce elevated ventricular wall tension, including cor pulmonale and acute pulmonary embolism. Falsely-low BNP levels can occur during the first 1 to 2 hours after symptom-onset in cases of flash pulmonary edema [20].

Emergency department management

Initial management of patients who experience CPE should focus on the "ABCs" of resuscitation. Large bore intravenous (IV) lines should be in place to administer needed medications. Patients should be placed in an upright sitting position attached to a cardiac monitor and pulse oximetry. Supplemental oxygen should be provided by way of a facemask with fraction of inspired oxygen of 1.0. If the patient remains persistently hypoxic despite the supplemental oxygen, or if the patient develops respiratory fatigue or a depressed level of consciousness, mechanical ventilation should be instituted (see section "Ventilatory Support"). An ECG should be obtained quickly to assess for bradydysrhythmias or tachydysrhythmias that may have precipitated the CPE. If a dysrhythmia has occurred, standard Advanced Cardiac Life Support measures should be performed. The ECG should also be assessed for evidence of acute myocardial ischemia or AMI, in which case appropriate anti-ischemia and reperfusion therapies should be used. A discussion of the acute management of acute coronary syndrome and MI is discussed elsewhere in this issue.

Most patients who experience CPE, however, do *not* have ECG evidence of an acute dysrhythmia or AMI. Treatment should therefore be aimed at redistributing the excessive pulmonary interstitial fluid into the systemic circulation, which improves alveolar oxygen-carbon dioxide exchange and hypoxia; therefore, pharmacologic agents that provide preload reduction and afterload reduction should be administered. In some cases, inotropic support is required also.

Pharmacologic therapy

Preload reduction

The first goal in pharmacologic treatment of CPE is preload reduction. Preload reduction reduces right heart and pulmonary venous return and, therefore, right-heart filling pressures and pulmonary capillary hydrostatic pressures, resulting in early symptomatic improvements in dyspnea. The typical medications used for preload reduction are nitroglycerin, morphine sulfate, and loop diuretics. More recently, a recombinant form of beta-natriuretic peptide known as nesiritide has been used for preload reduction also.

Nitroglycerin

The most effective and rapidly-acting preload-reducing medication is nitroglycerin (NTG) [21–25]. Multiple studies have demonstrated the superiority of NTG over furosemide [21,24,26–28] and morphine sulfate [28–30] for preload reduction, symptomatic improvement, and safety. NTG can be administered in sublingual, IV, or transdermal form, although the transdermal absorption can be erratic in the patient in extremis. NTG also has the benefit of a short half-life; therefore, if the patient develops a precipitous fall in blood pressure (generally uncommon in CPE patients), the blood pressure should return to previous values within 5 to 10 minutes of discontinuation of administration. Preload reduction and noticeable symptomatic improvements can be accomplished within 5 minutes of sublingual administration of NTG [31,32], and the dose can be repeated every 5 minutes during the first 10 to 15 minutes of presentation. If IV NTG is preferred, an initial dose of 10 to 20 μg/min should be titrated upwards rapidly until a dose of at least 100 μg/min is achieved. This type of aggressive administration of NTG also confers the benefit of afterload reduction [33,34], and therefore, NTG can function as an effective single agent therapy for patients who develop CPE. Unfortunately, many physicians are uncomfortable with administering these higher dosages of NTG for CPE and tend to use suboptimal dosages of the IV NTG infusion. Some investigators, therefore, recommend using *bolus* administration of IV NTG to insure adequate dosing [26,33]. In one study [26], 3 mg IV boluses of NTG were administered every 5 minutes to patients who had developed

CPE, a dose equivalent to a 600 μg/min infusion. This protocol was found to be safe, well-tolerated, and effective for these patients and associated with reduced need for mechanical ventilation and more rapid resolution of symptoms. Standard anti-anginal dosages of sublingual NTG with which most physicians are comfortable (ie, 400 μg every 5 minutes), has the bioequivalence of an IV NTG infusion of 60 to 80 μg/min. Physicians should, therefore, be comfortable with the safety of even higher dosages of NTG for patients who experience CPE and usually present in a hyper-adrenergic state with moderately-to-severely elevated blood pressures.

Tolerance may develop to IV infusions of NTG but rarely within the first 12 hours. Nitrates should be avoided if the patient is already hypotensive or becomes hypotensive. Nitrates should be avoided also in patients taking sildenafil or other related medications for erectile dysfunction because of reports of precipitous drops in blood pressure. Also, nitrates should be used with extreme caution, if at all, in patients who have developed aortic stenosis and pulmonary hypertension because of their dependence on preload to maintain adequate blood pressure.

Morphine sulfate

Morphine sulfate (MS) has been used as a standard preload-reducing medication for many years; however, despite decades of use in patients who have developed CPE, MS has not been studied in a randomized fashion to confirm hemodynamic benefits. MS probably exerts mild indirect hemodynamic benefits through anxiolysis, which results in a decrease in catecholamine production, indirectly resulting in vasodilation. Early studies demonstrated some evidence of vasodilation and venous pooling in the peripheral circulation (ie, in forearm and hand veins) after the administration of MS [35,36]; however, a consistent *central* preload-reducing effect (ie, reduction in pulmonary capillary wedge pressures [PCWP]) has not been found. In contrast, MS may be associated with adverse hemodynamic effects, including *increases* in left and right heart filling pressures [37] and reductions in cardiac index [29,37] caused by a direct myocardial depressant effect on the already-reduced contractile state of the ischemic heart [38]. The adverse hemodynamic effects are also apparent clinically. In one prehospital study [28] evaluating the use of various medications in patients who develop presumed CPE, 38% of patients who received MS had subjective deterioration (eg, increased dyspnea) in clinical status and 46% had objective deterioration (eg, increased respiratory rate). In another study of ED treatment of CPE [39], the use of MS was associated with a 5:1 odds ratio for need for intubation or ICU admission.

MS is sometimes administered to patients who present with CPE for its anxiolytic effect; however, MS has an undesirable side-effect profile, including nausea and vomiting, pruritis, rash, and urticaria. Any of these side effects can produce an increase in catecholamine output, which can exacerbate afterload. The authors prefer the use of low-dose benzodiazepines when patients require anxiolysis. Low-dose benzodiazepines have a more preferable side-effect profile and are not associated with myocardial or respiratory depression. Given the superiority of NTG for preload reduction and benzodiazepines for anxiolysis, little justification exists for the modern-day use of MS in patients who present with CPE.

Loop diuretics

IV loop diuretics, especially furosemide, have been used for many years as the cornerstone of treatment in patients who present with CPE. These medications produce a decrease in preload by inhibiting sodium chloride reabsorption in the ascending loop of Henle, which promotes increases in urine volume and excretion [2,40]; however, because patients who develop CPE have elevated systemic vascular resistance (afterload), renal perfusion is markedly diminished [41]. As a result, diuretics have a significantly delayed effect, often taking 45 to 120 minutes to produce effective diuresis [25,42–45]. Further complicating the use of diuretics in these patients is evidence that as many as 40% of patients who present with CPE have intravascular euvolemia or hypovolemia [41,46,47]. The use of diuretics in these patients may be associated with adverse effects, including electrolyte abnormalities and hypotension [28] caused by overdiuresis.

Also, diuretics are presumed to decrease preload through direct vascular effects. Early studies indicated that the use of furosemide produces rapid reductions in left and right heart filling pressures [25,48–52] in patients who are experiencing end-stage renal failure [50,53,54]. The evidence supporting this concept is far from convincing, however. Many other investigators have found that the acute use of furosemide in patients who have developed CPE is associated with initial adverse hemodynamic effects—including elevations of mean arterial pressure, heart rate, PCWPs, and left and right heart filling pressures (preload), and systemic vascular resistance (afterload)—and reductions in stroke volume and cardiac output [27,42,43,55–59]. The adverse effects seem to be related to an initial activation of the renin-angiotensin-aldosterone system and increased sympathetic activation [27,43,57] that occurs immediately after administration of furosemide. These adverse effects generally resolve once diuresis occurs, but often diuresis is significantly delayed because of depressed renal perfusion. The adverse hemodynamic changes may be blunted by administration of preload-reducing (eg, NTG) and afterload-reducing (eg, angiotensin-converting enzyme inhibitors) medications *before* furosemide [27].

Nesiritide

In recent years, a recombinant form of BNP has been suggested as an alternative to NTG for patients who develop acute left heart failure and CPE. Natriuretic peptides are hormonelike substances produced by the myocardium that modulate diuresis, natriuresis, venodilation, and vasodilation; however, when patients who develop chronic CHF develop acutely decompensated CHF and CPE, the ventricle's production of this substance is often inadequate; therefore, a recombinant form of BNP, "nesiritide," was manufactured for IV administration in patients who experience acutely decompensated CHF. Early manufacturer-supported human studies [60,61] demonstrated IV infusions of nesiritide-produced dose-related reductions in PCWP and increases in stroke volume and cardiac index. Symptomatic improvements were noted also, without an increase in heart rate or dysrhythmias. Beneficial effects were maintained throughout a 24-hour infusion (no evidence of tolerance). Occasional patients developed hypotension lasting up to 3 hours, but it was otherwise well-tolerated.

A more recent trial (the VMAC Study) compared the use of IV nesiritide with IV NTG [62]. In this manufacturer-supported study, patients receiving "standard treatment" were randomized to receive nesiritide (dose by protocol) or NTG (dose at the discretion of the treating physician). The patients receiving nesiritide were reported to have a greater decrease in PCWP compared with patients receiving NTG at 3 hours (decrease in PCWP by 5.8 mm Hg for nesiritide versus 3.8 mm Hg for NTG) and also at 24 hours (8.2 mm Hg for nesiritide versus 6.3 mm Hg for NTG). Patients receiving nesiritide were also reported to have greater improvement in "global clinical status" at 24 hours.

Many limitations in the VMAC study prevent simple extrapolation of the results to everyday ED practice [63]. Patients in the study received "standard treatment" before receiving the study drug. "Standard treatment" generally consists of MS and furosemide, neither one of which would be considered "*optimal* treatment" in the modern management of CPE. Some of the patients also received dopamine or dobutamine at the discretion of the treating physicians. Neither of these medications has been demonstrated to improve patient survival. Patients did not receive aggressive dosing of NTG (average doses of NTG were 30–40 μg/min), and investigators admitted knowledge that physicians generally tend to be reluctant to use high-dose NTG or to up-titrate NTG doses [64].

No indication existed that patients routinely received angiotensin-converting enzyme inhibitors or other vasodilators, and no indication that patients routinely received noninvasive positive pressure ventilation (NPPV), all of which have been shown to hasten resolution of CPE (see later discussion). The comparative improvements in PCWPs noted in the study between nesiritide and NTG were minimal (2.0 mm Hg difference at 3 hours; 1.9 mm Hg difference at 24 hours) and were not associated with any subjective improvement in dyspnea [62]. The "global clinical status" scale used in the study was undescribed and admitted to be a nonvalidated scoring system. No improvement in mortality occurred with nesiritide, and a trend occurred toward higher mortality at 90 days (19% for nesiritide, 13% for NTG, $P = .08$) [63]. A more recent pooled analysis of three randomized trials involving 485 patients receiving nesiritide versus 377 patients not receiving nesiritide also demonstrated an increased 30-day mortality associated with use of this medication (7.2% mortality in patients treated with nesiritide, 4.0% in patients not receiving nesiritide) [65]. Another recent concern is that the use of nesiritide seems to be associated with worsening renal function. An evaluation of five randomized studies involving 1269 patients demonstrated the following: (1) patients who experience acutely decompensated heart failure and were treated with nesiritide were more likely to have significant elevations in serum creatinine; in addition, they more often required medical intervention for worsening renal function than non–nesiritide-treated patients (11.1% versus 4.2%), although there was no increase in the need for hemodialysis [66]. Finally, questions exist regarding the cost-effectiveness of nesiritide because the cost is approximately 40 times that of NTG and patients in the study that received nesiritide had a 2-day longer duration of hospital stay [62].

Nesiritide may be useful for patients in whom NTG is contraindicated (eg, patients taking sildenafil) or in cases for which a prolonged infusion of NTG is needed because tolerance in these patients limits the efficacy of NTG; however, until future studies demonstrate (1) the safety of nesiritide in renal function and mortality and (2) the efficacy of nesiritide in patients who have received "*optimal* treatment" for decompensated CHF and CPE (ie, high-dose NTG, afterload-reducing medications, and NPPV) we cannot recommend routine ED administration of nesiritide for the early treatment of CPE.

Afterload reduction

Most patients who present with CPE have elevated catecholamine levels, which produce a marked increase in systemic vascular resistance—afterload. The already- compromised heart has difficulty producing an effective cardiac output against this increased resistance. Afterload reduction with vasodilator medications produces an increase in cardiac output and reduction in pulmonary interstitial edema. Another benefit is improved renal perfusion, which can lead to substantial improvements in diuresis even before administration of diuretics [67]. Afterload reduction can be accomplished using any one of several available medications. High-dose IV NTG effectively reduces afterload, but prolonged infusion can induce tolerance and limit its efficacy. Nitroprusside is a potent afterload-reducing medication, but it can induce labile fluctuations in blood pressure and requires intra-arterial hemodynamic monitoring. Reflex tachycardia can also occur when nitroprusside is used. Hydralazine is also an effective afterload-reducing agent; however, reflex tachycardia often occurs with hydralazine also.

Angiotensin converting enzyme inhibitors (ACEIs) are effective afterload-reducing agents have other acute hemodynamic benefits in patients who develop CPE. The administration of sublingual (captopril) or IV (captopril, enalapril) forms of ACEIs to patients who develop CPE is associated with reductions in systemic vascular resistance (afterload) and improvements in PCWP (preload), stroke volume, cardiac output, and mitral regurgitation without causing adverse changes in heart rate or mean arterial pressure [67–74]. These hemodynamic improvements and subjective improvements in dyspnea are noted within 6 to 12 minutes. Subjective and objective improvements are also noted when ACEIs are administered to patients who have already received other "standard" therapies, including MS, furosemide, and NTG [75], and in patients who have hemodialysis-dependent renal failure [76]. The use of ACEIs in patients who present with CPE has been shown to decrease rates of endotracheal intubation, intensive care unit (ICU) admission rates, and ICU length of stay [40,72], factors that are associated with reduced hospital costs. In the authors' experiences, regardless of whether a sublingual or IV form of ACEI is used, the single dose rarely needs to be repeated during the ED stay. ACEIs can be used safely in conjunction with NTG to provide combination preload and afterload reduction. Furthermore, because ACEIs seem to produce improvements in preload on their own, they can be used as an effective single agent in patients who cannot tolerate NTG (eg, if the patient has recently taken sildenafil).

Afterload-reducing agents should be avoided in patients who are hypotensive; however, these agents can be administered cautiously in conjunction with vasopressors in hypotensive patients. Preload- and afterload-reducing agents should be used with caution in patients who also have severe aortic stenosis. ACEIs specifically should be avoided in patients who have a previous history of ACEI-related angioedema.

Inotropic support

Although inotropic agents should improve outcomes in patients who present with CPE and depressed MI, routine use of inotropes is not recommended. Inotropic agents can cause tachycardia, dysrhythmias, increased myocardial oxygen demand, myocardial ischemia, and sometimes increased mortality [77,78]. Consequently, these medications should be reserved for patients who have hypotension and, therefore, are unable to tolerate the use of preload- and afterload-reducing medications noted earlier. When inotropic agents are used and have produced sufficient improvements in blood pressure, IV NTG or nitroprusside can then be added to provide the desired preload and afterload reduction to relieve pulmonary congestion [79,80]. These patients are best managed with pulmonary artery catheterization and invasive monitoring to closely track their hemodynamic status and allow precise titration of the medications [2,4,81]. Traditional agents used for inotropic support fall into two main classifications, catecholamines and phosphodiesterase inhibitors.

The catecholamine inotropes include dobutamine, dopamine, and norepinephrine. No studies to date have demonstrated a mortality benefit of these over the others in the ED setting. Dobutamine provides the advantage of inducing mild reductions in preload and afterload in addition to inotropic support; however, dobutamine occasionally causes a reduction in blood pressure also, precluding its continued use [82]. In this case, dobutamine should be discontinued and dopamine or norepinephrine can be used to support the patient's blood pressure. Dopamine and norepinephrine improve blood pressure by increasing systemic vascular resistance, which in turn can worsen cardiac output; therefore, when these agents are used, preload- and afterload-reducing medications should be added as soon as possible to improve LV performance and relieve pulmonary congestion.

One of the limitations of catecholamine inotropes is that their activity depends on adrenoreceptor sensitivity. Unfortunately, patients who develop CHF have chronically elevated levels of circulating catecholamines that produce adrenoreceptor tolerance. As a result, when catecholamine inotropes are administered, higher dosages than normal are required. High dosages of these medications are associated with increased adverse effects. Patients who experience CHF also develop tolerance to these medications more rapidly. Additionally, many patients who experience CHF are now treated chronically with beta-adrenergic receptor antagonists ("beta-blockers"). These medications antagonize the effects of catecholamine inotropes, causing a need for higher dosages of the inotropes.

Phosphodiesterase inhibitors (PDEIs) have the advantage over catecholamine inotropes of working independent of adrenoreceptor activity, so they are unaffected by circulating catecholamine levels or beta-blocker medications [83]. PDEIs work by increasing intracellular cyclic adenosine monophosphate levels, which produces a positive inotropic effect on the heart, induces peripheral vasodilation, and reduces pulmonary vascular resistance. As a result, PDEIs induce improvements in preload, afterload, and cardiac output [84]. Several studies have directly compared the use of milrinone, the most well-studied PDEI, with dobutamine in patients who experience severe acutely decompensated CHF and CPE [85–91]. Milrinone was consistently noted to produce similar or greater improvements in stroke volume, cardiac output, PCWP, and systemic vascular resistance. Milrinone was also associated with less tachycardia than dobutamine, is well-tolerated, and is not associated with sustained tachydysrhythmias [92,93]. Despite the apparent hemodynamic benefits, however, milrinone has not been demonstrated to improve hospital length of stay or mortality [90,91].

Levosimendan is a new IV medication classified as a "calcium sensitizer" that has recently been suggested as another alternative to dobutamine for patients who present with acutely decompensated heart failure [94,95]. A recent randomized double-blind trial compared 24-hour infusions of this agent with dobutamine in patients who presented with severe low-output heart failure [96]. Levosimendan produced more significant improvements in cardiac output and PCWP. Patients who received levosimendan also had a lower 180-day mortality rate (26% versus 38%) compared with patients who received dobutamine. Although the study demonstrated in-hospital and long-term benefits, further trials are needed to clarify whether levosimendan has a role in the acute ED management of patients who have developed CPE.

Ventilatory support

Noninvasive positive pressure ventilation

NPPV has been used successfully in patients who present with CPE and has gained popularity amongst acute care physicians. There are two types of NPPV, continuous positive airway pressure (CPAP) and bilevel positive airway pressure (BiPAP). In CPAP, the patient breaths against a continuous flow of positive airway pressure. In BiPAP, the patient receives additional positive pressure during inspiration. As a result, higher pressures can be applied during inspiration and lower pressures during expiration, allowing for greater patient comfort. Either form of NPPV assists patients who develop CPE by maintaining the patency of stiff fluid-filled alveoli and preventing them from becoming atelectatic during expiration. The work of breathing decreases becauseless energy is spent trying to reopen collapsed alveoli. The improved alveolar patency also results in improved oxygen and carbon dioxide exchange in the lung [2,97]. NPPV produces an increase in intrathoracic pressure, which leads to improvements in preload, afterload, and cardiac output [97–100].

CPAP and BiPAP use in patients who present with CPE are associated with a reduced need for endotracheal intubation (ETI) [97,101–106] and reduced ICU length of stay [76,107] and resulting reductions in hospital costs. Only one study has directly compared CPAP with BiPAP in patients who present with CPE [108]. The study was terminated prematurely because of safety concerns when it became apparent that more patients in the BiPAP group had MIs; however, the results of the study have been questioned because more patients in the BiPAP group had chest pain from the start. Subsequent studies comparing BiPAP with mask ventilation in patients who present with CPE [109] and BiPAP versus CPAP in acute respiratory failure of heterogeneous causes [110] failed to demonstrate an increase in MI or mortality in patients receiving BiPAP. In the latter study, a subgroup analysis focusing on the patients who presented with CPE also failed to demonstrate an increase in MI or mortality. Regardless of which form of NPPV is chosen, it must be administered early in the patient's course (ie, on arrival to the ED).

Mechanical ventilation

ETI and mechanical ventilation provides definitive airway support and allows for maximal oxygenation and ventilation. The decision to perform

ETI should be made on clinical grounds and should not wait for arterial blood gas testing. General indications for ETI in the patient who has developed CPE includes hypoxia despite maximal supplemental oxygenation, failed attempts at NPPV, decreased level of consciousness, worsening subjective or objective clinical appearance (eg, increasing fatigue, diaphoresis, anxiety, and so forth), and cardiogenic shock (CS) [2]. Once ETI is accomplished, positive end expiratory pressure (PEEP) should be added to the ventilator settings. The addition of PEEP produces the same hemodynamic benefits as NPPV, including improvements in preload, afterload, and cardiac output, and decreases the duration of mechanical ventilation [111].

Assisted circulation

Placement of an intra-aortic balloon pump (IABP) can be a life-saving intervention in patients who experience CS. Shock in these patients is usually the result of a large AMI or acute valvular disorder. The IABP serves as a temporizing measure while preparations for more definitive therapies are made. IABP counterpulsation provides blood pressure support while also providing improvements in coronary diastolic perfusion, afterload, and cardiac output. Definitive therapy for the patient who experiences CS caused MI involves angioplasty or cardiac bypass surgery. Definitive therapy for the patient with CS caused by acute valvular disorders involves emergent valvuloplasty or valve replacement. Placement of an IABP is usually performed by a cardiologist or cardiac surgeon.

Disposition

Although patients who experience mild CHF decompensations that are attributable to dietary indiscretions (excessive salt intake) or medication noncompliance can receive diuretics in the ED for symptomatic improvement and be discharged, patients who present with pulmonary edema should be admitted to a cardiac-monitored bed. Patients who require mechanical ventilation, experience acute valvular dysfunction, require inotropic support, and present with evidence of acute cardiac ischemia/infarction (based on ECG changes or elevated cardiac biomarkers) should be admitted to an ICU setting [112,113]. Other correlates of in-hospital mortality include advanced age, renal dysfunction, hypotension, digoxin use, chest pain, and anemia (Box 2) [114–118]. A recent analysis of a large registry (the Acute Decompensated Heart Failure National Registry, ADHERE) of patients hospitalized with decompensated heart failure identified (1) high admission levels of blood urea nitrogen (≥43 mg/dL) followed by (2) low admission systolic blood pressure (<115 mm Hg)

Box 2. Predictors of in-hospital mortality in patients who experience cardiogenic pulmonary edema

- Need for mechanical ventilation
- Acute valvular dysfunction
- Need for inotropic support
- Elevated cardiac biomarkers
- ECG evidence of ischemia or dysrhythmias
- Advanced age
- Renal dysfunction (serum elevations of blood urea nitrogen or creatinine)
- Hypotension
- Digoxin use
- Chest pain
- Anemia

followed by (3) high levels of serum creatinine ($\geq$2.75 mg/dL) as the best predictors for in-hospital mortality [117].

Emergent consultation of a cardiologist should be obtained if the cause of the acute CHF exacerbation is AMI or acute valvular dysfunction; or if the patient requires inotropic support. Consultation of a cardiac surgeon should also be considered if severe valvular dysfunction is present. The goal of admission should include symptomatic treatment of hypoxia and pulmonary edema and should also focus on discovering and treating the underlying cause.

Summary

CPE is a life-threatening condition associated with an in-hospital mortality rate of 15% to 20%. To minimize morbidity and mortality, physicians must be able to promptly diagnose and treat these patients. The use of BNP testing is associated with improvements in diagnostic ability beyond physical assessment and chest radiography. Treatment should focus on fluid redistribution through preload and afterload reduction rather than simply diuresis. The most effective and safest preload-reducing medication is NTG. Nesiritide shows promise as an effective preload-reducing medication for patients who present with CPE also, though recommendations for its routine use in the ED should await further studies.

Effective afterload reduction can be accomplished with high-dose NTG or ACEIs, either of which provides preload and afterload reduction, though the combination of medications is more effective than either one alone. ACEIs exert beneficial symptomatic and hemodynamic effects within minutes, and they have been demonstrated to reduce ICU use, intubation rates, and hospital costs.

Inotropes should not be used routinely in patients who present with CPE; however, in patients who develop CS or in patients who cannot tolerate preload- and afterload-reducing medications because of borderline blood pressure, the use of inotropes is often necessary. Milrinone provides greater hemodynamic benefits than traditional catecholamine inotropes, but a mortality difference is not apparent. Levosimendan is a new inotrope, still in investigation, which seems to provide greater hemodynamic benefits and mortality benefits compared with dobutamine. Ongoing studies should clarify its role in patients who have developed CPE.

Ventilatory support is critical in patients who present with CPE. NPPV should be used routinely in these patients. NPPV has been shown to produce improvements in oxygenation, preload, afterload, and cardiac output, and decreased ICU use, intubation rates, and hospital costs. Patients who fail NPPV or demonstrate evidence of respiratory fatigue and decreased level of consciousness require ETI and mechanical ventilation.

Patients who present with CPE should be admitted to a cardiac-monitored bed. Several factors have been found to be associated with increased in-hospital mortality. Emergency physicians should become familiar with these factors and admit these patients to an ICU.

References

[1] Fromm RE Jr, Varon J, Gibbs LR. Congestive heart failure and pulmonary edema for the emergency physician. J Emerg Med 1995;13:71–87.

[2] Mattu A. Cardiogenic pulmonary edema. Current Opinion in Cardiovascular, Pulmonary, and Renal Investigational Drugs 2000;2:9–16.

[3] Mattu A, Sharma S, Perkins AM, et al. Pulmonary edema, cardiogenic. eMedicine Journal 2002;3(2):http://www.emedicine.com/med/topic1955.htm.

[4] Gropper MA, Wiener-Kronish JP, Hashimoto S. Acute cardiogenic pulmonary edema. Clin Chest Med 1994;15:501–15.

[5] Dao Q, Krishnaswamy P, Kazanegra R, et al. Utility of B-type natriuretic peptide in the diagnosis of congestive heart failure in an urgent-care setting. J Am Coll Cardiol 2001;37: 379–85.

[6] Chait A, Cohen HE, Meltzer LE, et al. The bedside chest radiograph in the evaluation of incipient heart failure. Radiology 1972;105:563–6.

[7] Kostuk W, Barr JW, Simon AL, et al. Correlation between the chest film and hemodynamics in acute myocardial infarction. Circulation 1973;48:624–32.

[8] Chen JT. Radiographic diagnosis of heart failure. Heart Dis Stroke 1992;1:58–63.

[9] Badgett RG, Lucey CR, Mulrow CD. Can the clinical examination diagnose left-sided heart failure in adults? JAMA 1997;277:1712–9.

[10] Omland T. Heart failure in the emergency department: is B-type natriuretic peptide a better prognostic indicator than clinical assessment? J Am Coll Cardiol 2004;44:1334–6.

[11] McCullough PA, Hollander JE, Nowak RM, et al. Uncovering heart failure in patients with a history of pulmonary disease: rationale for the early use of B-type natriuretic peptide in the emergency department. Acad Emerg Med 2003;10:198–204.

[12] Pesola GR. The use of B-type natriuretic peptide (BNP) to distinguish heart failure from lung disease in patients presenting with dyspnea to the emergency department. Acad Emerg Med 2003;10:275–7.
[13] Remes J, Miettinen H, Reunanen A, et al. Validity of clinical diagnosis of heart failure in primary health care. Eur Heart J 1991;12:315–21.
[14] Maisel A, Hollander JE, Guss D, et al. Primary results of the rapid emergency department heart failure outpatient trial (REDHOT). J Am Coll Cardiol 2004;44:1328–33.
[15] Collins SP, Ronan-Bentle S, Storrow AB. Diagnostic and prognostic usefulness of natriuretic peptides in emergency department patients with dyspnea. Ann Emerg Med 2003; 41:532–45.
[16] Maisel AS, Krishnaswamy P, Nowak RM, et al. Rapid measurement of B-type natriuretic peptide in the emergency diagnosis of heart failure. N Engl J Med 2002;347:161–6.
[17] Ishii J, Nomura M, Nakamura Y, et al. Risk stratification using a combination of cardiac troponin T and brain natriuretic peptide in patients hospitalized for worsening chronic heart failure. Am J Cardiol 2002;89:691–5.
[18] Harrison A, Morrison LK, Krishnaswamy P, et al. B-type natriuretic peptide predicts future cardiac events in patients presenting to the emergency department with dyspnea. Ann Emerg Med 2002;39:131–8.
[19] Morrison LK, Harrison A, Krishnaswamy P, et al. Utility of a rapid B-natriuretic peptide assay in differentiating congestive heart failure from lung disease in patients presenting with dyspnea. J Am Coll Cardiol 2002;39:202–9.
[20] Silver MA, Maisel A, Yancy CW, et al. BNP consensus panel 2004: a clinical approach for the diagnostic, prognostic, screening, treatment monitoring, and therapeutic roles of natriuretic peptides in cardiovascular diseases. Congest Heart Fail 2004;10(5, Suppl 3): 1–30.
[21] Beltrame JF, Zeitz CJ, Unger SA, et al. Nitrate therapy is an alternative to furosemide/ morphine therapy in the management of acute cardiogenic pulmonary edema. J Card Fail 1998;4:271–9.
[22] Buseman W, Schupp D. Effect of sublingual nitroglycerin in emergency treatment of severe pulmonary edema. Am J Cardiol 1978;41:931–6.
[23] Dupuis J. Nitrates in congestive heart failure. Cardiovasc Drugs Ther 1994;8:501–7.
[24] Nelson GI, Silke B, Ahuja RC, et al. Haemodynamic advantages of isosorbide dinitrate over frusemide in acute heart-failure following myocardial infarction. Lancet 1983;1(8327): 730–3.
[25] Northridge D. Frusemide or nitrates for acute heart failure? Lancet 1996;347:667–8.
[26] Cotter G, Metzkor E, Kaluski E, et al. Randomized trial of high-dose isosorbide dinitrate plus low-dose furosemide versus high-dose furosemide plus low-dose isosorbide dinitrate in severe pulmonary oedema. Lancet 1998;351:389–93.
[27] Kraus PA, Lipman J, Becker PJ. Acute preload effects of furosemide. Chest 1990;98:124–8.
[28] Hoffman JR, Reynolds S. Comparison of nitroglycerin, morphine and furosemide in treatment of presumed pre-hospital pulmonary edema. Chest 1988;92:586–93.
[29] Timmis AD, Rothman MT, Henderson MA, et al. Haemodynamic effect of intravenous morphine in patients with acute myocardial infarction complicated by severe left ventricular failure. BMJ 1980;280:980–2.
[30] Sacchetti A, Ramoska E, Moakes ME, et al. Effect of ED management on ICU use in acute pulmonary edema. Am J Emerg Med 1999;17:571–4.
[31] Bussmann WD, Kaltenbach M. Sublingual nitroglycerin in the treatment of left ventricular failure and pulmonary edema. Eur J Cardiol 1976;4:327–33.
[32] Bussmann WD, Schupp D. Effect of sublingual nitroglycerin in emergency treatment of severe pulmonary edema. Am J Cardiol 1978;41:931–6.
[33] Haber HL, Simek CL, Bergin JD, et al. Bolus intravenous nitroglycerin predominantly reduces afterload in patients with severe congestive heart failure. J Am Coll Cardiol 1993; 22:251–7.

[34] Imhof PR, Ott B, Frankhauser P, et al. Differences in nitroglycerin dose response in the venous and arterial beds. Eur J Clin Pharmacol 1980;18:455–60.
[35] Vismara LA, Leaman DM, Zelis R. The effects of morphine on venous tone in patients with acute pulmonary edema. Circulation 1976;54:335–7.
[36] Zelis R, Mansour EJ, Capone RJ, et al. The cardiovascular effects of morphine. The peripheral capacitance and resistance vessels in human subjects. J Clin Invest 1974;54: 1247–58.
[37] Lappas DG, Geha D, Fischer JE, et al. Filling pressures of the heart and pulmonary circulation of the patient with coronary artery disease after large intravenous doses of morphine. Anesthesiology 1975;42:153–9.
[38] Amsterdam EA, Zelis R, Kohfeld DB, et al. Effect of morphine on myocardial contractility: negative inotropic action during hypoxia and reversal by isoproterenol. Circulation 1971; 43–4(Suppl II):135.
[39] Sacchetti A, Ramoska E, Moakes ME, et al. Effect of ED management on ICU use in acute pulmonary edema. Am J Emerg Med 1999;17:571–4.
[40] Gammage M. Treatment of acute pulmonary oedema: diuresis or vasodilatation? Lancet 1998;351:382–3.
[41] Figueras J, Weil MH. Blood volume prior to and following treatment of acute cardiogenic pulmonary edema. Circulation 1978;57:349–55.
[42] Ikram H, Chan W, Espiner EA, et al. Haemodynamic and hormone responses to acute and chronic frusemide therapy in congestive heart failure. Clin Sci 1980;59:443–9.
[43] Francis GS, Siegel RM, Goldsmith SR, et al. Acute vasoconstrictor response to intravenous furosemide in patients with chronic congestive heart failure. Ann Intern Med 1985;103:1–6.
[44] Nelson GI, Ahuja RC, Silke B, et al. Haemodynamic effects of frusemide and its influence on repetitive rapid volume loading in acute myocardial infarction. Eur Heart J 1983;4:706–11.
[45] Lal S, Murtagh JG, Pollock AM, et al. Acute haemodynamic effects of frusemide in patients with normal and raised left atrial pressures. Br Hear J 1969;31:711–7.
[46] Figueras J, Weil MH. Hypovolemia and hypotension complicating management of acute cardiogenic pulmonary edema. Am J Cardiol 1979;44:1349–55.
[47] Henning RJ, Weil MH. Effect of afterload reduction on plasma volume during acute heart failure. Am J Cardiol 1978;42:823–7.
[48] Biddle TL, Yu PN. Effect of furosemide on haemodynamic and lung water in acute pulmonary edema secondary to myocardial infarction. Am J Cardiol 1979;43:86–90.
[49] Dormans TPJ, Pickkers P, Russel FGM, et al. Vascular effects of loop diuretics. Cardiovasc Res 1996;32:988–97.
[50] Mukherjee SK, Katz MA, Michael UF, et al. Mechanisms of hemodynamic actions of furosemide: differentiation of vascular and renal effects on blood pressure in functionally anephric hypertensive patients. Am Heart J 1981;101:313–8.
[51] Pickkers P, Dormans TPJ, Smits P. Direct vasoactivity of frusemide. Lancet 1996;347: 1338–9.
[52] Pickkers P, Dormans TP, Russel FG, et al. Direct vascular effects of furosemide in humans. Circulation 1997;96:1847–52.
[53] Gehm L, Propp DA. Pulmonary edema in the renal failure patient. Am J Emerg Med 1989; 7:336–9.
[54] Schmieder RE, Messerli FH, deCarvalho JGR, et al. Immediate hemodynamic response to furosemide in patients undergoing chronic hemodialysis. Am J Kidney Dis 1987;9:55–9.
[55] Mond H, Hunt D, Sloman G. Haemodynamic effects of frusemide in patients suspected of having acute myocardial infarction. Br Heart J 1974;36:44–53.
[56] Fett DL, Cavero PG, Burnett JC Jr. Low-dose atrial natriuretic factor and furosemide in experimental acute congestive heart failure. J Am Soc Nephrol 1993;4:162–7.
[57] Kubo SH, Clark M, Laragh JH, et al. Identification of normal neurohormonal activity in mild congestive heart failure and stimulating effect of upright posture and diuretics. Am J Cardiol 1987;60:1322–8.

[58] Kiely J, Kelly DT, Taylor DR, et al. The role of furosemide in the treatment of left ventricular dysfunction associated with acute myocardial infarction. Circulation 1973;48: 581–7.
[59] Nishimura N, Kanbe N. The renal and hemodynamic effects of furosemide in acute myocardial infarction. Crit Care Med 1981;9:829–32.
[60] Colucci WS, Elkayam U, Horton DP. Intravenous nesiritide, a natriuretic peptide, in the treatment of decompensated congestive heart failure. N Engl J Med 2000;343:246–53.
[61] Mills RM, LeJemtel TH, Horton DP, et al. Sustained hemodynamic effects of an infusion of nesiritide (human b-type natriuretic peptide) in heart failure: a randomized, double-blind, placebo-controlled clinical trial. Natrecor Study Group. J Am Coll Cardiol 1999;34:155–62.
[62] Publication Committee for the VMAC Investigators. Intravenous nesiritide vs nitroglycerin for treatment of decompensated congestive heart failure: a randomized controlled trial. JAMA 2002;287:1531–40.
[63] Noviasky JA, Kelberman M, Whalen KM, et al. Science or fiction: use of nesiritide as a first-line agent? Pharmacotherapy 2003;23:1081–3.
[64] Elkayam U, Akhter MW, Singh H, et al. Comparison of effects of left ventricular filling pressure of intravenous nesiritide and high-dose nitroglycerin in patients with decompensated heart failure. Am J Cardiol 2004;93:237–40.
[65] Sackner-Bernstein JD, Kowalski M, Fox M, et al. Short-term risk of death after treatment with nesiritide for decompensated heart failure—a pooled analysis of randomized controlled trials. JAMA 2005;293:1900–5.
[66] Sackner-Bernstein JD, Skopicki HA, Aaronson KD. Risk of worsening renal function with nesiritide in patients with acutely decompensated heart failure. Circulation 2005;111: 1487–91.
[67] Barnett JC, Zink KM, Touchon RC. Sublingual captopril in the treatment of acute heart failure. Curr Ther Res 1991;49:274–81.
[68] Annane D, Bellissat E, Pussare E, et al. Placebo-controlled, randomized, double-blind study of intravenous enalaprilat efficacy and safety in acute cardiogenic pulmonary edema. Circulation 1996;94:1316–24.
[69] Haude M, Steffen W, Erbel R, et al. Sublingual administration of captopril versus nitroglycerin in patients with severe congestive heart failure. Int J Cardiol 1990;27:351–9.
[70] Langes K, Siebels J, Kuck KH. Efficacy and safety of intravenous captopril in congestive heart failure. Curr Ther Res 1993;53:167–76.
[71] Varriale P, David W, Chryssos BE. Hemodynamic response to intravenous enalaprilat in patients with severe congestive heart failure and mitral regurgitation. Clin Cardiol 1993;16: 235–8.
[72] Southall JC, Bissell DM, Burton JH, et al. ACE inhibitors in acutely decompensated congestive heart failure. Acad Emerg Med 2004;11:503.
[73] Brivet F, Delfraissy JF, Giudicelli JF, et al. Immediate effects of captopril in acute left ventricular heart failure secondary to myocardial infarction. Eur J Clin Invest 1981;11: 369–73.
[74] Tohmo H, Karanko M, Korpilahti K. Haemodynamic effects of enalaprilat and preload in acute severe heart failure complicating myocardial infarction. Eur Heart J 1994;15:523–7.
[75] Hamilton RJ, Carter WA, Gallagher EJ. Rapid improvement of acute pulmonary edema with sublingual captopril. Acad Emerg Med 1996;3:205–12.
[76] Sacchetti A, McCabe J, Torres M, et al. ED management of acute congestive heart failure in renal dialysis patients. Am J Emerg Med 1993;11:644–7.
[77] Felker GM, O'Connor CM. Between Scylla and Charybdis: the choice of inotropic agent for decompensated heart failure. Am Heart J 2001;142:932–3.
[78] Ewy GA. Inotropic infusions for chronic congestive heart failure: medical miracles or misguided medicinals? J Am Coll Cardiol 1999;33:572–5.
[79] Gagnon RM, Fortin L, Boucher R, et al. Combined hemodynamic effects of dobutamine and IV nitroglycerin in congestive heart failure. Chest 1980;78:694–8.

[80] Nohria A, Lewis E, Stevenson LW. Medical management of advanced heart failure. JAMA 2002;287:628–40.
[81] Eisenberg PR, Jaffe AS, Schuster DP. Clinical evaluation compared to pulmonary artery catheterization in the hemodynamic assessment of critically ill patients. Crit Care Med 1984;12:549–53.
[82] Keung EC, Siskind SJ, Senneblick EH, et al. Dobutamine therapy for acute myocardial infarction. JAMA 1981;245:144–6.
[83] Travill CM, Pugh S, Noble MI. The inotropic and hemodynamic effects of intravenous milrinone when reflex adrenergic stimulation is suppressed by beta-adrenergic blockade. Clin Ther 1994;16:783–92.
[84] Shipley JB, Tolman D, Hastillo A, et al. Milrinone: basic and clinical pharmacology and acute and chronic management. Am J Med Sci 1996;311:286–91.
[85] Colucci WS, Wright RF, Jaski BE, et al. Milrinone and dobutamine in severe heart failure: differing hemodynamic effects and individual patient responsiveness. Circulation 1986; 73(3):175–83.
[86] Grose R, Strain J, Greenberg M, et al. Systemic and coronary effects of intravenous milrinone and dobutamine in congestive heart failure. J Am Coll Cardiol 1986;7:1107–13.
[87] Karlsberg RP, DeWood MA, DeMaria AN, et al. Comparative efficacy of short-term intravenous infusions of milrinone and dobutamine in acute congestive heart failure following acute myocardial infarction. Milrinone-Dobutamine Study Group. Clin Cardiol 1996;19:21–30.
[88] Kawamura A, Yoshikawa T, Takahashi T, et al. Randomized trial of phosphodiesterase inhibitors versus catecholamines in patients with acutely decompensated heart failure. Jpn Circ J 2001;65:858–62.
[89] Mager G, Klocke RK, Kux A, et al. Phosphodiesterase III inhibition or adrenoreceptor stimulation: milrinone as an alternative to dobutamine in the treatment of severe heart failure. Am Heart J 1991;121:1974–83.
[90] Yamani MH, Haji SA, Starling RC, et al. Comparison of dobutamine-based and milrinone-based therapy for advanced decompensated congestive heart failure: hemodynamic efficacy, clinical outcome, and economic impact. Am Heart J 2001;142:998–1002.
[91] Cuffe MS, Califf RM, Adams KF Jr, et al. Short-term intravenous milrinone for acute exacerbation of chronic heart failure: a randomized controlled trial. JAMA 2002;287: 1541–7.
[92] Anderson JL, Askins JC, Gilbert EM, et al. Occurrence of ventricular arrhythmias in patients receiving acute and chronic infusions of milrinone. Am Heart J 1986;111:466–74.
[93] Varriale P, Ramaprasad S. Short-term intravenous milrinone for severe congestive heart failure: the good, bad, and not so good. Pharmacotherapy 1997;17:371–4.
[94] Nieminen MS, Akkila J, Hasenfuss G, et al. Hemodynamic and neurohumoral effects of continuous infusion of levosimendan in patients with congestive heart failure. J Am Coll Cardiol 2000;36:1903–12.
[95] Slawsky MT, Colucci WS, Gottlieb SS, et al. Acute hemodynamic and clinical effects of levosimendan in patients with severe heart failure. Circulation 2000;102:2222–7.
[96] Follath F, Cleland JG, Just H, et al. Efficacy and safety of intravenous levosimendan compared with dobutamine in severe low-output heart failure (the LIDO study): a randomized double-blind trial. Lancet 2002;360:196–202.
[97] Sacchetti AD, Harris RH, Paston C, et al. Bi-level positive airway pressure support system use in acute congestive heart failure: preliminary case series. Acad Emerg Med 1995;2:714–8.
[98] Bradley TD, Holloway RM, McLaughlin PR, et al. Cardiac output response to continuous positive pressure in congestive heart failure. Am Rev Respir Dis 1991;145:377–82.
[99] Baratz DM, Westbrook PR, Shah PK, et al. Effect of nasal continuous positive airway pressure on cardiac output and oxygen delivery in patients with congestive heart failure. Chest 1992;102:1397–401.

[100] Naughton MT, Rahman MA, Hara K, et al. Effects of continuous positive airway pressure on intrathoracic and left ventricular transmural pressures in patients with congestive heart failure. Circulation 1995;91:1725–31.
[101] Bersten AD, Holt AW, Vedig AE, et al. Treatment of severe cardiogenic pulmonary edema with continuous positive pressure delivered by face mask. N Engl J Med 1991;325:1825–30.
[102] Lin M, Yang YF, Chiang HT, et al. Reappraisal of continuous positive airway pressure therapy in acute cardiogenic pulmonary edema: short-term results and long-term follow-up. Chest 1995;107:1379–86.
[103] Masip J, Betbese AJ, Paez J, et al. Non-invasive pressure support ventilation versus conventional oxygen therapy in acute cardiogenic pulmonary oedema: a randomised trial. Lancet 2000;356:2126–32.
[104] Pang D, Keenan SP, Cook DJ, et al. The effect of positive pressure airway support on mortality and the need for intubation in cardiogenic pulmonary edema. Chest 1998;114:1185–92.
[105] Rasanen J, Heikklia J, Downs J, et al. Continuous positive airway pressure by face mask in acute cardiogenic pulmonary edema. Am J Cardiol 1985;55:296–300.
[106] Wigder HN, Hoffmann P, Mazzolini D, et al. Pressure support noninvasive positive pressure ventilation treatment of acute cardiogenic pulmonary edema. Am J Emerg Med 2001;19:179–81.
[107] Holt AW, Bersten AD, Fuller S, et al. Intensive care costing methodology: cost benefit analysis of mask continuous positive airway pressure for severe cardiogenic pulmonary oedema. Anaesth Intens Care 1994;22:170–4.
[108] Mehta S, Jay GD, Woolard RH, et al. Randomized, prospective trial of bilevel versus continuous positive airway pressure in acute pulmonary edema. Crit Care Med 1997;25:620–8.
[109] Levitt MA. A prospective, randomized trial of BiPAP in severe acute congestive heart failure. J Emerg Med 2001;21:363–9.
[110] Cross AM, Cameron P, Kierce M, et al. Non-invasive ventilation in acute respiratory failure: a randomized comparison of continuous positive airway pressure and bi-level positive airway pressure. Emerg Med J 2003;20:531–4.
[111] Grace MP, Greenbaum DM. Cardiac performance and response to PEEP in patients with cardiac dysfunction. Crit Care Med 1982;10:358–60.
[112] Hsieh M, Auble TE, Yealy DM. Predicting the future: can this patient with acute congestive heart failure be safely discharged from the emergency department? Ann Emerg Med 2002;39:181–9.
[113] Le Conte P, Coutant V, N'Guyen JM, et al. Prognostic factors in acute cardiogenic pulmonary edema. Am J Emerg Med 1999;17:329–32.
[114] Plotnick GD, Kelemen MH, Garrett RB, et al. Acute cardiogenic pulmonary edema in the elderly: factors predicting in-hospital and one-year mortality. South Med J 1982;75:565–9.
[115] Chin MH, Goldman L. Correlates of major complications or death in patients admitted to the hospital with congestive heart failure. Arch Intern Med 1996;156:1814–20.
[116] Brophy JM, Deslauriers G, Boucher B, et al. The hospital course and short term prognosis of patients presenting to the emergency room with decompensated congestive heart failure. Can J Cardiol 1993;9:219–24.
[117] Fonarow GC, Adams KF Jr, Abraham WT, et al. Risk stratification for in-hospital mortality in acutely decompensated heart failure. JAMA 2005;293:572–80.
[118] Felker GM, Gattis WA, Leimberger JD, et al. Usefulness of anemia as a predictor of death and rehospitalization in patients with decompensated heart failure. Am J Cardiol 2003;92:625–8.

ELSEVIER
SAUNDERS

Emerg Med Clin N Am
23 (2005) 1127–1139

EMERGENCY
MEDICINE
CLINICS OF
NORTH AMERICA

Management of Atrial Fibrillation in the Emergency Department

Arun V. Raghavan, MD, Wyatt W. Decker, MD*, Thomas D. Meloy, MD

Department of Emergency Medicine, Mayo Clinic College of Medicine, 200 First Street, SW, Rochester, MN 55905, USA

Emergency medicine physicians have the unique responsibility of being the point of first medical contact for patients presenting with atrial fibrillation (AF). Although atrial fibrillation is the most common cardiac arrhythmia [1], affecting approximately 2.2 million Americans [2], there is no accepted standard of practice with regard to the management of atrial fibrillation. The sequelae of atrial fibrillation range from none to devastating, including exercise intolerance, congestive heart failure, tachycardia-induced cardiomyopathy, and systemic emboli. The Framingham study [3] has revealed a 1.5 to 1.9 higher risk of death associated with chronic atrial fibrillation, attributable largely to thromboembolic stroke. This article reviews the pathophysiology and update management options for atrial fibrillation. Although each patient presenting to the emergency department with atrial fibrillation presents unique challenges, this article outlines effective management paths that will be of value in the acute management of this condition.

Pathophysiology

Atrial fibrillation is a supraventricular rhythm disorder that is usually the result of uncoordinated arrhythmogenic substrates. These substrates could include an ectopic focus, a single re-entry circuit, or multiple re-entrant circuits [4]. The lack of rhythm causes deterioration of atrial mechanical function and an irregular, usually rapid ventricular response depending on the atrioventricular (AV) node function. The loss of the atrial "kick," a rapid ventricular response, and ventricular irregularity can cause a decrease

* Corresponding author.
E-mail address: decker.wyatt@mayo.edu (W.W. Decker).

doi:10.1016/j.emc.2005.07.013 **emed.theclinics.com**

in cardiac output. In patients with underlying heart disease, such as valvular disease, diastolic dysfunction, cardiomyopathy, and coronary artery disease, the onset of atrial fibrillation can cause marked decreases in cardiac output and associated sequelae. The loss of atrial filling pressure explains common symptoms such as palpitations, shortness of breath, chest pain, weakness and near syncope caused by coronary insufficiency, congestive heart failure, hypotension, and shock. Atrial fibrillation also causes intra-atrial stasis, particularly in the atrial appendage, with the well-documented increased risk for thromboembolic events [5].

Causes

There are many precipitants for atrial fibrillation related to intrinsic atrial irritability [6], including contraction-excitation feedback, metabolic disorders, and cardiac and noncardiac disease [7]. For the emergency department physician, it is important to address likely underlying causes and risks related to the patient presenting with atrial fibrillation. It can be helpful to subcategorize causes into cardiopulmonary causes, systemic causes, and primary (lone) atrial fibrillation (Table 1).

History

Patients with atrial fibrillation may describe nonspecific symptoms such as palpitations, fatigue, or dyspnea. However, the history should focus on

Table 1
Etiology of atrial fibrillation

Serious cardiopulmonary causes	Other causes
Acute myocardial infarction or acute coronary syndrome	Hyperthyroidism
Pulmonary embolism	Ethanol use ("holiday heart")
Cardiomyopathy	Hypothermia
Restrictive heart disease	Drugs: sympathomimetrics, cocaine, amphetamine derivatives, ephedra
Chronic obstructive pulmonary disease	Metabolic causes: hypokalemia
Sleep apnea	Idiopathic: lone AF[a]
Hypertension	
Valvular heart disease	
Left ventricular hypertrophy	
Left ventricular diastolic dysfunction	
Congestive heart disease	
Sick sinus syndrome	
Pericarditis	
Post-cardiac surgery	

[a] Lone atrial fibrillation is most commonly found in younger population (age $\leq$ 65 yrs) with paroxysmal atrial fibrillation. Diagnosis includes absence of known causative factors and normal left ventricular function.

any triggering and potentially reversible causes of the dysrhythmia. Focused questioning needs to address the presence of chest pain or a history of coronary artery disease to suggest acute ischemia [8], fevers, or other constitutional symptoms associated with sepsis, acute volume shifts, alcohol ingestion, thyroid disorders, medications, alcohol, or drug use [9]. It is also important to determine the chronicity of the complaint [10]. Some patients may be able to describe an abrupt onset of their symptoms. Having the patient identify the time of onset of symptoms suggestive of atrial fibrillation has significant implications with regard to management. A recent article [11] that used extensive monitoring has documented that many episodes of atrial fibrillation were asymptomatic or "silent episodes," indicating that in patients with a history of atrial fibrillation, consideration must be given to the possibility that they may be unaware of the actual duration of their arrhythmia.

Physical examination

The initial focus of the physical examination must be the patient's vital signs, with the appropriate acute intervention to stabilize them if needed. The secondary focus is the cardiopulmonary examination and a focused neurologic and vascular examination to determine the possibility of embolic complications [12]. The hallmark of the initial rhythm is an irregular pulse with or without tachycardia. The cardiovascular examination should assess for evidence of congestive heart failure or significant valvular disease, such as murmurs, an S_3 gallop, jugular venous distension, pulmonary rales, or pedal edema.

Electrocardiogram

Although it is often identified on a cardiac monitor or single lead of a rhythm strip, the diagnosis of atrial fibrillation can be confirmed most easily using a standard electrocardiogram, which shows undulating low-amplitude fibrillary waves in place of discrete P waves and a consequent irregular ventricular response. Although a narrow complex tachycardia is typical, some patients may present with wide QRS complexes because of an underlying or rate-related conduction aberrancy or pre-excitation in patients with Wolff-Parkinson-White (WPW) syndrome. It is important that the physician ensures that there are no delta waves suggestive of WPW syndrome because the use of AV nodal blocking agents such as calcium channel blockers, β-blockers, and adenosine can lead to a rapid ventricular rate that may degenerate into ventricular fibrillation and sudden cardiac death [13]. Additionally, ST-segment and T-wave changes consistent with ischemia or infarction should be noted and addressed.

Laboratory evaluation and additional testing

Laboratory evaluation and additional testing needs are dictated by the history, physical examination, the individual patient presentation, and a likely differential diagnosis. An initial ECG should be obtained, and, if available, a comparison with previous ECG tracings can be helpful. The evaluation of the ECG should focus on identifying ischemic changes, rate and rhythm, QRS duration, and evidence of aberrancy. Additional laboratory testing includes a complete blood count, an electrolyte panel, glucose and thyroid function testing, and a chest radiograph, which are reasonable studies for the initial evaluation. More extensive immediate testing may be indicated for the unstable patient to evaluate for serious underlying causes. Causes may include cardiac biomarkers (for possible acute coronary syndrome), CT scan of the chest (for suspicion of pulmonary embolism), or an arterial blood gas assay (to evaluate for carbon monoxide exposure, hypercarbia, shock, or acidemia) [9]. Transthoracic echocardiography may be helpful to assess for left ventricular function and wall motion abnormalities, as well as chamber size, valvular function, and the presence of pericardial fluid. Although it is generally recommended in the assessment of a patient with atrial fibrillation at some point in their evaluation, formal echocardiography is usually not required acutely in the ED. Transesophageal echocardiography has been well substantiated to be more sensitive than transthoracic echocardiography for the assessment of intra-atrial thrombus. It is helpful in assessing thrombotic risk in elective cardioversion [14] but currently has a limited role in the management of acute atrial fibrillation in the ED.

Management of atrial fibrillation

Management of the patient with atrial fibrillation is dictated by the acuity of onset, associated symptoms, stability (or instability) of vital signs, and the duration of the dysrhythmia. It is helpful for management to categorize patients into three general classes: (1) the hemodynamically unstable patient; (2) atrial fibrillation of less than 48 hours; and (3) atrial fibrillation of more than 48 hours (Fig. 1).

Management of atrial fibrillation in the hemodynamically unstable patient

In significant hemodynamic instability or life-threatening complications such as myocardial infarction, pulmonary edema, hypotension, or decompensated heart failure, the patient needs immediate attention to the airway, breathing, and circulation. Urgent rate and rhythm control are the immediate goals for the patient presenting with rapid atrial fibrillation and severe cardiopulmonary symptoms or hemodynamic instability. Emergent synchronized cardioversion is indicated [15]. In patients with atrial fibrillation

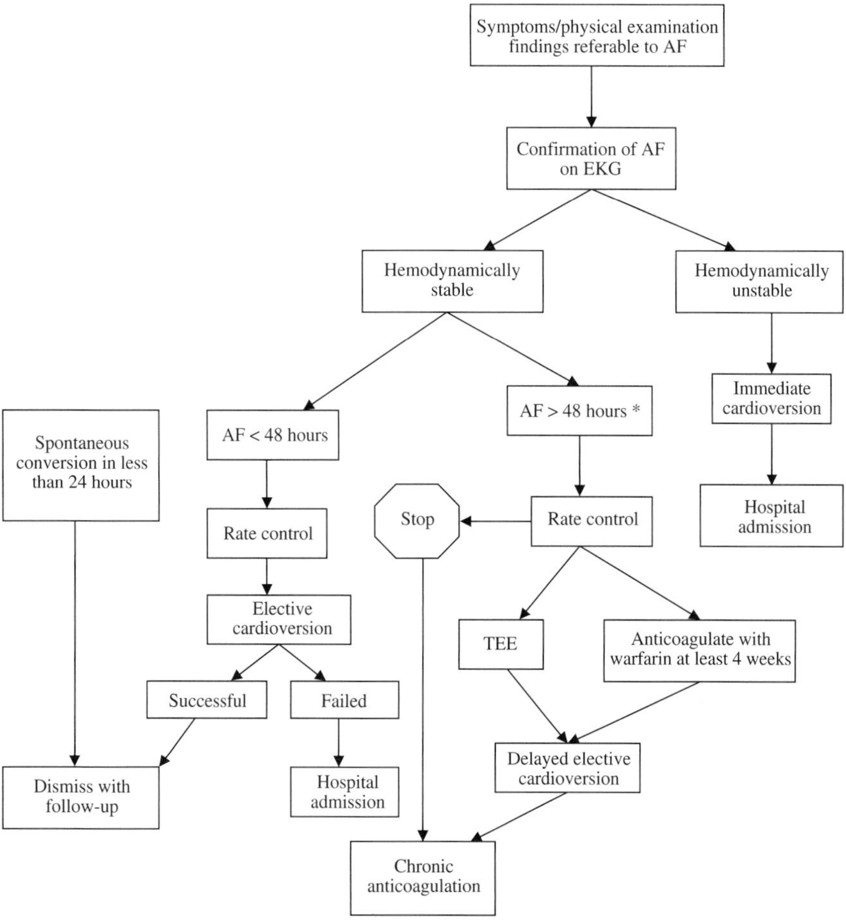

Fig. 1. Algorithm for acute management of atrial fibrillation. *AF of greater than 48 hours requires hospital admission in most settings to initiate rate control and anticoagulation. TEE, transesophageal echocardiogram.

with normal or bradycardic rates, who have severe cardiopulmonary symptoms or hypotension, the physician should be cautious in assuming that atrial fibrillation is the cause of the acute symptoms. These patients need to be treated symptomatically according to the likely underlying cause. These patients will require admission and further cardiovascular evaluation.

Temporal considerations in the management of the hemodynamically stable patient

There are a number of different management options for patients without severe cardiopulmonary symptoms or hemodynamic instability, who present with a new onset (less than 48 hours) of atrial fibrillation. Recent literature has been helpful in clarifying the options for many patients, but controversy remains concerning the best strategy for each individual patient. The issues are: (1) rate control versus rhythm control; (2) rhythm control: electrical cardioversion versus anti-arrhythmic drugs; (3) anticoagulation; and (4) patient disposition: admission, observation, or outpatient management. It is beyond the scope of this discussion to specifically address all of these issues, but recent published literature can clarify some of these management options.

Rate control

The initial management of atrial fibrillation in patients who are hemodynamically stable, regardless of duration, is adequate rate control. In the presence of a rapid ventricular rate not believed to be WPW, rate control with pharmacologic agents that depress atrioventricular node conduction is indicated [9]. β-blockers, calcium channel blockers, and digoxin can be used for rate control in atrial fibrillation. None of these agents has been shown to convert atrial fibrillation to normal sinus rhythm or to maintain normal sinus rhythm. Selecting the appropriate drug depends on the individual patient profile and presentation. β-blockers such as metoprolol, propranolol, and esmolol prolong the conduction time through the AV node because they act at the level of β-adrenergic receptors and may offer additional benefit in the setting of concomitant ischemia or infarction [16]. Contraindications to β-blockers are primarily the presence of chronic obstructive pulmonary disease and asthma. However, it has been shown that an esmolol drip may be used successfully in the acute setting in patients with obstructive lung disease [17]. Calcium channel blockers such as diltiazem and verapamil are effective in rate control but must be used cautiously in the setting of congestive heart failure, with close monitoring for hypotension [16]. The hypotensive effects of calcium channel blockers may be decreased with the use of parenteral calcium. Digoxin has a limited role in the acute rate control management of atrial fibrillation in the ED because the onset of action and effect may take hours. Digoxin also has been shown recently in the VERDICT trial [18] to exacerbate the electrical component of atrial remodeling and may potentiate susceptibility to AF after conversion. Another complicating issue concerns the patient with ECG findings or a history that identifies WPW syndrome. β-blockers, calcium channel blockers, or digoxin should be avoided because they facilitate anterograde conduction through the accessory pathway and can cause severe decompensation and hypotension by precipitating dysrhythmias, particularly, rapid atrial fibrillation or atrial flutter [13]. In the case of known or possible WPW, synchronized cardioversion is the treatment of choice. Pharmacologic options include procainamide and amiodarone.

Rhythm control

For the long-term management of patients with AF, the rate-versus-rhythm control controversy has been clarified for some patients as a result of the RACE [19] and AFFIRM [20] trials. In patients with persistent AF, the RACE trial has concluded that rate control was not inferior to rhythm control at the end of 12 months with regard to the composite primary endpoint, including cardiovascular death, congestive heart failure (CHF), transient ischemic attack/cerebrovascular accident, and bleeding. Women and hypertensive patients had worse outcomes with rhythm control.

The AFFIRM trial [20] further addressed the issue of rate versus rhythm control with a primary endpoint of mortality. Inclusion criteria included patients who were at least 65 years of age or who had other risk factors for stroke or death, and who had a history of atrial fibrillation for at least 6 hours in the past 6 months. There was trend toward an increase in deaths in the rhythm control arm, although it was not statistically significant ($P = .07$). Rates for the composite endpoint (death, disabling stroke, disabling anoxic encephalopathy, major bleeding, or cardiac arrest) demonstrated no difference between the two groups. Results from these trials suggest that, if ventricular rate and the patient's symptoms could be adequately controlled, the option of rate control could be the preferred choice for the long-term management of these patients. All patients received long-term anticoagulation in these trials, according to the current practice guidelines [9]. In addition to the clinical outcomes, a cost analysis from the AFFIRM trial has shown a cost benefit to the rate control approach, with a higher cost associated with rhythm control, ranging from $2189 to $5481 more per patient than rate control [21].

The longer a patient is in atrial fibrillation, the less likely it is that sinus rhythm can be restored and maintained, with some studies demonstrating only 9% to 14% of patients remaining in sinus rhythm for a significant period after cardioversion [22,23].

In discussing rhythm control for patients with atrial fibrillation, it is important to recognize that major trials to date have not included a number of important groups of patients, including younger patients with lone atrial fibrillation (up to 15% of AF patients), patients with highly symptomatic atrial fibrillation, patients with significant CHF, and patients with contraindications for anticoagulation or rate control. Up to 50% of all atrial fibrillation patients are classified in this large group of patients, and management decisions must be made based on individual patient presentation and characteristics. Rhythm control with cardioversion may be the most appropriate management for many of these patients. Furthermore, none of the studies addresses new onset atrial fibrillation, which is still generally believed to warrant attempts at rhythm control.

A reasonable approach for the new onset atrial fibrillation patient without severe symptoms or hemodynamic compromise is to assess the time of onset, age, previous cardioversion attempts and success, and to initiate parenteral calcium channel blockers or β-blockers for rate control. If the onset is clearly less than 48 hours (low likelihood of atrial thrombus) and there are no contraindications, then cardioversion may be considered [10]. The proper timing of cardioversion has not been answered definitively. It may be performed immediately in the ED or after a period of observation, because approximately 50% of patients spontaneously cardiovert within 24 hours [24], with the goal of attaining normal sinus rhythm within a 48-hour window to decrease risk of thromboembolic complications. Patients may then be monitored for a short period of time or admitted if there are complications or other indications for admission. Generally, patients should be examined promptly for further cardiovascular evaluation, if they are dismissed. In a single-center prospective study [25], patients who were randomized to an ED observation unit and cardioverted after 6 hours showed no increased risk, and their length of stay was found to decrease substantially, compared with routine hospital admission.

Cardioversion: chemical versus electrical

Cardioversion can be attempted chemically with antidysrhythmic medications or electrically with direct-current (DC) cardioversion. There are advantages and disadvantages to each approach. Chemical cardioversion avoids the necessity for sedation; however, it generally will take longer for onset and has a proarrhythmic potential (approximately 3%–5%), and it often requires monitoring period of up to 12 hours for the assessment of dysrhythmias or high-risk electrocardiographic findings [26]. Moreover, chemical cardioversion has a lower success rate (approximately 50%) compared with electrical cardioversion (89%) [27].

Antiarrhythmic drug therapy in conjunction with rate control to maintain sinus rhythm after successful cardioversion may be indicated with cardiology consultation. The appropriate choice of an antiarrhythmic agent for long-term treatment of atrial fibrillation is determined largely by the patient's symptoms, the underlying heart disease, the presence of QTc abnormalities, and whether the drug in question will warrant admitting the patient to the hospital for prolonged electrocardiographic monitoring to address proarrhythmic potential.

Electrical DC cardioversion has the advantage of a greater success rate, but it requires additional personnel for the conscious sedation and the performance of the DC cardioversion. The patient is sedated, and synchronized DC cardioversion is initiated with increasing energy levels if it is initially unsuccessful. DC cardioversion should be aborted if there is a failure to convert despite maximum energy settings or if there is repeated rapid recurrence of atrial fibrillation despite initial successful cardioversion. Biphasic waveform shock cardioversion has been shown to be more effective than the older monophasic cardioversion [28]. These patients may require antidysrhythmic therapy for successful outcome. Complications can include failure to convert the rhythm, cardiac damage, dysrhythmias, and anesthetic complications, although these complications are rare. The effectiveness of the cardioversion can be increased by pretreatment with some antidysrhythmic agents such as ibutilide [29]. However, this can increase the post-event duration of cardiac monitoring and is associated with complications including ventricular dysrhythmias.

Anticoagulation

Atrial fibrillation is associated with an increased risk for thromboembolism and stroke in patients in atrial fibrillation for over 48 hours. Hence, patients with atrial fibrillation of more than 48 hours should be treated with anticoagulant therapy for at least 3 to 4 weeks before cardioversion, with the alternative of undergoing transesophageal echocardiography to determine the presence of atrial thrombus, and if none is found, proceed directly to cardioversion [30]. The risk of thromboembolism in patients with new onset atrial fibrillation with a duration of less than 48 hours is less than 1%, obviating the need for prior anticoagulant treatment [31].

An effective tool to risk-stratify those patients who require chronic anticoagulation is the CHADS 2 scoring system (Table 2) [32,33]. Patients who have a score of 0 are at low risk and may be managed effectively with aspirin therapy for prophylaxis. A score of 1 to 2 correlates with intermediate risk, and the decision to anticoagulate with aspirin versus warfarin is left to the clinician's discretion, weighing risks and benefits. Patients who have a score grater than or equal to 3 should be treated with warfarin in the absence of contraindications. The stroke rate per 100 patient-years without antithrombotic therapy was shown to increase by a factor of 1.5 (95% CI, 1.3-1.7) for each 1-point increase in the CHADS 2 score.

Other treatment options

There are a number of other treatment options available for complicated atrial fibrillation that has not responded to standard rate or rhythm management. Although these options are not applicable to emergency department management, it is important to have a knowledge of additional management options. These may include radiofrequency, microwave, or surgical maze ablation [34–36]. Internal atrial defibrillation remains experimental [37].

Disposition

Do all patients with acute onset of atrial fibrillation require hospitalization? Which patients can be dismissed from the emergency department?

Table 2
CHADS 2 score

CHADS 2 score	95% CI	Yearly risk of stroke (%)
0	<1.2-3.0>	1.9
1	<2.0-3.8>	2.8
2	<3.1-5.1>	4.0
3	<4.6-7.3>	5.9
4	<6.3-11.1>	8.5
5	<8.2-17.5>	12.5
6	<10.5-27.4>	18.2

Yearly risk of stroke in patients with chronic atrial fibrillation without antithrombotic therapy. Prior stroke, 2 points; congestive heart failure, 1 point; hypertension, 1 point; diabetes, 1 point; age 75 years or older, 1 point.

The management of the patient with new onset atrial fibrillation must be dictated by the acuity of symptoms, the presence of cardiopulmonary complications, and the presence of comorbidities. Decisions regarding disposition must take into account these same issues, including the short-term risk of complications and the patient's response to therapy. Patients with significant comorbidities, hemodynamic instability, or acute coronary syndrome will require admission to the hospital. In the absence of these complications and for the patient who responds well to therapy or converts to normal sinus rhythm, it may be appropriate to observe the patient for a few hours in the emergency department or an observation unit, with subsequent dismissal if there are no complications. These patients should be scheduled for follow-up with their primary care physician or cardiologist.

Summary

Given the lack of standardization in the treatment and disposition of patients presenting to the emergency department with complaints referable to atrial fibrillation, it is necessary to adopt a framework that is evidence-based. Greater than half of the patients presenting with acute atrial fibrillation will convert spontaneously to sinus rhythm within a 24-hour period. In patients who are hemodynamically stable, identifying the time of onset of atrial fibrillation is critical with regard to the initiation of anticoagulation and the decision as to whether cardioversion, either electrical or chemical, should be attempted. For chronic atrial fibrillation, a conservative approach with rate control and anticoagulation remains a safe, effective and often preferable mode of management. Those patients who are hemodynamically unstable must undergo immediate cardioversion. The patient's disposition depends ultimately on the chronicity of atrial fibrillation, symptoms, and presence of underlying structural abnormalities. It is expected that, as our approach to patients presenting with atrial fibrillation becomes more clearly delineated, a greater subset of these patients may be managed safely and discharged from the emergency department setting with appropriate longitudinal follow-up.

Acknowledgments

The authors wish to express their gratitude to Dr. Win-Kuang Shen for his expert review of this article as well as Ms. Susan Puetz for her tireless assistance in its preparation.

References

[1] Connors S, Dorian P. Management of supraventricular tachycardia in the emergency department. Can J Cardiol 1997;13(Suppl A):19A–24A.

[2] Ryder KM, Benjamin EJ. Epidemiology and significance of atrial fibrillation. Am J Cardiol 1999;84(9A):131R–8R.

[3] Benjamin EJ, Wolf PA, D'Agostino RB, et al. Impact of atrial fibrillation on the risk of death: the Framingham Heart Study. Circulation 1998;98(10):946–52.

[4] Nattel S. New ideas about atrial fibrillation 50 years on. Nature 2002;415(6868):219–26 [review].

[5] Atrial Fibrillation Investigators. Risk factors for stroke and efficacy of antithrombotic therapy in atrial fibrillation: analysis of pooled data from five randomized control trials. Arch Intern Med 1994;154:1449–57.

[6] Ortiz J, Niwano S, Abe H, et al. Mapping the conversion of atrial flutter to atrial fibrillation and atrial fibrillation to atrial flutter: insights into mechanisms. Circ Res 1994;74(5): 882–94.

[7] Prystowsky EN. Tachycardia-induced tachycardia: a mechanism of initiation of atrial fibrillation. In: DiMarco JP, Prystowsky EN, editors. Atrial arrhythmias: state of the art. Armonk (NY): Furtura Publishing Co, 1995. p. 81–95.

[8] Kannel WB, Abbott RD, Savage DD, et al. Coronary heart disease and atrial fibrillation: the Framingham Study. Am Heart J 1983;106(2):389–96.

[9] Fuster V, Ryden LE, Asinger RW, et al. ACC/AHA/ESC guidelines for the management of patients with atrial fibrillation: executive summary a report of the American College of Cardiology/American Heart Association Task Force on Practice Guidelines and the European Society of Cardiology Committee for Practice Guidelines and Policy Conferences (Committee to Develop Guidelines for the Management of Patients with Atrial Fibrillation) developed in collaboration with the North American Society of Pacing and Electrophysiology. Circulation 2001;104(17):2118–50.

[10] Jung F, DiMarco JP. Treatment strategies for atrial fibrillation. Am J Med 1998;104(3): 272–86.

[11] Page R, Tilsch TW, Connolly SJ, et al. Aymptomatic or "silent" atrial fibrillation: frequency in untreated patients and patients receiving azimilide. Circulation 2003;107:1141–5.

[12] Wolf PA, Kannel WB, McGee DL, et al. Duration of atrial fibrillation and imminence of stroke: the Framingham study. Stroke 1983;14(5):664–7.

[13] Hamada T, Hiraki T, Ikeda H, et al. Mechanisms for atrial fibrillation in patients with Wolff-Parkinson-White syndrome. J Cardiovasc Electrophysiol 2002;13(3):223–9.

[14] Klein AL, Grimm RA, Murray RD, et al for the Assessment Of Cardioversion Using Transesophageal Echocardiography Investigators. Use of transesophageal echocardiography to guide cardioversion in patients with atrial fibrillation. N Engl J Med 2001;344(19): 1411–20.

[15] American Heart Association. Part 6: Advanced cardiovascular life support: section 7: algorithm approach to ACLS emergencies: 7C: a guide to the international ACLS algorithms. Circulation 2000;102(Suppl I):S158–65.
[16] Elam K, Bolar-Softich KL. Dilemmas in the acute pharmacologic treatment of uncontrolled atrial fibrillation. Am J Emerg Med 1997;15(4):418–9.
[17] Barbier GH, Shettigar UR, Appunn DO. Clinical rationale for the use of an ultra-short acting beta-blocker: esmolol. Int J Clin Pharmacol Ther 1995;33(4):212–8.
[18] Van Noord T, Van Gelder IC, Tieleman RG, et al. VERDICT: the Verapamil versus Digoxin Cardioversion Trial: a randomized study on the role of calcium lowering for maintenance of sinus rhythm after cardioversion of persistent atrial fibrillation. J Cardiovasc Electrophysiol 2001;12(7):766–9.
[19] Van Gelder IC, Hagens VE, Bosker HA, et al for the Rate Control versus Electrical Cardioversion for Persistent Atrial Fibrillation Study Group. A comparison of rate control and rhythm control in patients with recurrent persistent atrial fibrillation. N Engl J Med 2002;347(23):1834–40.
[20] Wyse DG, Waldo AL, DiMarco JP, et al for the Atrial Fibrillation Follow-up Investigation of Rhythm Management (AFFIRM) Investigators. A comparison of rate control and rhythm control in patients with atrial fibrillation. N Engl J Med 2002;347(23):1825–33.
[21] Marshall D, Levy AR, Vidaillet H, et al. Cost-effectiveness of rhythm versus rate control in atrial fibrillation. Ann Intern Med 2004;141:653–60.
[22] Fynn SP, Todd DM, Hobbs WJ, et al. Clinical evaluation of a policy of early repeated internal cardioversion for recurrence of atrial fibrillation. J Cardiovasc Electrophysiol 2002; 13(2):135–41.
[23] Bertaglia E, D'Este D, Zerbo F, et al. Success of serial external electrical cardioversion of persistent atrial fibrillation in maintaining sinus rhythm: a randomized study. Eur Heart J 2002;23(19):1522–8.
[24] Danias PG, Caulfield TA, Weigner MJ, et al. Likelihood of spontaneous conversion of atrial fibrillation to sinus rhythm. J Am Coll Cardiol 1998;31(3):588–92.
[25] Decker WW, Goyal DG, Boie ET, et al. A prospective, randomized trial of an emergency department observation unit for acute onset atrial fibrillation. Acad Emerg Med 2003;10(5): 543–4 [abstract: 358].
[26] Flaker GC, Blackshear JL, McBride R, et al for the Stroke Prevention in Atrial Fibrillation Investigators. Antiarrhythmic drug therapy and cardiac mortality in atrial fibrillation. J Am Coll Cardiol 1992;20(3):527–32.
[27] Michael JA, Stiell IG, Agarwal S, et al. Cardioversion of paroxysmal atrial fibrillation in the emergency department. Ann Emerg Med 1999;33(4):379–87.
[28] Page RL, Kerber RE, Russell JK. Biphasic versus monophasic shock waveform for conversion of atrial fibrillation. JACC 2002;39(12):1956–63.
[29] Van Noord T, Van Gelder IC, Crijns HJ. How to enhance acute outcome of electrical cardioversion by drug therapy: importance of immediate reinitiation of atrial fibrillation. J Cardiovasc Electrophysiol 2002;13(8):822–5.
[30] Stoddard MF, Dawkins PR, Prince CR, et al. Transesophageal echocardiographic guidance of cardioversion in patients with atrial fibrillation. Am Heart J 1995;129(6):1204–15.
[31] Weigner MJ, Caulfield TA, Danias PG, et al. Risk for clinical thromboembolism associated with conversion to sinus rhythm in patients with atrial fibrillation lasting less than 48 hours. Ann Intern Med 1997;126(8):615–20.
[32] Go AS, Hylek EM, Chang Y, et al. Anticoagulation therapy for stroke prevention in atrial fibrillation: how well do randomized trials translate into clinical practice? JAMA 2003; 290(20):2685–92.
[33] Gage BF, Waterman AD, Shannon W, et al. Validation of clinical classification schemes for predicting stroke: results from the National Registry of Atrial Fibrillation. JAMA 2001; 285(22):2864–70.

[34] Cox JL, Canavan TE, Schuessler RB, et al. The surgical treatment of atrial fibrillation: II: intraoperative electrophysiologic mapping and description of the electrophysiologic basis of atrial flutter and atrial fibrillation. J Thorac Cardiovasc Surg 1991;101:406–26.

[35] Swartz JF, Pellersels G, Silvers J, et al. A catheter-based curative approach to atrial fibrillation in humans. Circulation 1994;90(Suppl I):I335 [abstract].

[36] Man KC, Daoud E, Knight B, et al. Right atrial radiofrequency catheter ablation of paroxysmal atrial fibrillation. J Am Coll Cardiol 1996;27(Suppl A):188A [abstract].

[37] Murgatroyd FD, Slade AKB, Sopher SM, et al. Efficacy and tolerability of transvenous low energy cardioversion of paroxysmal atrial fibrillation in humans. J Am Coll Cardiol 1995;26: 1347–53.

ELSEVIER
SAUNDERS

Emerg Med Clin N Am
23 (2005) 1141–1158

EMERGENCY
MEDICINE
CLINICS OF
NORTH AMERICA

Severe Hypertension in the Emergency Department Patient

Rachel M. Gilmore, MB, MRCPI,
Stephan J. Miller, MD, Latha G. Stead, MD, FACEP*

Department of Emergency Medicine, Mayo Clinic College of Medicine, 200 First Street, SW, Rochester, MN 55905, USA

Hypertension affects approximately 50 million people in the United States and over one billion people worldwide. One third of hypertensive patients remain undiagnosed. Despite the availability of effective antihypertensive therapies, two thirds of hypertensive patients fail to achieve satisfactory control [1].This theme is consistent worldwide. A survey in the United Kingdom indicated only 6% of hypertensive patients had their blood pressure lowered consistently below 140/90 mmHg [2,3]. Aging of the population will be inevitably associated with further increases in the prevalence of this disorder [1,4].

Hypertension-related Emergency Department (ED) visits may account for over one quarter of all acute medical emergencies in busy urban areas [5]. Many more patients who have unrelated complaints are found to have markedly raised blood pressure readings while they are in the ED. Despite this finding, there is no clear consensus on the most appropriate management of these patients. This, at least in part, reflects the great heterogeneity of this population. The challenge facing emergency physicians is to discern rapidly those patients who require aggressive blood pressure reduction and to provide tailored therapy based on physiologic goals that go beyond mere reduction in numbers.

By convention, severely elevated blood pressure is defined as a systolic blood pressure (SBP) greater than 180 mmHg or diastolic blood pressure (DBP) of over 120 mmHg [6,7]. This arbitrary cutoff is of little relevance to the emergency physician because the majority of these patients do not require emergent blood pressure reduction. Conversely, patients who have

* Corresponding author.
E-mail address: stead.latha@mayo.edu (L.G. Stead).

0733-8627/05/$ - see front matter
doi:10.1016/j.emc.2005.07.012

mild blood pressure elevation may require immediate antihypertensive therapy as part of a life-saving treatment [8,9]. The patient with thoracic aortic dissection and a blood pressure of 140/90 mmHg would constitute such an emergency, whereas the chronically hypertensive patient with a pressure of 200/130 mmHg but no acute end-organ compromise would not.

In this context, the triage of patients who have severely elevated blood pressure is best determined by searching for the presence of acute target organ damage. If present, this clinical scenario is defined as a *hypertensive emergency* that requires immediate reduction in blood pressure within 1 hour. There is more ambiguity in relation to the optimal classification of patients who have severely elevated blood pressure who are not experiencing target organ compromise. *Hypertensive urgencies* involve patients who may not be in immediate danger but for whom continued severe hypertension poses a significant short-term threat [6] and for whom the urgent initiation of oral therapy and perhaps even a period of inpatient observation may be warranted. All other patients with blood pressures over 180/120 mmHg are defined as having *severe uncontrolled hypertension*. Although these patients undoubtedly would benefit from long-term blood pressure control, they have a low short-term risk for end-organ damage and do not need emergent antihypertensive therapy or inpatient monitoring.

Causes

Hypertensive emergencies and urgencies can be associated with any disorder that leads to increased blood pressure. Some diseases such as pheochromocytoma or renovascular hypertension have a greater tendency to precipitate such a crisis. Essential hypertension accounts for the majority of cases of hypertension; thus, most hypertensive emergencies are seen in this setting. Inadequate blood pressure control and noncompliance are common precipitants [8,10]. The incidence of hypertensive crises (hypertensive emergencies and urgencies) is higher among African Americans and the elderly [11,12]. Nonetheless, less than 1% of patients who have primary hypertension go on to develop the accelerated malignant phase. *Accelerated hypertension* is defined as severely elevated blood pressure associated with grade-3 retinopathy on fundoscopy. Malignant hypertension denotes the presence of papilledema. This incidence of malignant hypertension has remained constant over the last quarter of a century despite the evolution of a wide range of highly effective therapies [13].

Pathogenesis

An appreciation of the mechanisms underlying normal blood pressure regulation is vital for the correct interpretation of the many forms of hypertensive crisis and may guide the clinician in selecting the most appropriate therapy. Blood pressure (*BP*) is the product of cardiac output (*CO*) and peripheral vascular resistance (*PVR*), where BP = CO × PVR. Cardiac output is itself determined by heart rate and stroke volume, in which the latter is dependent on intrinsic myocardial contractility and the preload of the heart. For any increase in BP to occur, an imbalance in these variables is required. Most commonly, either a disproportionate increase in peripheral vascular resistance or intravascular volume is responsible, which is offset inadequately by feedback mechanisms that regulate blood pressure homeostasis. These fundamental principles apply equally to uncomplicated chronic hypertension and to a hypertensive crisis [14,15].

Markedly elevated blood pressure is a cause for concern in any clinical context. However, the single most important factor leading to the development of a hypertensive crisis is not the absolute change in blood pressure but the rate at which mean arterial pressure (MAP) rises [16,17]. Patients with chronically elevated blood pressure undergo adaptive vascular changes, which, although in the long-term may be detrimental, may serve to protect end organs from acute increases in blood pressure. In contrast, patients who develop acutely elevated blood pressure without pre-existing hypertension suffer end-organ damage even at relatively lower blood pressure levels [16].

When blood pressure rises, it exerts a mechanical stress on the vessel wall. Under normal circumstances, the blood vessel will respond by vasoconstriction, supporting the vascular endothelium and minimizing acute injury. This phenomenon is known as *autoregulation*. In severe, rapidly evolving hypertensive states, this ability to autoregulate is overwhelmed, local vasodilation ensues, and the shear forces are transmitted to the endothelium. Endothelial damage leads to enhanced vascular permeability and leakage, with deposition of plasma proteins and fibrinogen in vessel walls. Mediators of coagulation and cell proliferation also are activated, with adverse short- and long-term consequences [18]. Fibrinoid necrosis is the pathologic lesion characteristic of this type of arteriolar injury. This disruption of the arteriolar wall causes obstruction of the vessel and downstream ischemia. These changes are visible directly in the retina as linear hemorrhages dissecting along nerve fibers associated with cotton-wool spots of swollen, ischemic axons.

An important driver of many acute hypertensive emergencies is the renin-angiotensin-aldosterone system. Under normal circumstances, this system plays a valuable role in the regulation of blood pressure and sodium homeostasis [14]. Renin produced by the kidney stimulates the formation of angiotensin II, a potent vasoconstrictor. This in turn promotes aldosterone release and consequently the avid retention of salt and water. Significant increases in both peripheral vascular resistance and intravascular volume combine to produce an elevation in blood pressure. In situations such as acute intravascular volume depletion, this may be a life-saving system.

However, when it is dysregulated, this system may play a central role in exacerbating hypertensive crises [16]. Regardless of the cause of the initial abrupt rise in blood pressure, if renovascular injury and ischemia ensue, this system will be activated, generating a feedback loop of further rises in blood pressure, which result in yet more renovascular insult. This vicious cycle will lead inevitably to progressive end-organ damage if left unchecked [7,16,18].

Clinical evaluation

The medical history should focus on symptoms of target organ compromise, including headache, chest pain, dyspnea, interscapular pain, visual disturbance, and altered mental status. The medical history should also clearly document the duration and severity of pre-existing hypertension, the quality of blood pressure control, compliance, and the presence of previous end-organ damage. The patient's current medications may provide important clues to the underlying cause of their condition. In addition, the use of monoamine oxidase inhibitors and any illicit drugs may play a critical role in the development of hypertensive crisis.

Persistently elevated blood pressure should be confirmed in both upper limbs with an appropriately sized cuff. The physical examination should focus on the commonly affected target organs, retina, heart, brain, and kidneys, seeking evidence of acute or chronic injury. Fundoscopic examination is important, looking in particular for the presence of new hemorrhages, hard exudates, or papilledema. Evidence of cardiovascular compromise includes signs of pulmonary edema (S_3, pulmonary rales, and elevated jugular venous pressure) or signs of aortic dissection (pulse discrepancy among limbs and new aortic regurgitation murmur). Neurologic assessment should include mental status, visual fields, and focal neurologic signs to exclude hypertensive encephalopathy, intracranial hemorrhage, and acute ischemic stroke.

A complete blood count, electrolytes, blood urea nitrogen, creatinine level, and a urinalysis are valuable first-line investigations in patients presenting with severely elevated BP. For those with chest/back pain or shortness of breath, chest radiography findings of mediastinal widening or pulmonary edema should be sought. A 12-lead ECG should be obtained and examined for evidence of myocardial ischemia or hypertrophy. The ECG has been shown to be abnormal in over 20% of asymptomatic ED patients who have a diastolic blood pressure greater than 115 mmHg [19]. CT of the head is indicated in patients who have altered mental status or focal neurologic signs. If there is a suspicion of illicit drug use, urine toxicology for cocaine and amphetamines may be helpful in confirming the diagnosis. Some practitioners advocate reserving a serum sample for a renin assay before commencing therapy, which may be valuable in guiding the long-term management of the patient [7].

Autoregulation

The safe management of hypertensive emergencies requires an understanding of vascular autoregulation of vital organs. The brain, kidneys, and heart exhibit mechanisms that protect from ischemic damage when blood pressure drops abruptly, a mechanism that has been described most extensively in the brain [20].

When aortic blood pressure rises, cerebral vasoconstriction occurs. Conversely, when blood pressure falls, intracerebral vessels dilate. This ensures that cerebral blood flow remains constant over a wide range of mean arterial pressures. Although individuals with normal cerebral vasculature can tolerate rapid reductions in blood pressure, this is not true of the majority that suffers hypertensive crises. Chronic hypertension, cerebral vascular disease, and aging tend to impair normal cerebral autoregulation. When antihypertensive drugs lower the blood pressure too quickly, chronically hypertensive individuals may not tolerate the reduction and experience cerebral hypoperfusion. Symptoms include weakness and dizziness, but if this relative hypotension is sustained, there is a risk of ischemia and infarction. Standgaard [21] has reported that the lower limit of autoregulation occurred at an average MAP of 113 mmHg in chronic hypertensive subjects, compared with 73 mmHg in normotensive controls. A reduction in MAP of 15% to 20% is felt to be safe when treating most hypertensive emergencies. In the setting of stroke, greater caution is warranted as acute cerebral ischemia is associated with further impairment of cerebral autoregulation. A reduction of less than 2% in this setting may lead to an extension of the infarcted area [14].

Management of hypertensive emergencies

As defined above, hypertensive emergencies are clinical scenarios that require immediate blood pressure reduction (not necessarily to the normal range) to prevent or limit target organ damage (Fig. 1). Patients presenting to the ED with critical elevation in blood pressure and signs of end-organ damage require prompt treatment to avoid catastrophic injury to the central nervous system, the heart, or the kidneys. It is equally important to avoid overzealous treatment leading to an excessively rapid drop in blood pressure. Hypertensive emergency patients should be placed on a cardiac monitor, and intravenous access should be established. An arterial line may be placed to confirm the cuff readings and to guide therapy.

Goals

The Seventh Report of the Joint National Committee (JNC-7) on Prevention, Detection, Evaluation, and Treatment of High Blood Pressure [1] recommends an initial reduction of mean arterial pressure by no more

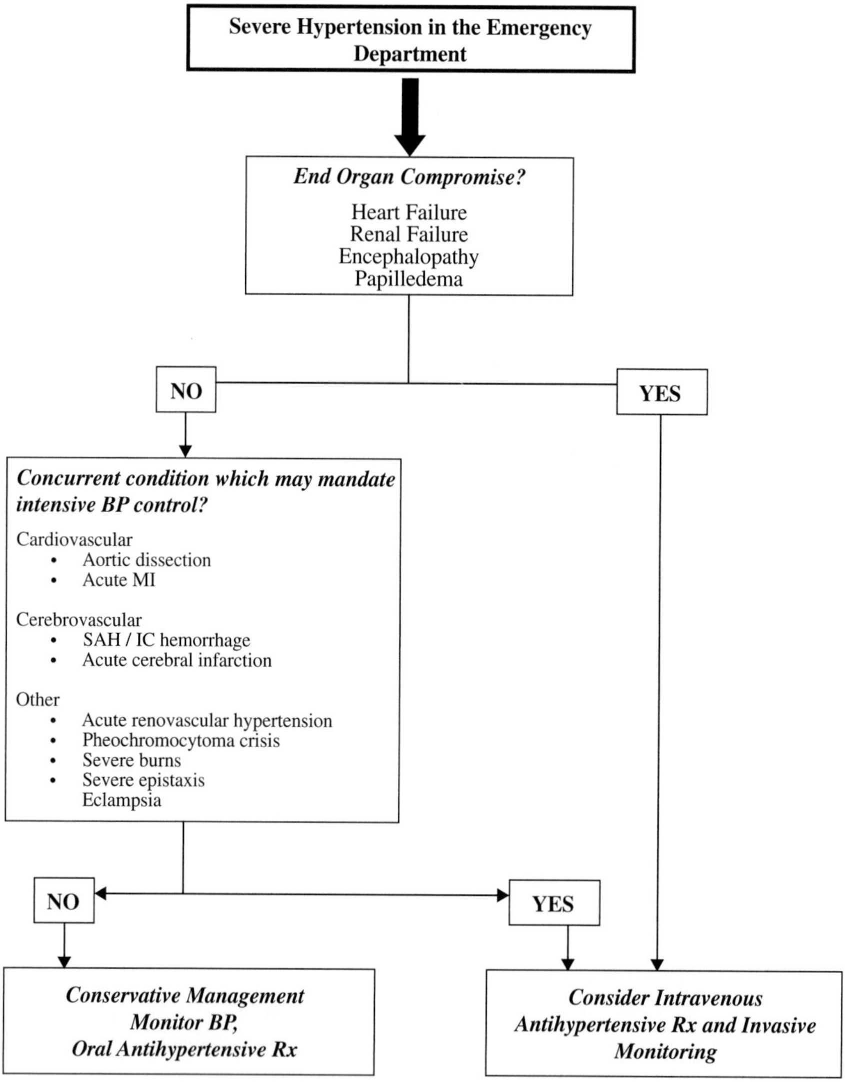

Fig. 1. Management of severe hypertension in the ED.

than 25%, within a range of minutes to 1 hour. If the patient is stable, this initial reduction should be followed by further reduction toward a goal of 160/100 mmHg within 2 to 6 hours. A gradual reduction toward a normal BP may be pursued over the next 8 to 24 hours if the patient is stable.

Drug treatment

There have been no large clinical trials investigating optimum therapy in patients presenting with hypertensive emergencies. The choice of pharmacologic therapy is based on the underlying medical condition and end organ involved. Generally, parenteral drug therapy is recommended because of the faster onset of action, ease of titration, and the fact that treatment can be can be discontinued readily in the event of hypotension. Some of the more important pharmacologic agents used in hypertensive emergencies are discussed here and summarized in Table 1.

Sodium nitroprusside is a powerful vasodilator with a direct effect on the smooth muscle of both resistance and capacitance vessels. Its very rapid onset and cessation of action when stopped make it the drug of choice for most hypertensive emergencies. Hemodynamic effects include a decrease in MAP, afterload and preload, and an increase in renal blood flow. Cardiac output generally is not affected, but it may improve in patients who have heart failure. However, because sodium nitroprusside acts as an arteriolar

Table 1
Parental drugs for treatment of hypertensive emergency

Drug	Dosage	Onset/Duration	Adverse effects
Vasodilators			
Nitroprusside	0.25–10 μg/kg/min as IV infusion	Instantaneous/ 1–2 min	Nausea, vomiting, muscle twitching, thiocyanate and cyanide poisoning
Nitroglycerin	5–100 μg/min as IV infusion	1–5 min/ 3–5 min	Flushing, headache, vomiting, methemoglobinemia
Nicardipine	5–15 mg/h IV	5–10 min/1–4 h	Tachycardia, headache, nausea, flushing; avoid in heart failure
Hydralazine	10–20 mg IV	5–15 min/3–8 h	Marked hypotension, tachycardia, flushing; avoid in aortic dissection and MI
	10–40 mg IM	20–30 min	
Enalapril	1.25–5 mg q6 h	30 min/6 h	Marked hypotension in high renin states, renal failure, hyperkalemia
Fenoldopam	0.1–0.3 μg/kg per min IV infusion	5 min/ 10–15 min	Tachycardia, headache, flushing, nausea
Adrenergic inhibitors			
Labetalol	20–80 mg IV bolus every 10 min, 2 mg/min IV infusion	5–10 min/3–6 h	Heart block, orthostatic hypotension; avoid in heart failure and asthma
Esmolol	200–500 μg/kg/min for 4 min, then 150–300 μg/kg/min IV	1–2 min/ 10–20 min	Hypotension; avoid in heart failure and asthma
Phentolamine	5–15 mg IV	1–2 min/ 3–10 min	Tachycardia, flushing, headache

Abbreviations: IV, intravenous; MI, myocardial infarction.

dilator, it may increase intracranial pressure (ICP) secondary to increased blood flow [22]. In many cases, however, this increase is counteracted by decreased mean arterial pressure, with an overall neutralizing effect on ICP. Prolonged use, for greater than 3 to 4 days, may lead to cyanide toxicity, particularly in patients who have renal or hepatic dysfunction.

Labetalol is an excellent treatment for many hypertensive emergencies. As an adrenergic antagonist that combines α- and non-cardioselective β-blocking properties, labetalol effectively reduces peripheral vascular resistance without reflex tachycardia. It has little effect on the cerebral vasculature, hence, it is an attractive option in cases with raised ICP. The main disadvantage of labetalol is its relatively long duration of action. The usual precautions of β-blocking medication also apply.

Intravenous calcium-channel blockers can be useful in most situations. Sublingual nifedepine, a powerful antihypertensive, however, should be avoided. Although nifedepine has been used widely in the past, numerous serious adverse effects related to uncontrolled hypotension have been reported [12,23–28]. Intravenous nicardipine has been found to provide responses similar to nitroprusside, with very few side effects [29].

Volume depletion is common in patients who have hypertensive emergency because of pressure natriuresis and may lead to an excessive fall in blood pressure during treatment. In fact, there have been some reports of volume expansion with saline leading to a reduction in BP [30,31]. Therefore, diuretics should be avoided unless they are specifically indicated. Other useful drugs in the management of hypertensive emergencies include hydralazine, nitroglycerin, and fenoldopam.

Hypertensive encephalopathy

Hypertensive encephalopathy results from hyperperfusion of the brain when the upper limit of cerebral autoperfusion is exceeded, resulting in cerebral edema, petechial hemorrhages, and microinfarcts [6,20,32,33]. Today, this reaction is uncommon because even a minor reduction in blood pressure with antihypertensive therapy seems to be protective. Hypertensive encephalopathy is more likely to occur in normotensive individuals who experience a rapid rise in blood pressure, such as a child with acute renal failure caused by acute glomerulonephritis. The symptoms include severe headache, nausea, vomiting, visual disturbances, confusion, and focal or generalized weakness. Signs include disorientation, seizures, and focal neurologic signs. Neuroimaging is important to rule out other intracranial pathology such as intracerebral or subarachnoid bleeding.

Hypertensive encephalopathy is reversible with the reduction of blood pressure, but if it is left untreated, it may result in coma and even death. The goal of therapy is to reduce the mean arterial pressure by no more than 25% or the diastolic blood pressure to 100 mmHg (whichever represents the lesser reduction) in the first hour of treatment [16,34]. Deterioration in neurologic function with blood pressure reduction should prompt consideration of stopping or lowering the dose of the infusion. Sodium nitroprusside has been the mainstay of treatment for hypertensive encephalopathy in the past. However, because nitroprusside is a powerful arteriolar dilator, a rise in ICP may rarely be precipitated. Therefore, other parenteral agents such as labetalol, fenoldopam, and nicardipine are now used more widely.

Intracerebral hemorrhage

Hypertension is the most important risk factor for intracerebral hemorrhage (ICH) [35] and is seen commonly in the acute post-hemorrhage period [36]. This blood pressure rise tends to be more severe and less likely to resolve spontaneously compared with hypertension following cerebral infarction [37,38]. An elevated blood pressure immediately after ICH is associated with hematoma expansion and poorer outcomes [39]. However, it remains unclear whether the elevated blood pressure is primarily a cause or consequence of this association.

Cerebral perfusion pressure (*CPP*) depends on the mean arterial pressure and intracranial pressure, where CPP = MAP − ICP. As the intracranial pressure rises, the MAP also must rise if sufficient cerebral perfusion pressure is to be maintained. However, as the MAP rises so too, theoretically, does the risk of re-bleeding from ruptured small arteries and arterioles. A prospective observational study [40] that measured baseline blood pressure and growth in the volume of ICH has not confirmed such concerns, but the frequent early use of antihypertensive agents in this series may have obscured the true nature of this relationship. This issue is further complicated by recognizing that the cerebral autoregulation curve of patients who have chronic hypertension is in many cases permanently altered, making these patients less likely to tolerate aggressive lowering of blood pressure.

Controversy remains, and the current guidelines from the American Heart Association (AHA) recommend decreasing the blood pressure when the MAP is greater than 130 mmHg or when the SBP is greater than 220 mmHg [41].

Subarachnoid hemorrhage

Severe hypertension also is a common feature in the acute phase of subarachnoid hemorrhage (SAH) [42,43]. In common with ICH, the management of blood pressure must balance the risk of re-bleeding with the risk of cerebral ischemia. Nimodipine has been shown to significantly improve outcomes following SAH [42]. This is likely because of a reduction in vasospasm caused by chemical irritation of arteries by blood in the subarachnoid space. It is not recommended, however, for routine blood pressure reduction because of a high incidence in transient hypotension [44,45].

The patient's cognitive status may be a useful guide to the state of cerebral perfusion pressure. If the patient is alert, then CPP probably is adequate, and careful blood pressure lowering could be considered. The management of patients who have a severely impaired level of consciousness should be more circumspect. Direct ICP monitoring allows MAP to be titrated with greater precision in these cases.

If blood pressure reduction is required in the acute phase of ICH or SAH, intravenous esmolol or labetalol is the agent of choice because it allows rapid and safe titration. Intravenous nitroprusside should be considered to be a second-line agent because of the risk of increasing ICP.

Acute ischemic stroke

The elevation in arterial blood pressure occurs in over 80% of all acute ischemic strokes (AIS) [38]. This elevation may be caused by an acute sympathetic response or by chronic hypertension, which is a major risk factor for AIS.

A similar basic physiology in respect to cerebral perfusion applies, as discussed above in the context of intracranial bleeding. However, in the setting of an acute cerebral infarct, specific considerations are a little different. On the one hand, high blood pressure may be associated with an increased risk of cerebral edema and hemorrhagic transformation of the infarct [43]. On the other hand, the elevation in ICP not matched by an increased MAP risks extension of the infarct to involve the so-called ischemic penumbra. Furthermore, in patients who have AIS, the cerebral perfusion pressure beyond the acute obstruction is low. The distal vessels become dilated, and with ongoing ischemia, their ability to autoregulate is diminished. An abrupt restoration of brisk perfusion in this setting may run an increased risk of vascular compromise and hemorrhage and has been a significant factor limiting the overall success of reperfusion therapy in this context.

Blood pressure reduction after a stroke tends to be challenging, with even minimal intervention often leading to precipitous drops in pressure. Expectant management may be most appropriate because blood pressure often declines spontaneously in the first few hours [46]. A decline to prestroke values within 4 days of the acute event is documented frequently [47]. In the literature, high blood pressure after a stroke has been associated with both good [48,49] and poor outcomes [50,51]. Recent observational studies also demonstrate low blood pressure to be associated with poor outcome [52–55]. A Cochrane review that examines 65 randomized controlled trials comprising 11,500 patients concludes that there is insufficient evidence to evaluate the effect of altering blood pressure on outcome after an acute stroke. Consequently, current AIS guidelines from the AHA recommend that BP be reduced only if the SBP exceeds 220 mmHg, or the DBP exceeds 120 mmHg, or if there is evidence of end-organ damage believed to be related to the elevation in blood pressure [56]. If blood pressure must be reduced after an AIS, labetolol or sodium nitroprusside is the agent suggested by both the AHA and the European stroke initiative [57]. Patients who are being considered for thrombolysis must have a blood pressure less than 185/110 mmHg, and labetolol is the agent recommended to achieve and maintain this goal [56].

Aortic dissection

Acute aortic dissection is a rare but potentially catastrophic illness. In the Emergency Department, the immediate reduction in blood pressure and, particularly, in shear stress (the ratio of change in blood pressure [Δp] with change in time [Δt]) is essential to limit the extent of dissection while surgical treatment is being considered or arranged. Initial therapeutic goals should include the elimination of pain and reduction of systolic blood pressure to 100 to 120 mmHg or the lowest level commensurate with adequate vital organ perfusion [34,58]. Blood pressure reduction should proceed in tandem with reduction in the force of left ventricular contraction (Δp/Δt). Sodium nitroprusside used in combination with a β-blocker such as propranolol is a good first-line therapy. Labetalol is an excellent alternative because it combines α- and β-adrenergic receptor blocking properties, achieving reductions in both shear stress and arterial pressure with a single agent [59].

Myocardial ischemia or infarction

Acute myocardial ischemia may be complicated by hypertension because of pain, anxiety, and increased sympathetic tone. An elevation in blood pressure increases afterload, resulting in greater myocardial work and oxygen requirements. In addition, increased wall stress is associated with impairment of subendocardial tissue perfusion, leading to further imbalance in myocardial oxygen supply and demand.

Combined with reperfusion and antithrombotic therapies, the reduction in blood pressure and heart rate can serve to minimize the extent of myocardial injury sustained. β-blockers are the antihypertensive of choice because they reduce heart rate and blood pressure while also elevating the threshold for ventricular fibrillation. Nitroglycerin is a useful adjunct for patients who have ongoing pain, especially if blood pressure remains elevated. Beta-blockers and ACE inhibitors have been shown to reduce mortality in patients who have myocardial infarction [60,61]. Pure vasodilators (such as nitroprusside) should be used with caution because they can induce reflex tachycardia and hence aggravate myocardial ischemia. BP should be aggressively controlled in patients who have ST-elevation MI who are being considered for thrombolytic therapy [23].

Acute left ventricular failure

Patients who present with acute pulmonary edema often have marked hypertension. After treatment, many of these patients are found to have a normal ejection fraction on echocardiogram. Long-standing hypertension frequently results in myocardial hypertrophy, which leads to impaired left ventricular filling and consequent elevation in pulmonary venous pressures. Further acute rise in blood pressure in this setting may be enough to precipitate an episode of pulmonary edema or diastolic heart failure [62]. These patients require a rapid reduction in blood pressure. Intravenous nitroprusside or nitroglycerin is very useful in this situation. Titrate the dose until the blood pressure is controlled and the signs of heart failure are alleviated.

Left ventricular systolic dysfunction may also be associated with hypertension because of markedly increased sympathetic tone. Reduction in afterload and preload of the heart with nitroprusside or nitroglycine is again the mainstay of therapy in this context.

Renal insufficiency

Renal insufficiency is both an important cause and consequence of rapidly progressive hypertension. Both primary renal diseases (glomerulonephritis, renal artery stenosis, and vasculitis) and the medications used to treat them (steroids, cyclosporin), can cause severe elevations in BP. Conversely, chronic hypertension accounts for 30% of cases of end-stage renal disease.

The primary goal in treating patients who have new onset renal disease is prevention of further renal damage through blood pressure control. Therapy should be directed toward reducing systemic blood pressure while maintaining adequate renal blood flow. Sodium nitroprusside is effective, as are IV calcium antagonist such as nicarpidine [12].

Hypertensive urgencies

Hypertensive urgencies have traditionally been described as situations where severe elevations in blood pressure are not causing immediate end-organ damage, but should be controlled within 24 hours [6,7,63,64]. However, there have been no clinical trials to clearly define which patients are at greatest risk of developing complications if left untreated over this time period. Accordingly, this is probably the most difficult category of patient to identify within the ED.

It has been well documented that long-term treatment of hypertension reduces cardiovascular morbidity and mortality [65,66]. Over the years, the threshold for treatment and the targets sought have steadily fallen. The recent Hypertension Optimal Treatment (HOT) randomized trial demonstrated a treatment benefit all the way down to a DBP of 82 mmHg [67].

There is very little evidence however to support a significant short-term benefit of blood pressure control [68]. A landmark study of hypertension published in the 1960's provides useful insights in this context. It compared placebo with drug treatment in patients who have severe hypertension, defined as DBPs between 115 and 130 mmHg. No difference in adverse events within the first 3 months was demonstrated. Furthermore, there is a growing body of evidence to suggest the practice of urgently lowering blood pressure in patients who have uncontrolled severe hypertension may actually be associated with increased risk to the patient [69].

Shayne and Pitts [19], in a recent review of this topic, have suggested that patients who have evidence of previous end-organ damage but who are not acutely compromised should be defined as having a hypertensive urgency and merit closer monitoring and follow-up. Other investigators have argued for a simpler classification of just two categories, hypertensive emergency and uncontrolled severe hypertension, with all patients in the latter class receiving close follow-up until a gradual reduction in blood pressure to target levels has been achieved.

Most antihypertensive drugs with a relatively short onset of action have been shown to be effective in the treatment of severely elevated BP. The more commonly used oral agents are described here and are summarized in Table 2. Captopril is the fastest acting oral angiotensin-converting enzyme (ACE) inhibitor. At low doses it rarely causes marked hypotension, although this potential exists particularly among those who are volume-depleted or who have renal artery stenosis [70]. Clonidine also is widely used in this setting, and the dose can be repeated hourly to safely and effectively reduce very high blood pressure. Clonidine has similar efficacy to nifedipine but a more favorable safety profile [71]. Side effects include rebound hypertension and sedation. Short-acting nifedipine is not recommended because patients are subjected to possible uncontrolled hypotension [1,12]. Labetalol is available in an oral preparation, which can be given in hourly doses and has been shown to be highly effective in the acute reduction of blood pressure [72].

Table 2
Oral drugs for hypertensive urgencies

Drug	Dosage	Onset/ Duration	Indications	Adverse effects
Captopril	6.25–25mg q6 h	15–30 min/6 h	Well tolerated in most scenarios	Hypotension in high renin states
Clonidine	0.1–0.2 mg hourly, to max 0.8 mg in 24 h	30–60 min/ 6–12 h	Severe uncomplicated hypertension	Sedation, bradycardia, dry mouth
Labetalol	100–200 mg q12 h	30–120 min/ 8–12 h	Well tolerated in most scenarios	Heart failure, heart block, bronchospasm

Uncontrolled severe hypertension

The treatment of uncontrolled severe hypertension is probably best initiated by the patient's regular physician, who will monitor the effect of such therapy over time. Treatment usually is lifelong, and compliance is a major issue. In some situations however, the decision to initiate treatment is made in the ED. Thus, it may be useful for emergency physicians to be familiar with current guidelines for the management of hypertension.

The JNC-7 report amended the previous classification of hypertension, adding a new category designated "prehypertension." This category includes patients who have a SBP of 120 to 139 mmHg or a DBP of 80 to 89 mmHg. Stage-1 hypertension is defined as a SBP of 140 to 159 mmHg or a DBP of 90 to 99 mmHg. Stage-2 hypertension includes all values greater than 160/100 mmHg. Patients are categorized according to risk profiles, and appropriate initial drug therapy regimens are suggested [1].

Treatment should be started and long-term follow up arranged in collaboration with the patient's regular physician. The chosen agent should be easy to take, well tolerated, and affordable to maximize compliance. Thiazide diuretics have a long history in the treatment of hypertension [73] and remain virtually unsurpassed in preventing the cardiovascular complications of this disease [1]. They should be used as the initial therapy for most patients who have hypertension. Diuretics are especially useful in older patients and African Americans, who tend to have lower renin levels and do not respond particularly well to β-blocker or ACE inhibitor monotherapy [74,75]. For other patients, comorbid conditions may govern the choice of tailored antihypertensive therapy. ACE inhibitors, for instance, appear to have several mechanisms of benefit beyond lowering blood pressure in diabetes and are considered first-line agents for these patients. β-blockers may be more suitable for the patient with a history of angina or myocardial infarction.

Summary

Severe hypertension is a problem encountered on a daily basis by emergency physicians. Patients with this condition cover a wide spectrum, from those who are critically ill to those who have isolated blood pressure elevation but low short-term risk of adverse events. The key to correct management is the reliable identification of patients who have hypertensive emergencies. The appropriate intervention must take underlying pathology into account and should be tempered by the avoidance of overzealous blood pressure reduction. Hippocrates' admonishment "primum non nocere" (the first thing [is] to do no harm) was never more relevant than in the care of these patients.

References

[1] Chobanian AV, Bakris GL, Black HR, et al. The seventh report of the Joint National Committee on Prevention, Detection, Evaluation, and Treatment of High Blood Pressure: the JNC 7 report. JAMA 2003;289(19):2560–72.
[2] Colhoun HM, Dong W, Poulter NR. Blood pressure screening, management and control in England: results from the health survey for England 1994. J Hypertens 1998;16(6):747–52.
[3] Mancia G, Sega R, Milesi C, et al. Blood-pressure control in the hypertensive population. Lancet 1997;349(9050):454–7.
[4] Vasan RS, Beiser A, Seshadri S, et al. Residual lifetime risk for developing hypertension in middle-aged women and men: the Framingham Heart Study. JAMA 2002;287(8):1003–10.
[5] Zampaglione B, Pascale C, Marchisio M, et al. Hypertensive urgencies and emergencies: prevalence and clinical presentation. Hypertension 1996;27(1):144–7.
[6] The sixth report of the Joint National Committee on prevention, detection, evaluation, and treatment of high blood pressure. Arch Intern Med 1997;157(21):2413–46.
[7] Kaplan N, Norman M, Lieberman E. Hypertensive crises. In: Kaplan's clinical hypertension. Philadelphia: Lippincott and Wilkins; 2002. p. 339–56.
[8] Bennett NM, Shea S. Hypertensive emergency: case criteria, sociodemographic profile, and previous care of 100 cases. Am J Public Health 1988;78(6):636–40.
[9] Gifford RW Jr. Management of hypertensive crises. JAMA 1991;266(6):829–35.
[10] Kaplan NM. Treatment of hypertensive emergencies and urgencies. Heart Dis Stroke 1992; 1(6):373–8.
[11] Lip GY, Beevers M, Potter JF, et al. Malignant hypertension in the elderly. QJM 1995;88(9): 641–7.
[12] Varon J, Marik PE. The diagnosis and management of hypertensive crises. Chest 2000; 118(1):214–27.
[13] Lip GY, Beevers M, Beevers G. The failure of malignant hypertension to decline: a survey of 24 years' experience in a multiracial population in England. J Hypertens 1994;12(11): 1297–305.
[14] Blumenfeld JD, Laragh JH. Management of hypertensive crises: the scientific basis for treatment decisions. Am J Hypertens 2001;14(11 Pt 1):1154–67.
[15] Laragh JH. Laragh's 25 lessons in pathophysiology and 12 clinical pearls for treating hypertension [abstract, closing summary, and table of contents]. Am J Hypertens 2001; 14(12):1173–7.
[16] Vaughan CJ, Delanty N. Hypertensive emergencies. Lancet 2000;356(9227):411–7.
[17] Finnerty FA Jr. Hypertensive encephalopathy. Am J Med 1972;52(5):672–8.
[18] Kitiyakara C, Guzman NJ. Malignant hypertension and hypertensive emergencies. J Am Soc Nephrol 1998;9(1):133–42.
[19] Shayne PH, Pitts SR. Severely increased blood pressure in the emergency department. Ann Emerg Med 2003;41(4):513–29 [comment] 530–1.
[20] Strandgaard S, Olesen J, Skinhoj E, et al. Autoregulation of brain circulation in severe arterial hypertension. BMJ 1973;1(5852):507–10.
[21] Strandgaard S. Autoregulation of cerebral blood flow in hypertensive patients: the modifying influence of prolonged antihypertensive treatment on the tolerance to acute, drug-induced hypotension. Circulation 1976;53(4):720–7.
[22] Cottrell JE, Patel K, Turndorf H, et al. Intracranial pressure changes induced by sodium nitroprusside in patients with intracranial mass lesions. J Neurosurg 1978;48(3):329–31.
[23] American Heart Association [and] the International Liaison Committee on Resuscitation. Guidelines 2000 for cardiopulmonary resuscitation and emergency cardiovascular care: part 7: the era of reperfusion: acute stroke [section 2]. Circulation 2000;102(Suppl 8):I204–16.
[24] Grossman E, Messerli FH, Grodzicki T, et al. Should a moratorium be placed on sublingual nifedipine capsules given for hypertensive emergencies and pseudoemergencies? JAMA 1996;276(16):1328–31.

[25] Impey L. Severe hypotension and fetal distress following sublingual administration of nifedipine to a patient with severe pregnancy induced hypertension at 33 weeks. BJOG Br J Obstet Gynaecol 1993;100(10):959–61.
[26] O'Mailia JJ, Sander GE, Giles TD. Nifedipine-associated myocardial ischemia or infarction in the treatment of hypertensive urgencies. Ann Intern Med 1987;107(2):185–6.
[27] Schwartz M, Naschitz JE, Yeshurun D, et al. Oral nifedipine in the treatment of hypertensive urgency: cerebrovascular accident following a single dose. Arch Intern Med 1990;150(3): 686–7.
[28] Wachter RM. Symptomatic hypotension induced by nifedipine in the acute treatment of severe hypertension. Arch Intern Med 1987;147(3):556–8.
[29] Neutel JM, Smith DH, Wallin D, et al. A comparison of intravenous nicardipine and sodium nitroprusside in the immediate treatment of severe hypertension. Am J Hypertens 1994;7 (7 Pt 1):623–8.
[30] Baer L, Parra-Carrilo JZ, Radichevich I, et al. Detection of renovascular hypertension with angiotensin II blockade. Ann Intern Med 1977;86(3):257–60.
[31] Kincaid-Smith P. Management of severe hypertension. Am J Cardiol 1973;32(4):575–81.
[32] Gifford RW Jr, Westbrook E. Hypertensive encephalopathy: mechanisms, clinical features, and treatment. Prog Cardiovasc Dis 1974;17(2):115–24.
[33] Lassen NA, Agnoli A. The upper limit of autoregulation of cerebral blood flow on the pathogenesis of hypertensive encepholopathy. Scand J Clin Lab Invest 1972;30(2):113–6.
[34] Garcia JY Jr, Vidt DG. Current management of hypertensive emergencies. Drugs 1987; 34(2):263–78.
[35] Brott T, Thalinger K, Hertzberg V. Hypertension as a risk factor for spontaneous intracerebral hemorrhage. Stroke 1986;17(6):1078–83.
[36] Qureshi AI, Tuhrim S, Broderick JP, et al. Spontaneous intracerebral hemorrhage. N Engl J Med 2001;344(19):1450–60.
[37] Adams RE, Powers WJ. Management of hypertension in acute intracerebral hemorrhage. Crit Care Clin 1997;13(1):131–61.
[38] Wallace JD, Levy LL. Blood pressure after stroke. JAMA 1981;246(19):2177–80.
[39] Carlberg B, Asplund K, Hagg E. The prognostic value of admission blood pressure in patients with acute stroke. Stroke 1993;24(9):1372–5.
[40] Brott T, Broderick J, Kothari R, et al. Early hemorrhage growth in patients with intracerebral hemorrhage. Stroke 1997;28(1):1–5.
[41] Broderick JP, Adams HP Jr, Barsan W, et al. Guidelines for the management of spontaneous intracerebral hemorrhage: a statement for healthcare professionals from a special writing group of the Stroke Council, American Heart Association. Stroke 1999;30(4):905–15.
[42] Feigin VL, Rinkel GJ, Algra A, et al. Calcium antagonists in patients with aneurysmal subarachnoid hemorrhage: a systematic review. Neurology 1998;50(4):876–83.
[43] Powers WJ. Acute hypertension after stroke: the scientific basis for treatment decisions. Neurology 1993;43(3 Pt 1):461–7.
[44] Porchet F, Chiolero R, de Tribolet N. Hypotensive effect of nimodipine during treatment for aneurysmal subarachnoid haemorrhage. Acta Neurochir (Wien) 1995;137(1–2):62–9.
[45] Radhakrishnan D, Menon DK. Haemodynamic effects of intravenous nimodipine following aneurysmal subarachnoid haemorrhage: implications for monitoring. Anaesthesia 1997; 52(5):489–91.
[46] Broderick J, Brott T, Barsan W, et al. Blood pressure during the first minutes of focal cerebral ischemia. Ann Emerg Med 1993;22(9):1438–43.
[47] Brott T, Lu M, Kothari R, et al. Hypertension and its treatment in the NINDS rt-PA Stroke Trial. Stroke 1998;29(8):1504–9.
[48] Kaste M, Fogelholm R, Erila T, et al. A randomized, double-blind, placebo-controlled trial of nimodipine in acute ischemic hemispheric stroke. Stroke 1994;25(7):1348–53.

[49] Semplicini A, Maresca A, Boscolo G, et al. Hypertension in acute ischemic stroke: a compensatory mechanism or an additional damaging factor? Arch Intern Med 2003; 163(2):211–6.
[50] Ahmed N, Wahlgren G. High initial blood pressure after acute stroke is associated with poor functional outcome. J Intern Med 2001;249(5):467–73.
[51] Leonardi-Bee J, Bath PM, Phillips SJ, et al. Blood pressure and clinical outcomes in the International Stroke Trial. Stroke 2002;33(5):1315–20.
[52] Castillo J, Leira R, Garcia MM, et al. Blood pressure decrease during the acute phase of ischemic stroke is associated with brain injury and poor stroke outcome. Stroke 2004;35(2): 520–6.
[53] Stead LG. Evidence-based emergency medicine: blood pressure control in acute stroke. Ann Emerg Med 2004;43(1):129–32.
[54] Vlcek M, Schillinger M, Lang W, et al. Association between course of blood pressure within the first 24 hours and functional recovery after acute ischemic stroke. Ann Emerg Med 2003; 42(5):619–26.
[55] Stead LG, Decker WW, Weaver AL, et al. Does emergency department blood pressure determine survival following acute ischemic stroke? Acad Emerg Med 2004;11:539b–40b.
[56] Adams HP Jr, Brott TG, Crowell RM, et al. Guidelines for the management of patients with acute ischemic stroke: a statement for healthcare professionals from a special writing group of the Stroke Council, American Heart Association. Stroke 1994;25(9):1901–14.
[57] Klijn CJ, Hankey GJ. Management of acute ischaemic stroke: new guidelines from the American Stroke Association and European Stroke Initiative. Lancet Neurol 2003;2(11): 698–701.
[58] Ram CV. Hypertensive crises. Prim Care 1983;10(1):41–61.
[59] Isselbacher EM. Heart Disease: A Textbook of Cardiovascular Medicine. 6th edition. In: Braunwald E, Zipes DP, Libby P, editors. Philadelphia: WB Saunders; 2001. p. 1431–46.
[60] Blumenfeld JD, Sealey JE, Mann SJ, et al. Beta-adrenergic receptor blockade as a therapeutic approach for suppressing the renin-angiotensin-aldosterone system in normotensive and hypertensive subjects. Am J Hypertens 1999;12(5):451–9.
[61] Gottlieb SS, McCarter RJ, Vogel RA. Effect of beta-blockade on mortality among high-risk and low-risk patients after myocardial infarction. N Engl J Med 1998;339(8):489–97.
[62] Gandhi SK, Powers JC, Nomeir AM, et al. The pathogenesis of acute pulmonary edema associated with hypertension. N Engl J Med 2001;344(1):17–22.
[63] Calhoun DA, Oparil S. Treatment of hypertensive crisis. N Engl J Med 1990;323(17): 1177–83.
[64] Houston MC. Pathophysiology, clinical aspects, and treatment of hypertensive crises. Prog Cardiovasc Dis 1989;32(2):99–148.
[65] Collins R, Peto R, MacMahon S, et al. Blood pressure, stroke, and coronary heart disease: part 2: short-term reductions in blood pressure: overview of randomised drug trials in their epidemiological context. Lancet 1990;335(8693):827–38.
[66] Hansson L. The benefits of lowering elevated blood pressure: a critical review of studies of cardiovascular morbidity and mortality in hypertension. J Hypertens 1996;14(5):537–44.
[67] Hansson L, Zanchetti A, Carruthers SG, et al for the HOT Study Group. Effects of intensive blood-pressure lowering and low-dose aspirin in patients with hypertension: principal results of the Hypertension Optimal Treatment (HOT) randomised trial. Lancet 1998;351(9118): 1755–62.
[68] Chiang WK, Jamshahi B. Asymptomatic hypertension in the ED. Am J Emerg Med 1998; 16(7):701–4.
[69] Zeller KR, Von Kuhnert L, Matthews C. Rapid reduction of severe asymptomatic hypertension: a prospective, controlled trial. Arch Intern Med 1989;149(10):2186–9.
[70] Postma CT, Dennesen PJ, de Boo T, et al. First dose hypotension after captopril; can it be predicted? a study of 240 patients. J Hum Hypertens 1992;6(3):205–9.

[71] Jaker M, Atkin S, Soto M, et al. Oral nifedipine vs oral clonidine in the treatment of urgent hypertension. Arch Intern Med 1989;149(2):260–5.

[72] McDonald AJ, Yealy DM, Jacobson S. Oral labetalol versus oral nifedipine in hypertensive urgencies in the ED. Am J Emerg Med 1993;11(5):460–3.

[73] Psaty BM, Smith NL, Siscovick DS, et al. Health outcomes associated with antihypertensive therapies used as first-line agents: a systematic review and meta-analysis. JAMA 1997;277(9): 739–45.

[74] Ramsay LE, Wallis EJ, Yeo WW, et al. The rationale for differing national recommendations for the treatment of hypertension. Am J Hypertens 1998;11(6 Pt 2):79S–88S [discussion: 95S–100S].

[75] Abate G, Zito M, Di Iorio A, et al. Treatment of hypertension in the elderly. Cardiologia 1999;44(5):427–32.

ELSEVIER
SAUNDERS

Emerg Med Clin N Am
23 (2005) 1159–1177

EMERGENCY
MEDICINE
CLINICS OF
NORTH AMERICA

Challenges, Controversies, and Advances in Aortic Catastrophes

Luis H. Haro, MD[a,*], Michelle Krajicek, MD[b], Joseph K. Lobl, MD[a]

[a]*Department of Emergency Medicine, Mayo Clinic Rochester, Mayo Clinic College of Medicine, 200 First Street, Rochester, MN 55901, USA*

[b]*Department of Emergency Medicine, Mayo Clinic College of Medicine, Mayo School of Graduate Education, 200 First Street, Rochester, MN 55901, USA*

This article reviews the recent advances in the pathogenesis, presentation, and management of PAUs, IMH, and their relationship with AD. The authors provide the most recent data on the clinical presentation of ruptured abdominal aortic aneurysm (AAA) and AD, including the controversies and misconceptions of the physical examination findings. This article discusses challenges and advances in serum markers for AD, and advances in the management of these entities relevant to the emergency physician are reviewed. The authors hope that it helps reduce the uncertainty and helps the physician maximize outcomes for these patients.

Penetrating aortic ulcer and intramural hematoma

Until recently, considering the diagnosis of AD in patients who presented with acute chest or back pain in the emergency department (ED) was sufficient. With the widespread use of newer imaging techniques, it has become more apparent that several different causes of acute pain related to the aorta exist. Over the past 20 years, physicians increasingly have recognized penetrating aortic ulcer (PAU) and intramural hematoma (IMH) as etiologies of acute aortic pain, in addition to classic AD. Analogous to the advancements in pathophysiology that led to the replacement of the diagnosis "rule-out myocardial infarction (MI)" with "acute coronary syndrome (ACS)", the authors agree with the proposal to label the intense, tearing, migratory chest, neck, or back pain "acute aortic syndrome (AAS)" [1], replacing the less complete "rule-out AD." Using AAS as a diagnosis reminds the clinician that

* Corresponding author.
E-mail address: haro.luis@mayo.edu (L.H. Haro).

doi:10.1016/j.emc.2005.07.010 *emed.theclinics.com*

patients who present with PAU or IMH can be clinically indistinguishable from patients who present with AD. Currently, most experts recommend similar treatments for these varied conditions, but the recognition of these separate entities likely will lead to more specific treatment regimes.

Pathophysiology

Although the clinical presentation of PAU and IMH can be identical to AD, the pathophysiology of each entity is different. AD is characterized classically by a tear in the lining of the aorta, with the subsequent creation of a "false lumen" that extends longitudinally within the wall of the aorta. An intimal flap and associated hemorrhage into the false lumen, essentially creating a double-lumen aorta, are the other features of dissection. The location of the intimal tear is often associated with areas of higher wall tension within the aorta, such as the right lateral wall of the ascending aorta or the proximal segment of the descending thoracic aorta [1].

IMH is considered a variant of acute dissection, with hemorrhage within the wall of the aorta but lacking an intimal tear or visible flap. This lack of an intimal tear suggests that the bleeding within the aortic wall likely comes from tearing of the small penetrating blood vessels, the vaso vasorum, of the aortic wall. With no tears in the aortic lining, this localized hematoma has no Doppler flow seen on echocardiogram and no enhancement with contrast administration on CT scan. In some cases, however, IMH can rupture into the aortic lumen, essentially creating an AD. IMH can also progress by rupturing outward into the adventitia, or through the entire aortic wall, leading to aortic rupture.

PAU also seems to have a unique origin. These lesions are usually small ruptures of aortic atherosclerotic plaques, with penetration into the media of the aortic wall, which usually appears as a localized divot in the lining of the aorta. Sometimes an associated leakage of blood exists longitudinally, essentially creating a variant of IMH. This process may occasionally continue, leading to what looks like an acute dissection or to further penetration and aortic rupture. PAUs are usually found in the descending thoracic aorta. When these progress into what seem to be acute dissections, the location of the entrance tear may be a clue that PAU was the initiating feature, and the "flap" appears thicker, more calcified, and static, compared with "true" aortic dissections.

Fig. 1 demonstrates the pathologic difference between PAU, IMH, and aortic dissection.

Natural history

In recent years, the natural history of IMH and PAU have also been better defined, though are still controversial. Historically, 10% to 29% of patients initially believed to have acute AD are found on further

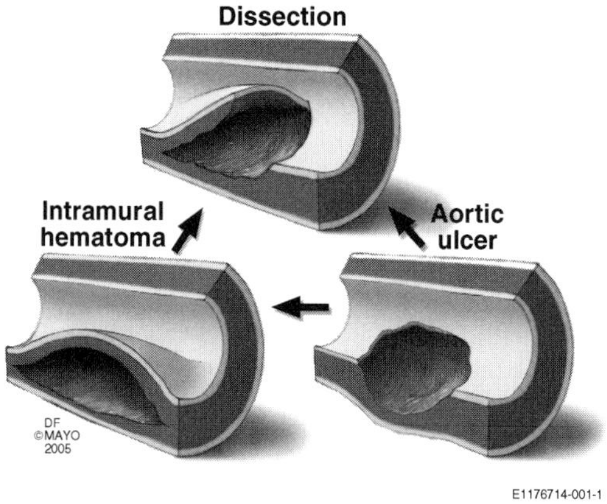

Fig. 1. Schematic representation of the layers of the aorta and the relationship between Aortic dissection, Intramural hematoma and penetrating Aortic ulcer. Used with permission from Mayo Foundation.

investigation to have IMH. Earlier reports of retrospective analyses of series of patients who present with IMH showed high acute mortality rates (up to 80%) with medical treatment alone, particularly with those involving the ascending aorta. This promoted the idea that patients who present with proximal IMH should be treated similarly to those who present with proximal acute dissection, with emergent surgery. Recent reports [2] have challenged this recommendation, with significantly lower mortality rates reported (7%) with medical treatment of proximal IMH. The reason for the discrepancy between studies is unclear. Investigators have postulated that early diagnosis with prompt initiation of aggressive medical care may have contributed to better outcomes. Another theory speculates that the much lower mortality seen in newer studies, which have come from Asia, may indicate a different disease process or different genetic or environmental factors in this subpopulation compared with the prior studies, which reported on patients in Europe and the United States.

Current work is ongoing to elaborate risk factors for rupture of IMH. A maximal aortic diameter of greater than 50 mm in one study [3], or maximal aortic diameter greater than 40 mm, along with a maximum aortic wall thickness of greater than 10 mm in another study [4] seemed to be independent predictors of risk for rupture in patients with IMH. Currently, most experts still advocate emergent surgery for proximal IMH, but clearly the final word is not yet in on this topic. In contrast, widespread support exists for the initial medical management of descending aortic IMH, as survival in most series is virtually identical with initial medical versus surgical therapy.

PAU is somewhat less common than IMH, with studies showing 7% to 10% of patients initially believed to have acute dissection actually having PAU instead. Most (87%) of PAU occur in the descending aorta. Current views regarding the natural history of PAU have also been controversial. The "rediscovery" of PAU in the 1980s [5] seemed to indicate a particularly poor prognosis with initial medical treatment, leading to recommendations to treat these patients with aggressive surgical management. Further studies [6] demonstrated that medical management could be successful, but this has been disputed [7]. Most recently, the largest series to date [7] has demonstrated that initial nonsurgical management frequently leads to successful outcomes, leading the authors to suggest aggressive medical management as initial treatment for all patients with PAU. With such divergent opinions in the literature, the best treatment advice currently would be to initiate aggressive medical management, similar to that for acute dissection, for all patients who develop PAU and expedite transport to a medical center with cardiovascular surgeons experienced in caring for these patients.

Acute aortic dissection

AD is one of the most common and serious diseases of the aorta [8–10]. This cardiovascular catastrophe has high morbidity and mortality [8–12]. AD also has a high likelihood of legal implications if missed. EPs have one of the most difficult challenges in the medical field when it comes to making the diagnosis of AD; no other specialty comes across as frequently as the dilemma of working up a patient chest pain for AD. A main reason is the ratio of chest pain to AD presentations, whereas the incidence of AD is reported to be 2000 new cases per year in the United States. Approximately 4.6 million patients per year present to the ED with chest pain (8.2% of all ED visits) [11]. The other reason is the poor sensitivity and specificity of the clinical presentation; "classic" findings, such as ripping interscapular back pain, diastolic murmur, and a wide mediastinum are present in less than one third of the cases [9,11,13,14]. Not surprisingly, when initially evaluating patients with AD, physicians correctly suspect the diagnosis in as few as 15% to 43% of the cases [9–11]. Diagnostic delays of more than 24 hours after hospitalization are not uncommon and occur in up to 39% of the cases (31% for proximal AD and 53% for distal AD) [15]. Finally, many times when the diagnosis is made, an incidental discovery is made during an advanced imaging procedure requested to assess for other diagnoses.

Clinical manifestations of AD are often dominated by the pathoanatomic characteristics of a malperfusion syndrome from dissection-related side branch obstruction [14]. These characteristics range from abrupt onset pain with or without stroke (carotid occlusion), heart failure (aortic valve insufficiency), syncope (tamponade, CNS ischemia and stroke), buttock and leg pain (femoral artery occlusion), back and flank pain (renal artery occlusion), abdominal pain (mesenteric ischemia or celiac trunk involvement), to the patient with trivial chest pain and the infamous painless AD. The range in presentations decides which imaging modality to use, but this *is not* the most difficult part of the work-up of these patients. These decisions are commonly based on availability and stability and frequently are CT and transesophageal echocardiography (TEE) [13]. But who should be imaged? The ratio of chest pain to AD prohibits performing advanced imaging on every patient with severe chest pain. Most importantly, if one becomes complacent and has the misfortune of missing or misdiagnosing AD, it could have disastrous consequences. Decisions are dependent acutely on the clinical history, examination, and, to a lesser degree, plain chest radiograph, to determine which patients require further study. The EP should have the best clinical information available and consider the clinical presentation in detail to avoid unpleasant surprises.

Over the last decade many studies have evaluated the predictive value of several historical clues and physical examination findings in AD. Particularly useful is Klompas's comprehensive review of the literature [11] and the International Registry of Aortic Dissection (the IRAD database) whose inception and structure is based on 18 large referral centers in six countries [13]. Following are some of the most recent advances in the clinical presentation of AD based on these and other studies.

Aortic dissection in the young patient: who is at risk and who is not?

Traditionally, AD is present in patients in the later decades of life, 95% are older than 40 years old, mean age at presentation is 65 years old [9,11,13]; however, EPs are faced frequently with a patient of younger than aged 40 with abrupt onset of chest pain. Who is at risk and who is not? Januzzi and colleagues [16] evaluated 1078 patients with AD from IRAD 69 (6.4%) were younger than 40 years old, traditional risk factors, such as hypertension and atherosclerosis were lower significantly. Marfan's syndrome, bicuspid aortic valve, and prior aortic valve surgery were significantly higher ($P < .0001$). Other clinical factors, such as symptoms at presentation, physical examination findings, and type of AD were not statistically different; therefore, EPs should have a lower threshold to image patients younger than 40 years old who present with chest pain or back pain in the setting of these high risk predisposing factors (Table 1).

Characteristics of pain

Severe pain is the most common presenting symptom, 74% to 84% of the patients recall an abrupt onset [9,11,13]. This symptom alone should trigger suspicion of an AD. Anterior chest pain is more frequent in patients who experience AD involving the aortic arch (Stanford type A) whereas patients who experience AD distal to the left subclavian (Stanford type B) more often experience back pain and abdominal pain [13]. However, it is difficult to predict what type of AD the patient has based on location of symptoms. Contrary to common belief, pain is described as sharp more often than tearing or ripping pain. Pain that migrates throughout the chest is present in

Table 1
Risk factors associated with aortic dissection

Risk factor	AD > 40 y	AD < 40 y	P value
Marfan syndrome	2%	49%	<.001%
Hypertension	74%	35%	<.001%
Bicuspid valve	3%	16%	<.001%
Prior aortic valve replacement	5%	13%	<.01%
Atherosclerosis	31%	2%	<.001%

28% of the patients with no difference between type A or type B. Abdominal pain is present in 29% of all patients with AD (42% of the cases with type B) [13]. Unfortunately, abdominal pain characteristics have not been described in detail in the literature and therefore one should consider the diagnosis when a patients presents with abrupt onset of generalized abdominal pain and findings of acute abdomen, especially if combined with chest, back, or other pain syndromes (Table 2) [15].

Other associated clinical findings

Syncope

The presence of syncope as a symptom in AD has been documented in 8% to 13% of the cases [11,13]. By 2001, IRAD had captured 728 patients who developed AD, syncope was found in 96 (13%) patients, including 24 (3%) who described it in isolation without any symptoms of chest or back pain [16].

Syncope is more frequent in type A than type B (19% versus 3% $P > .001$). Those with syncope were more likely to have cardiac tamponade (28% versus 8% $P > .001$); stroke (18% versus 4% $P > .001$) and other neurological deficits, such as decreased level of consciousness, coma, and spinal cord ischemia (25% versus 14% $P > .005$). Forty-six percent did not have the presence of any of the prior. The intense discomfort from the dissection itself can induce a vasovagal mediated syncope or the AD can cause direct stretching of the baroreceptors in the aortic wall and cause syncope (Table 3).

Table 2
Pain characteristics in aortic dissection

Pain characteristic	IRAD database	Klompas review	Mayo clinic 1980–1990
Abrupt severe onset	84.4%	84%	74%
Migrating	16%	31%	21%
Posterior chest/back pain	28.3%	N/R	19%
Abdominal pain	29.5% (42% B)	23%	8%–15%
No pain reported	4.5%	N/R	15%

Table 3
Causes of syncope in aortic dissection

	AD with syncope	AD without syncope
Type A	19%	81%
Type B	3%	97%
Cardiac tamponade	28%	8%
Stroke	18%	4%
Other neurological deficits	25%	14%
Unknown	46%	

Syncope in AD alone is a prognostic indicator of high mortality. Patients who presented with syncope were more likely to die in the hospital than those without syncope (34% versus 23% $P > .01$), which may be second as a result of a higher frequency of type A AD. The presence of syncope in AD is often associated with cardiovascular catastrophes and requires prompt diagnosis and intervention. The uncommon patient (3%) that presents with syncope without chest or back pain is always a challenge, a careful physical examination and review of the chest radiographs might provide clues toward the diagnosis of AD. In some cases, missing the diagnosis might be inevitable and remains a challenge for all.

Neurological deficits

Transient ischemic attack (TIA) symptoms, and other focal neurological complaints, are pooled into one category in most of the AD case series. These findings are documented in 4.7% to 17% of the cases [9,11,13]. Neurological abnormalities are found more often in patients who present with proximal AD as a result of occlusion of the carotid artery; they are also found in distal dissections caused by global ischemia and other occlusive syndromes. A neurological complaint or deficit associated with abrupt onset chest or back pain, whether present or not at the time of evaluation in the ED, should prompt the EP to evaluate expeditiously for AD.

Focal deficits are present in only 17% of the cases; however, this finding paired with chest pain has one of the highest likelihood ratios of being AD (positive liklihood ratio (LR) 6.6–33) [11]. Unfortunately, when a focal neurologic deficit is absent it does not alter the negative likelihood of AD and, therefore, is not useful in excluding AD.

Helpful physical examination findings

Physical examination findings associated with AD are typically present in less than half of the cases [11]. Amongst the most useful signs able to predict AD is:

Pulse deficit

The presence of a pulse deficit between the carotid, radial, or femoral arteries is infrequent (25%–30%), but when present the finding is suggestive strongly of AD in the setting of chest or back pain (positive LR ratio of 5.7; 95% CI 1.4–23.0) [11]. This finding can predict in-hospital complications and mortality in patients who present with acute type A AD and has been studied in detail by Bossone and colleagues [17]. In their evaluation, pulse deficit was defined as decreased or absent carotid or peripheral pulses as noted by clinicians and later confirmed by diagnostic imaging at surgery or at autopsy. The in-hospital mortality was 41% versus 25%, and mortality was raised significantly with the number of pulses that were absent [17]. In the midst of a busy ED when evaluating patients with chest pain, it is frequently forgotten to check pulses; many believe that it has a low yield. However, in the setting of a suspected AD, noting a pulse deficit is sure to increase your pretest probability and warrants further imaging even if your initial work up (frequently CT or TEE) results negative or equivocal.

Unhelpful physical examination findings

Diastolic murmur

Diastolic murmur in a patient who presents with chest pain does not help in predicting AD. One third of the patients with AD have a diastolic murmur (sensitivity 28%). The positive LR for this finding is 1.4 and negative LR is 0.9 and, therefore, should not be considered helpful. One could consider that a *new* murmur might be useful; however, to most practicing EPs all patients are new and discerning new from old is nearly impossible.

Blood pressure on presentation

A patient's blood pressure on presentation also does not seem to be helpful. Although approximately half of the patients present with elevated blood pressure, an equal proportion is hypertensive or normotensive (Table 4) [10,11,13].

Based on the prior data, the only significant physical findings helpful in predicting AD are that of a pulse deficit and that of a focal neurologic deficit; the palpation of pulses and targeted neurologic examination is an essential part of the evaluation of a patient who is experiencing chest pain and is at risk for AD.

Table 4
Frequency of classic findings of aortic dissection

Physical findings	IRAD database	Klompas review
Hypertension on presentation	49%	49%
Shock	8%	19%
Aortic murmur	31.6%	28%
Focal neurologic deficit	4.7%	17% (Positive LR 6.6–33)
Pulse deficit	15%	31% (Positive LR 5.7)

Serum markers in the work up of aortic dissection

The lack of symptoms or signs that have a good negative predictive value (NPV) has forced investigators to look at serologic means to diagnose AD. This concept is particularly attractive to EPs because a serum test with a good NPV would obviate the need to image. Theoretically, it would also improve survival because it could lead to prompt a diagnosis, especially when considering AD type A mortality of 1% per hour in the first 24 hours. The last decade has been particularly exciting as several efforts have been made toward this goal. The main focus of serologic diagnoses are in soluble elastic compounds, D-dimer, and smooth muscle myosin heavy chain (SMMHC).

SMMHC is a major component of smooth muscle; this marker has been shown to be present and elevated in the first 24 hours of patients with AD. Katoh and Suzuki [18] first described the use of SMMHC in AD in Japan in 1995, their assay showed 100% reactivity with the aorta smooth muscle myosin, whereas with platelet, ventricle, and skeletal muscle myosin it was 0.1%. SMMHC has been tested in serum of healthy subjects who have levels of 0.9 ± 0.9 ng/mL and in four patients who presented with AD confirmed by surgery with all four demonstrating levels elevated at presentation (>7 ng/mL) dropping to normal values after 24 hours. Particularly useful is that in 10 patients with acute myocardial infarction (AMI), no elevation occurred in serum levels.

This immunoassay has shown sensitivity of 90% in the first 12 hours of onset of symptoms with a specificity of 97%. Most recently, Suzuki and colleagues [19] documented 25 patients enrolled in the IRAD (12 type A, 13 type B) that had SMMHC measured, which showed elevated levels of 19.6 ± 56.6 ng/mL (normal < 2.5 ng/mL) with a presentation time of 6.1 hours ± 4.5 hours. This study showed superior diagnostic performance in the early hours after onset (>90% sensitivity in the first 3 hours after onset); however, the sensitivity decreases to 44% after 3 hours and most significantly after 6 hours. The investigators' conclusion is that patients who come to the ED within hours of the onset of symptoms of AD has elevated levels with high sensitivities, therefore, facilitating diagnosis and early treatment [19]. Another potential use is with the patient who has a low pretest probability and present early to the ED. Unfortunately, later presentations and the fact that SMMHC is also present in the intestine and uterus and the NPV is lost in patients who have diseases, such as Crohn's, ulcerative colitis, pelvic inflammatory disease, and other inflammatory disease of the intestine and uterus.

Elastin is one of the major components of the arterial wall. An enzyme linked immunosorbent assay to measure soluble elastin fragments (sELAF), a product of human aortic elastin was developed by Shinohara. Twenty-five patients with AD, 50 with AMI, and 474 subjects were studied. Sixteen patients who present with AD had elevated sELAF; unfortunately, all patients without patent false lumen had normal levels and yet, obviously, had AD. Patients who presented with a patent pseudo lumen had elevated levels in 88.9% of the cases [20]. Although the authors conclude that the test might be helpful in the diagnosis and screening of AD, one patient who experienced AMI had elevated levels, the study was retrospective, and, finally, the NPV was poor and, therefore, not useful to exclude AD.

D-dimer is used frequently to exclude thromboembolic disease in low-risk patients, Weber and colleagues [21] prospectively tested D-dimer levels in 10 patients who presented with suspected AD; in addition, 14 patients who had developed proven AD were reviewed and 35 patients served as a control group. D-dimer was elevated in all AD patients. The investigators concluded that in the setting of a negative D-dimer, the presence of AD is unlikely [21]. This provoking thought is being evaluated currently in a multicenter study along with sELAF and SMMHC (Haro LH, personal communication, 2004).

Bedside specific biomarkers are not yet in clinical use, although biochemical diagnosis of AD might be available in the future. It is a promising area of research that will help the clinician tremendously in this particular disease.

ECG abnormalities in aortic dissection: does this patient need a surgeon or a fibrinolytic?

EPs are challenged frequently with a patient that presents with chest pain that radiates to the back and an ECG with ST elevation suggestive of an AMI. In these cases, delay in therapy is not uncommon because patients often go to CT or are transferred without fibrinolytic therapy for "rule-out dissection". The frequency of ST elevation and Q waves suggestive of an AMI in AD is well documented in the literature. In the initial IRAD publication the finding was documented in 4.6% of type A and in 0.7% of type B [13]. In Komplan's review new MI on ECG was present in 7% of the cases (95% CI 4–14).

The low frequency of AD with ST elevation compared with actual ST elevation myocardial infarction (STEMI), would argue for selected and infrequent need for imaging. Approximately 2000 new dissections per year, 62% of these are type A. Those with type A have an incidence of 5% to 7% of ST abnormalities suggestive of a STEMI, representing approximately 25 cases in the United States a year. Tens of thousands of patients per year in the United States develop STEMI. Further, coronary artery involvement (CAI) in AD and ST abnormalities in the ECG do not go hand-in-hand. Bossone and colleagues [22] evaluated the clinical characteristics and outcomes of 475 patients who developed AD and 64 (13.5%) of the patients had CAI. When they reviewed the ECGs, patients with CAI were more likely to show new Q wave or ST elevation on ECG (16.7% versus 4.3%, P = .0001); however, these ECG findings were present in only one of six

CAI patients; therefore, ST elevation in AD seems to be uncommon and even when AD with CAI is present frequently, the ECG is not diagnostic.

In general, in the setting of a patient who presents with chest pain and ST elevation in the ECG, one should assume STEMI and treat accordingly. An exception would be of course uncommon findings highly suggestive of AD, such as a focal deficit, pulse deficit, or a chest radiograph highly suggestive of AD.

Isolated arch dissection

No guidelines exist in the literature for the management of isolated arch dissection, typically classified as Stanford type A. Most EPs consider this a surgical entity, however, this specific dissection subtype has been approached on a case-by-case basis, heavily influenced by the surgeons experience, the patients age, hemodynamic status, comorbid states and, of course, the patients personal preference. Barbara Richartz and colleagues [23] published the international experience with isolated arch dissections. Amongst 989 patients, 92 (9%) had isolated arch dissection, 39 (42%) were treated surgically, and 53 (58%) were treated medically. Thirty-day mortality was 17% (23% with surgery and 13% with medical management) and, therefore, much lower than typical type A dissections (35% with surgery and 65% with medical management). Complications were the same. The conclusion was that isolated arch dissections are best managed conservatively and represent an exception to classic type A dissection. EPs should not be surprised when these patients are managed without surgical intervention.

Percutaneous management of aortic dissection

Complicated type B dissections have been subject to novel percutaneous therapies, such as percutaneous fenestration (restores flow to the true lumen by creating a tear in the dissection flap between the true and false lumen) and percutaneous stent-graft placement. With these techniques compromised flow can be restored in 90% of the cases (range 70%–100%). If a patient survives the intervention, postoperative average 30-day mortality is 10% (range 0%–25%) and rarely is additional surgical intervention needed [24]. Percutaneous endovascular balloon fenestration of a dissecting aortic membrane to treat mesenteric ischemia in type B AD is particularly promising. Patients with this complication in AD have a mortality of 87%, operative fenestration mortality is up to 61%, percutaneous fenestration is becoming popular for this complication and is demonstrating promising results and decreased mortality.

Depressurization and shrinking of the false lumen is the main goal of stent-graft therapy. This therapy is being used successfully in patients who present with compression of the true aortic lumen by an enlarging false lumen, by placing these stents with or without percutaneous fenestration, interventionalists have increased the flow successfully to the true lumen, therefore, establishing flow to compromised aortic branches. Obstructions of aortic branches can be overcome with endovascular stents across the vessel origin; however, stent-graft placement across the celiac superior mesenteric and renal arteries is discouraged strongly for empirical reasons and has not been studied extensively. Postprocedure mortality of these percutaneous interventions is dependent largely on the severity and duration of ischemia before the procedure; therefore, timely percutaneous management is highly desirable.

Finally, recent reports have suggested that percutaneous stent placement for type B AD is safer and produces better results than surgical intervention and particularly decrease the rates of paraplegia to an extremely rare event. Table 5 lists a summary of the current treatment options in AD.

Abdominal aortic aneurysm: challenges, controversies, and advances

In 1905 Sir William Osler noted the difficulties in diagnosis and management of abdominal aortic aneurysm (AAA) [25]. One hundred years later, these problems. In addition, the incidence of AAA is increasing. One research group looked at the incidence over a 30-year period and noted that more aneurysms occurred in the last decade studied than in the previous two decades combined. The size of AAA at time of diagnosis increased over the three decades [26]. With the incidence and size of AAAs increasing, changes should be evaluated continually.

Misdiagnosis of ruptured AAA remains a serious challenge to all practitioners. Lederle and colleagues [27] looked at the magnitude of the problem in the ED at a Veterans Affairs hospital. They found that in 14 cases (61%), ruptured AAA was missed on initial diagnosis. In 9 of these patients who were hemodynamically stable at presentation, diagnosis was not made until shock developed. Researchers found that urinary tract obstruction or infection, spinal disease, and diverticulitis were the most frequent misdiagnoses [27]. Another study looked at patients with symptomatic AAA presenting to a county ED. Twenty-four of 134 (18%) of these patients were diagnosed initially with nephrolithiasis. Furthermore, 14 of the patients studied had ex-tensive diagnostic work-up, delaying the time to diagnosis by

Table 5
Management of aortic dissection

Surgery	Medical therapy	Interventional therapy
• Type A AD	Uncomplicated type B AD	Unstable Type B AD
• Type B with:	Stable, isolated arch AD	Malperfusion syndrome
Retrograde extension into the ascending aorta		
Marfan's syndrome		
Rupture or impending rupture		
Progression with compromise of vital organs		

greater than 5 hours [28]. Misdiagnosis is a serious problem because it leads to significant morbidity and mortality. In Lederle's study, diagnosis was delayed frequently until shock set in. Of the patients who subsequently underwent surgery, 7 of 8 with preoperative shock died, whereas only 2 of 9 without shock died ($P < .02$) [27]. In Borrero's study [28], all patients who had extensive diagnostic evaluation lasting more than 5 hours died. The frequency of misdiagnosis challenges clinicians to seek historical clues, physical examination signs, and diagnostic aids.

The diagnosis of ruptured AAA requires a high index of suspicion. Some historical clues have a well-established relationship with AAA. These clues include advanced age, cardiovascular disease, and risk factors. In one study, 56% of patients who presented with AAA had evidence of occlusive arterial disease including MI, angina, peripheral vascular disease, and cerebrovascular disease [29]. Other historical data has been studied recently. Data from the SMART study linked cerbrovascular disease and AAA pathophysiology to increased arterial stiffness determined by ultrasound measurement of carotid artery stiffness [30]. Calcium channel blockers have been found to increase aortic wall stiffness and to be an independent risk factor for AAA presence [31]. The data on arterial wall stiffness and calcium channel blockers is promising but remains controversial and requires further study.

Recent advances in identifying those at risk for AAA have come in the fields of genetics and molecular biology. Attention has been given to the study of aortic inflammation and the upregulation of proteases and dysfunctional tissue-turnover [32]. Engstrom and colleagues [33] studied five inflammation-sensitive plasma proteins (ISPs) and noted an association with fatal or surgically repaired AAA in patients who experience increasing numbers of ISPs. Presence of susceptibility loci for AAA have been identified by Shibamura and colleagues [34] on chromosomes 19q13 and 4q31. These discoveries show promise for earlier identification of patients at risk.

Despite advances and controversies in identifying patients at risk, the problem of correctly diagnosing the acute ruptured AAA remains. With or without the knowledge of a patient's risk factors, the clinician must turn to the bedside examination as the next step in the process of this time-sensitive diagnosis. The classic examination finding is a pulsatile, exspansile abdominal mass. The accuracy of the physical examination in diagnosis of ruptured and nonruptured AAA remains highly controversial. For bedside identification of AAA by physical examination, the sensitivity rates range from 33% to 100% and specificity rates range from 75% to 100% [35]. Lederle and Simel [36] report that sensitivity of abdominal palpation increases with size of the aneurysm. They report 29% sensitivity for 3.0–3.9 cm AAAs, 50% for 4.0–4.9 cm, and 76% for 5.0 cm or greater [36]. With such varied reports, the clinician cannot rely accurately on physical examination alone to exclude the diagnosis of abdominal aortic aneurysm.

With physical examination unreliable and historical clues only helpful if present, the clinician must turn to other diagnostic tools. Portable abdominal films and ultrasound are available typically at the patient's bedside in the ED. The technology and availability of the plain abdominal radiograph has changed little in recent years. Despite the lack of change, it can be helpful in diagnosis. In a retrospective review of 31 patients with ruptured AAA, 65% had aneurysm calcification, 67% had complete loss of one or both psoas outlines, 78% has complete loss of one or both renal outlines, and 25% had renal displacement [37]. Although these numbers are promising, they certainly leave room for error and missed diagnosis. Many have made the argument that advances in bedside ultrasound in the ED have replaced the need for abdominal plain films.

Numerous studies have confirmed ultrasound as a significant advance in the timely diagnosis of ruptured AAA. Kuhn and colleagues [38] report a study of 68 scans performed by EPs, which, on confirmation by CT scan, formal ultrasonography, angiography, laparotomy, or radiologist review of recorded ED ultrasound, were 100% accurate. EP ultrasound of the abdominal aorta was also evaluated by Tayal, Graf, and Gibbs [39]. One hundred and twenty-five scans performed by EPs had 100% sensitivity and 98% specificity for AAA on confirmatory testing with radiology ultrasound, abdominal CT, abdominal MRI, or laparotomy [39]. In a study assessing the ability of EPs to perform ultrasound for diagnosis of various diseases, Schlager and colleagues [40] found a 100% specificity and 100% sensitivity for AAA. The evaluation of screening for AAA using a handheld device has also been explored in the office setting. Lin and colleagues [41] reported sensitivity of 93% and specificity of 97% when hand-held ultrasound by vascular surgeon was compared with formal radiology ultrasound. The accuracy of a "quick screen" ultrasound compared with a full conventional study was compared by Lee and colleagues [42] and found to be 100%. This study also determined the quicker version to be more cost efficient [42]. One study specifically addressed the EPs ability to visualize the entire abdominal aorta by way of ultrasound. Blaivas and Theodoro [43] determined that in 8% of patients scanned a significant portion (one third or greater) of the abdominal aorta could not be visualized. Although confirmatory studies showed that no AAAs were missed by the EPs, this study points out that there is still room for error. Ultrasonography of the abdominal aorta by EPs is a fast and accurate test. It should be the first line in imaging in patients for whom the diagnosis is suspected. It can aid significantly in expediting the trip to the operating room, therefore reducing morbidity and mortality. Indeed, Valentine and colleagues [44] report that in patients taken to the operating room for suspected ruptured AAA, finding an intact aortic aneurysm is rare. Even when this is found, 90% of these patients have other abdominal pathologies that required operative treatment [44].

Although ultrasound is ideal for identifying AAA, it is typically poor for identifying the presence of leaking. In unstable patients, hemodynamic instability plus identification of AAA by ultrasound is an indication for laporotomy; however, in stable patients, further imaging may be necessary to determine if the finding of AAA is causal or incidental. CT findings in patients with ruptured AAA include retroperitoneal hematoma, focal discontinuity in circumferential calcification, high-attenuating peripheral crescent, indistinct aortic wall, and frank contrast medium extravasation [45]. In addition to better identification of a leak, a CT scan aids in diagnosis of other causes of intra-abdominal pathology. Although the CT scan provides more information, the accuracy for diagnosing AAA rupture has been questioned. In 74 patients who underwent CT scanning because of doubt of ruptured AAA on clinical grounds alone, 22 of 28 patients were diagnosed correctly and 30 of 39 patients were excluded correctly, a sensitivity of 79% and specificity of 77%. The investigators, Adam and colleagues [46], conclude that CT adds little additional diagnostic value [46]; however, as endovascular aneurysm repair of ruptured AAA is becoming more popular, vascular surgeons may prefer further imaging before proceeding to the operating room. In a study performed by Lloyd and colleagues [47], time to death (studied in non-operative candidates) in patients who present with ruptured AAA was reported to be over 2 hours in 87.5% of patients. The authors conclude that most patients with a ruptured AAA who survive to the hospital are, therefore, stable enough to undergo CT scanning before surgery [47]. The use of CT in the diagnosis and evaluation of the patient who presents with suspected ruptured AAA remains controversial. On one hand, it is a risk to allow the potentially unstable patient to leave the ED for a test and to delay the transport to the operating room. On the other hand, CT is more sensitive for aneurysm leakage and can provide a better road map for endovascular repair when compared with ultrasound alone.

Magnetic resonance angiography (MRA) has been praised for ability to provide essential anatomic information in AAA, including size and character, and the status of celiac, mesenteric, renal and iliac arteries [48], an advance in preoperative screening for the patient with AAA. This test is time-consuming (1 hour in the above study), however, typically far from the ED, and often unavailable emergently. MRA imaging, therefore, is not practical or appropriate for patients with suspected ruptured AAA.

Management

Challenges, controversies, and advances have emerged in the management of ruptured AAA. The definitive management, surgical repair, is not debated; however, issues in ED management and surgical technique still exist.

The typical ED management includes type and cross for 10 units of packed red blood cells and aggressive resuscitation of the hemodynamically unstable patient; however, the extent of fluid resuscitation has been debated highly. Myers [49] reports that numerous animal model studies of uncontrolled hemorrhage have shown increased mortality in animals resuscitated with large fluid volumes compared with little to no fluid administration. The increase in mortality has been attributed to increased blood loss prolonging the period of shock [49]. Currently, no published prospective clinical studies investigating preoperative fluid resuscitation in ruptured AAA exist. Brimacombe and Berry [50] report that several retrospective studies have addressed this topic, and the results have varied. Several of the early studies supported minimal fluid administration, but later studies failed to confirm these findings [50]. This topic remains controversial, and more investigation is warranted.

Over the last decade, endovascular aneurysm repair (EVAR) has emerged as an advance in elective repair of AAA. Proponents of this method praise the improved peri-operative morbidity and mortality rates, whereas opponents question the long-term effectiveness of the grafts [51]. Recently, several case series have reported the use of EVAR for ruptured AAA. Doss and colleagues [52] deployed six emergent endovascular stent grafts in the abdominal aorta, with successful deployment in all cases. The report decreased morbidity and mortality from traditional repair with two MI deaths in the postoperative period, two endoleaks, one in-stent stenosis, one temporary renal failure, and one episode of myocardial ischemia [52]. In this study, and the other recent studies, all patients were imaged before surgery by way of spiral CT scan. The other trials report similar decrease in morbidity and mortality; however, critics argue that the better outcomes in EVAR are a result of patient selection. Typically, the patients selected to undergo EVAR are stable hemodynamically [53]. A recent randomized trial compared complication rates of EVAR with traditional open repair for nonruptured AAA. These investigators found the operative mortality rate of 4.6% in the open-repair group and 1.2% in the endovascular-repair group [54]. Whether these results can be applied to ruptured AAA remains to be seen.

From misdiagnosis to surgical repair, the care of patients who present with ruptured AAA remains challenging. Some major advances, including breakthroughs in understanding the disease process leading to better identification, ultrasound identification in the ED, and endovascular aneurysm repair have changed the way physicians care for patients who present with ruptured AAA. Despite advances, many controversies still exist. These include reliability of physical examination, usefulness of abdominal plain film, role of CT scanning, and endovascular versus open repair. In this disease that has increasing prevalence and high mortality, the challenges, controversies, and advances need to be evaluated continually.

References

[1] Vilacosta I, Roman JA. Acute aortic syndrome. Heart 2001;85(4):365–8.

[2] Song JK, Kim HS, Song JM, et al. Outcomes of medically treated patients with aortic intramural hematoma. Am J Med 2002;113(3):181–7.

[3] Kaji S, Nishigami K, Akasaka T, et al. Prediction of progression or regression of type A aortic intramural hematoma by computed tomography. Circulation 1999;100(Suppl 19): II281–6.
[4] Sueyoshi E, Imada T, Sakamoto I, et al. Analysis of predictive factors for progression of type B aortic intramural hematoma with computed tomography [comment]. J Vasc Surg 2002;35: 1179.
[5] Stanson AW, Kazmier FJ, Hollier LH, et al. Penetrating atherosclerotic ulcers of the thoracic aorta: natural history and clinicopathologic correlations. Ann Vasc Surg 1986;1(1): 15–23.
[6] Coady MA, Rizzo JA, Hammond GL, et al. Penetrating ulcer of the thoracic aorta: what is it? How do we recognize it? How do we manage it? J Vasc Surg 1998;27(6):1006–16.
[7] Cho KR, Stanson AW, Potter DD, et al. Penetrating atherosclerotic ulcer of the descending thoracic aorta and arch. J Thorac Cardiovasc Surg 2004;127(5):1393–401.
[8] Clouse DW, Halleti JW, Schaff HV, et al. Acute aortic dissection: population-based incidence compared with degenerative aortic aneurysm rupture. Mayo Clin Proc 2004;79: 176–80.
[9] Spitell PC, Spitell JA, Joyce JW, et al. Clinical features and differential diagnosis of aortic dissection: experience with 236 cases (1980–1990). Mayo Clin Proc 1993;68:542–651.
[10] Meszaros I, Morocz J, Szlavi J, et al. Epidemiology and clinicopathology of aortic dissection: a population-based longitudinal study over 27 years. Chest 2000;117:1271–8.
[11] Klompas M. Does this patient have an acute thoracic aortic dissection? JAMA 2002;287(17): 2262–72.
[12] Park SW, Hutchinson S, Mehta RH, et al. Association of painless aortic dissection with increased mortality. Mayo Clin Proc 2004;79(10):1252–7.
[13] Hagan PG, Nienaber CA, Isselbacher EM, et al. The international registry of acute aortic dissection (IRAD): new insights into an old disease. JAMA 2000;283:897–903.
[14] Nienamber CA, Eagle KA. Aortic dissection: new frontiers in diagnosis and management. Circulation 2003;108:628–35.
[15] Viljanen T. Diagnostic difficulties in aortic dissection: retrospective study of 89 surgically treated patients. Ann Chir Gynaecol 1986;75:328–32.
[16] Januzzi JL, Isselbacher EM, Fatorri R, et al. Characterizing the young patient with aortic dissection: results from the international registry of aortic dissection (IRAD) [abstract 1081–154]. J Am Coll Cardiol 2003;41(6):235A.
[17] Bossone E, Vincenzo R, Nienamber CA, et al. Usefulness of pulse deficit to predict in-hospital complications and mortality in patients with type A aortic dissection. Am J Cardiol 2002;89:851–5.
[18] Katoh H, Suzuki T. A novel immunoassay of smooth muscle myosin heavy chain in serum. J Immanuol Methods 1995;185:57–63.
[19] Suzuki T, Trimarchi S, Smith D, et al. Early diagnosis of acute aortic dissection: identification of clinical variables associated with early diagnosis and determination of the usefulness of biochemical diagnosis as shown by the international registry of acute aortic dissection (IRAD) database. Circulation 2004;110(17):III-370.
[20] Shinohara T, Suzuki K, Okada M, et al. Soluble elastin fragments are elevated in acute aortic dissections. Art Throm and Vasc Biol J of the AHA 2003;23:1839–44.
[21] Weber T, Hogler S, Auer J, et al. D-dimer in acute aortic dissection. Chest 2003;123(5): 1375–8.
[22] Bossone E, Mehta RH, Trimarchi S, et al. Coronary involvement in patients with acute type A aortic dissection. J Am Coll Cardiol 2003;235A:1034–141.
[23] Richartz B, Schiller F, Bossone E, et al. Aortic arch dissection as a distinct entity: lessons learned from IRAD. Circulation 2002;106:473.
[24] Nienaber CA, Eagle KA. Aortic dissection: new frontiers in the diagnosis and management. Part II: therapeutic management and follow-up. Circulation 2003;108:772–8.
[25] Osler W. Aneurysm of the abdominal aorta. Lancet 1905;2:1089–96.

[26] Bickerstaff LK, Hollier LH, Van Peenen HJ, et al. Abdominal aortic aneurysms: the changing natural history. J Vasc Surg 1984;1(1):6–12.
[27] Lederle F, Parenti C, Chute E. Ruptured abdominal aortic aneurysm: the internist as diagnostician. Am J Med 1994;96(2):163–7.
[28] Borrero E, Queral LA. Symptomatic abdominal aortic aneurysm misdiagnosed as nephroureterolithiasis. Ann Vasc Surg 1988;2(2):145–9.
[29] Lloyd GM, Newton JD, Norwood M, et al. Patients with abdominal aortic aneurysm: are we missing the opportunity for cardiovascular risk reduction? J Vasc Surg 2004;40(4):691–7.
[30] Dijk JM, van der Graf Y, Grobbee DE, et al. Increased arterial stiffness is independently related to cerebrovascular disease and aneurysms of the abdominal aorta: the second manifestations of arterial disease (SMART) study. Stroke 2004;35:1642–6.
[31] Wilmink A, Vardulaki K, Hubbard C, et al. Are antihypertensive drugs associated with abdominal aortic aneurysms? J Vasc Surg 2002;36(4):751–7.
[32] Belsley SJ, Tilson MD. Two decades of research on etiology and genetic factors in the abdominal aortic aneurysm (AAA): with a glimpse into the 21st century. Acta Chir Belg 2003;103(2):187–96.
[33] Engstrom G, Borner G, Bengt L, et al. Incidence of fatal or repaired abdominal aortic aneurysm in relation to inflammation-sensitive plasma proteins. Arterioscler Thromb Vasc Biol 2004;24:337–41.
[34] Shibamura H, Olson J, van Vlijmen-van Keulen C, et al. Genome scan for familial abdominal aortic aneurysm using sex and family history as covariates suggests genetic heterogeneity and identifies linkage to chromosome 19q13. Circulation 2004;109:2103–8.
[35] Lynch R. Accuracy of abdominal examination in the diagnosis of non-ruptured abdominal aortic aneurysm. Accid Emerg Nurs 2004;12:99–107.
[36] Lederle F, Simel D. Does this patient have abdominal aortic aneurysm? JAMA 1999;281(1): 77–82.
[37] Loughran CF. A review of the plain abdominal radiograph in acute rupture of abdominal aortic aneurysms. Clin Radiol 1986;37(4):383–7.
[38] Kuhn M, Bonnin R, Davey M, et al. Emergency Department ultrasound scanning for abdominal aortic aneurysm: accessible, accurate, and advantageous. Ann Emerg Med 2000; 36(3):219–23.
[39] Tayal V, Graf C, Gibbs M. Prospective study of accuracy and outcome of emergency ultrasound for abdominal aortic aneurysm over two years. Acad Emerg Med 2003;10(8): 867–71.
[40] Schlager D, Lazzareschi G, Whitten D, et al. A prospective study of ultrasonography in the ED by emergency physicians. Am J Emerg Med 1994;12(2):185–9.
[41] Lin P, Bush R, McCoy S, et al. A prospective study of a hand-held ultrasound device in abdominal aortic aneurysm evaluation. Am J Surg 2003;186:455–9.
[42] Lee TY, Heller JA, Kilaru S, et al. The cost-effectiveness of a 'quick-screen' program for abdominal aortic aneurysms. Surgery 2002;132(2):399–407.
[43] Blaivas M, Theodoro D. Frequency of incomplete abdominal aorta visualization by emergency department bedside ultrasound. Acad Emerg Med 2004;11(1):103–5.
[44] Valentine RJ, Barth MJ, Myers SI, et al. Nonvascular emergencies presenting as ruptured abdominal aortic aneurysms. Surgery 1993;113(3):286–9.
[45] Bhalla S, Menias C, Heiken J. CT of acute abdominal aortic disorders. Radiol Clin North Am 2003;41(6):1153–69.
[46] Adam DJ, Bradbury AW, Stuart WP, et al. The value of computed tomography I the assessment of suspected ruptured abominal aortic aneurysm. J Vasc Surg 1998;27(3):431–7.
[47] Lloyd GM, Bown M, Norwood M, et al. Feasibility of preoperative computer tomography in patients with ruptured abdominal aortic aneurysm: a time-to-death study in patients without operation. J Vasc Surg 2004;39(4):788–91.
[48] Prince MR, Narasimham DL, Stanley JC, et al. Gadolinium-enhanced magnetic resonance angiography of abdominal aortic aneurysms. J Vasc Surg 1995;21(4):656–69.

[49] Myers C. Fluid resuscitation. Eur J Emerg Med 1997;4(4):224–32.
[50] Brimacombe J, Berry A. Haemodynamic management in ruptured abdominal aortic aneurysm. Postgrad Med J 1994;70(822):252–6.
[51] Hinchliffe RJ, Hopkinson BR. Current concepts and controversies in endovascular repair of abdominal aortic aneurysm. J Cardiovasc Surg (Torino) 2003;44(4):481–502.
[52] Doss M, Martens S, Hemmer W. Emergency endovascular interventions for ruptured thoracic and abdominal aortic aneurysms. Am Heart J 2002;144(3):481–502.
[53] Hinchliffe RJ, Braithwaite BD, Hopkinson BR. The endovascular management of ruptured abdominal aortic aneurysms. Eur J Vasc Endovasc Surg 2003;25:191–201.
[54] Prinssen M, Verhoeven E, Buth J, et al. A randomized trial comparing conventional and endovascular repair of abdominal aortic aneurysms. N Engl J Med 2004;351(16):1607–18.

ELSEVIER
SAUNDERS

Emerg Med Clin N Am
23 (2005) 1179–1194

EMERGENCY
MEDICINE
CLINICS OF
NORTH AMERICA

Emergency Department Ultrasound and Echocardiography

Alice Tang, DO, MPH*, Brian Euerle, MD, RDMS

Division of Emergency Medicine, University of Maryland School of Medicine, 110 South Paca Street, Sixth Floor, Suite 200, Baltimore, MD 21201, USA

Real-time bedside ultrasonography is rapidly becoming an important component of the emergency physician's skill set. Because the emergency physician uses ultrasonography in a focused manner and early in the patient's evaluation, it becomes an extension of the physical examination and can provide timely information on entities such as cholecystitis, hemoperitoneum, abdominal aortic aneurysm, and ectopic pregnancy.

Echocardiography refers to the use of ultrasound to evaluate the heart. This modality is ideal for the use in the emergency department because it is rapid, accurate, and noninvasive and allows repeat examinations [1]. In one of the earliest reports of the routine use of real-time echocardiography by emergency physicians, Mayron and colleagues [2] describe the use of ultrasonography in patients with pericardial tamponade, electromechanical dissociation, pulmonary embolus, and unexplained hypotension. Although further uses of echocardiography have since been developed and continue to be studied, these applications remain at the core of echocardiography as currently practiced by emergency physicians. More recent studies have confirmed that emergency physicians are able to practice bedside echocardiography with a high degree of overall accuracy [3].

Emergency medicine residency programs and the Residency Review Committee for Emergency Medicine have stressed the importance of ultrasonography in the training curriculum [4,5]. As more practicing emergency physicians come to possess these skills, more patients will benefit from the potentially life-saving diagnoses and interventions it offers.

* Corresponding author.
E-mail address: atang002@umaryland.edu (A. Tang).

doi:10.1016/j.emc.2005.07.015 **emed.theclinics.com**

Anatomy

The views obtained of the heart with echocardiography are less intuitive than those obtained of other areas of the body with ultrasonography. For this reason, it is helpful for the physician to have a good understanding of the anatomy of the heart. The heart is located within the mediastinum, posterior to the sternum and anterior to the spine. The lungs are adjacent to the sides of the heart. The great vessels are located superiorly and the diaphragm inferiorly. The long axis of the heart is oriented along a line from the patient's right shoulder to the left hip. When viewed from the front, it can be seen that the right heart border is formed by the right atrium and the left heart border by the left ventricle (Fig. 1). The lateral view shows that the right ventricle is located the most anteriorly, directly behind the sternum (Fig. 2) [6].

The heart is surrounded by two layers of fibrous pericardium [7]. The visceral pericardium is adherent to the outside surface of the heart, while the parietal pericardium lines the cavity in which the heart sits. In the normal state, these two layers oppose each other and appear as a single structure.

All four chambers of the heart can be visualized by echocardiography, and the differences between them are obvious. The ventricles are more muscular and thicker walled than the atria. In the normal heart, the left ventricle is larger than the right. The heart valves also can be visualized, most commonly the mitral, tricuspid, and aortic. The proximal aortic root can be seen in conjunction with the aortic valve. One additional structure of the heart that is often visualized and can help with orientation is the thick, muscular septum that separates the right from the left ventricle.

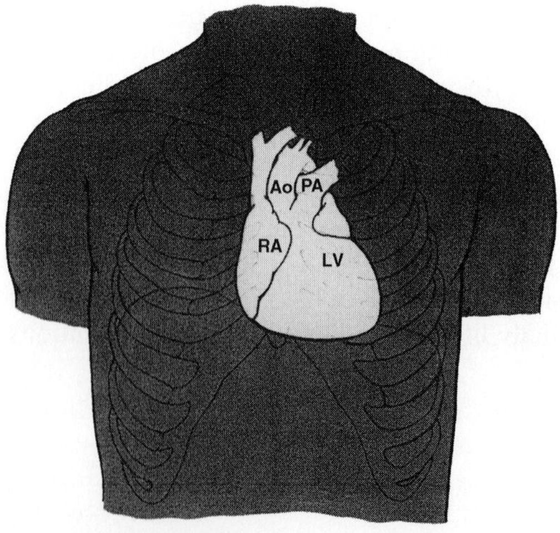

Fig. 1. Anterior view of the heart. Ao, aorta; LV, left ventricle; PA, pulmonary artery; RA, right atrium. (*Adapted from* Salcedo E. Atlas of echocardiography. 2nd edition. Philadelphia: WB Saunders; 1985. p. 3; with permission.)

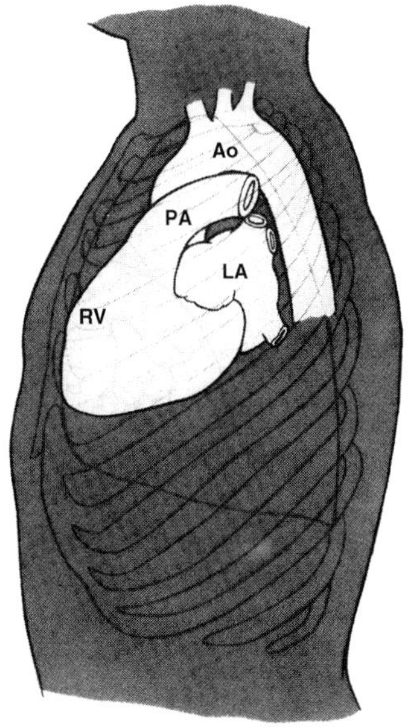

Fig. 2. Lateral view of the heart. Ao, aorta; LA, left atrium; PA, pulmonary artery; RV, right ventricle. (*From* Salcedo E. Atlas of echocardiography. 2nd edition. Philadelphia: WB Saunders; 1985. p. 3; with permission.)

Ultrasound theory

Physics

A basic understanding of ultrasound physics is beneficial to the emergency physician performing echocardiography. Ultrasonography uses high frequency sound waves, which are emitted by the transducer, travel through the body, and are reflected back to the transducer by various structures within the body. The ultrasound machine then processes this signal and displays it on the screen. The first important concept is that the brightness level of an object on the screen is related to the strength of the reflected signal. Blood and other fluids within the body are not strong reflectors and thus appear black or dark gray on the ultrasound screen.

Another important concept is the frequency of the sound wave. A higher frequency sound wave produces a better quality image but, because of attenuation, does not penetrate as deeply into the body. A lower frequency sound wave has the opposite characteristics, a poorer quality image but deeper penetration. A typical transducer used by an emergency physician for echocardiography has a frequency range between 2 and 5 MHz. Generally, the physician should select the highest frequency possible that gives adequate depth of penetration because this will result in the highest quality image. Various approaches or views vary widely in their depth requirements.

The final basic physics concept that is important for the emergency physician is temporal resolution. Ultrasound imaging of the heart differs from imaging other parts of the body in that the object of interest is a moving, dynamic structure. Temporal resolution involves the accuracy of an image over time, from one moment to another. For reasons beyond the scope of this discussion, temporal resolution can be optimized by selecting the minimum depth of field that is needed to visualize all structures adequately. If the physician finds that only the topmost portion of the ultrasound screen is being used, the depth of field setting should be decreased until the majority of the screen is filled with the object of interest. This will maximize the temporal resolution.

B mode

Ultrasound machines offer a selection of modes and settings. For the emergency physician, the setting used most often is the brightness (B) mode. The B mode produces the standard two-dimensional gray-scale images that most clinicians associate with ultrasonography. The brightness of any object on the screen is related to its strength as a reflector of ultrasound waves. The strength of an object as a reflector is related to its acoustic impedance as well as the acoustic impedance of surrounding objects.

When echocardiography is performed, three general types of tissue are encountered: the bone of the sternum and ribs, soft tissue such as heart muscle and liver, and blood. Of these tissues, bones are the strongest reflector and will be very bright (white). Soft tissue is a moderate reflector and will be a shade of gray. Liquid (eg, unclotted blood) is the weakest reflector and will appear dark gray or black. Because of the importance of B mode, it is the default setting for most ultrasound machines.

M mode

Motion (M) mode is an ultrasound machine setting that examines the movement of structures over time and produces a one-dimensional tracing [7]. The display in M mode is typically a split screen: one screen shows a typical gray-scale image, and the other displays a scrolling tracing that represents the movement of structures along a single scan line of the gray-scale image. This setting, which is of limited use to the emergency physician, is used mainly to measure left ventricular size and function [7]. The M mode is more important during obstetric scanning, where it is used to obtain an accurate measurement of fetal heart rate [8].

Doppler

Doppler ultrasound is based on the Doppler shift, which is a change in the frequency of reflected sound when objects are moving toward or away from each other. In the human body, the circulating red blood cells serve as the moving reflector. The Doppler shift is measured by the ultrasound machine, and calculations are made to determine the speed and direction of blood movement. This information can be provided in a variety of ways, including intensity and choice of specific colors, as in color flow Doppler. Doppler ultrasound can help emergency physicians assess a variety of conditions, but its use in echocardiography is an advanced technique, so it is generally not used for this purpose in the emergency department.

Equipment

Several issues must be considered concerning the suitability of an ultrasound machine for use in the emergency department. The first issue is the size and portability of the unit. One of the fundamental principles of emergency ultrasound is that the examination is performed at the patient's bedside, that is, the machine is brought to the patient, not vice versa. A machine that is too heavy, bulky, or difficult to move will not serve this purpose well. Personal experience has shown that a machine in the 300-lb range approaches the upper limit of what can be moved easily. This is a trade-off, however, because the larger machines offer more capabilities in terms of data storage and image capture. Several recent studies highlight the use of small hand-carried ultrasound machines for echocardiography [9–12]. These machines generally weigh less than 10 lbs and offer the ultimate in portability. Theses machines have great promise for the future as technology continues to improve and techniques such as remote data storage are refined.

Another issue to consider is the start-up or warm-up time of the machine, which can range from 20 seconds to several minutes for the more advanced computer-based units. This is not a concern for non-urgent scans; however, in other situations, especially the critically ill hypotensive patient, this delay may be a factor. Proper planning can help in this regard: the machine can be warmed up when advanced notification of the patient's arrival is received. Another strategy is to store the machine in the acute resuscitation bay, turned on, and ready to use, if this does not contradict the manufacturer's recommendations.

The method of image capture is also important. The recording of static images, generally by a thermal printer or digital storage, is a basic capability of nearly all ultrasound machines. Because of the dynamic nature of echocardiography, however, the ability to record moving images is especially useful. This can be accomplished by a standard videocassette recorder or the digital storage of video clips. The availability of these methods will greatly add to the quality assurance and educational aspects of an emergency echocardiography program.

The last aspect of echocardiography equipment to be considered is the transducer. All standard indications for echocardiography can be performed with the standard convex probe found on many machines used for emergency ultrasonography. The same probe can be used for other applications, including abdominal and focused assessment with sonography for trauma (FAST) scanning. The available frequencies will generally range from 2 to 5 MHz.

The disadvantage of using the standard convex probe for echocardiography is that, when assessing several of the cardiac windows, the relatively large footprint (ie, area of contact) of this probe can cause rib shadows throughout the image, which can hinder interpretation. However, this can be overcome in a variety of ways, such as by repositioning the probe. A micro-convex or cardiac transducer can eliminate the issue of rib shadows because its smaller footprint allows easy access between the ribs.

Scanning techniques

The emergency physician can use several approaches or acoustic windows when performing echocardiography. These approaches use the three image planes of the heart [13].

- The long-axis plane extends from the left ventricular apex through the center of the left ventricular base.
- The short-axis plane is perpendicular to the long-axis and produces a cross-sectional image of the left ventricle.
- The four-chamber plane perpendicular to the other two views produces an image of all four heart chambers.

All ultrasound transducers have a marker along one edge, which allows the ultrasonographer to orient the transducer in such a way as to produce images with a consistent orientation. The confusing factor here is that some ultrasound machines, when they are in the "cardiac" setting or mode, may invert the image 180° from what would normally be expected. This situation is made more confusing by the fact that emergency medicine physicians can be inconsistent in their scanning modes. For example, if the heart is being examined as part of a FAST examination, the machine will likely be in the "abdominal" or "general" mode, which does not flip the image; if the heart is being examined on its own, the "cardiac" mode may be selected, which may or may not flip the image, depending on the machine. To avoid confusion, the physician must be aware of (1) the mode being used for a particular examination and (2) whether the machine flips images 180° when it is in the "cardiac" mode. The following comments about transducer orientation are based on the assumption that the image is not being flipped 180° by the machine.

Subcostal

The subxiphoid (subcostal) view should be the standard, default view for the emergency physician performing echocardiography. It is easily learned, accessible, and repeatable, and it gives important information concerning pericardial fluid and cardiac activity [1,7]. The transducer is placed in a subxiphoid location, slightly to the right of midline, and directed toward the left shoulder (Fig. 3). The marker should be oriented toward the patient's right side. It is important that the transducer be placed at a very shallow angle to the patient's upper abdomen. To facilitate this position, the physician should hold the transducer with the hand over the top of the transducer, rather than below it. This window will likely require the deepest depth setting of any scans that the emergency physician performs. In many cases, image quality can be improved by asking the cooperative patient to take and hold a deep breath, which will pull the heart and diaphragm downward, closer to the transducer. This window produces a view of all four heart chambers, the mitral and tricuspid valves and the pericardium (Fig. 4).

A variation of this view, which may be preferred by some physicians in the FAST examination, is the subcostal long-axis view [7]. The transducer is placed in a longitudinal orientation, with the marker toward the patient's head. This position produces an image of the heart, liver, and inferior vena cava. It is especially useful for visualizing pericardial fluid between the heart and liver.

Parasternal long

The parasternal window is located immediately to the left of the sternum, in the second, third, or fourth intercostal space (see Fig. 3). To obtain the long-axis view, the transducer is oriented along the long axis of the heart, from the right shoulder to the left hip, with the marker toward the left hip. The depth setting should be at the lower range because the heart is located quite close to the anterior chest wall. Parasternal images are nearly always enhanced by placing the patient in a left lateral position, which should be done whenever circumstances permit. This image provides views of the left atrium and ventricle, a portion of the right ventricle, the mitral and aortic valves, the aortic root, the pericardium, and the descending aorta (Fig. 5).

Parasternal short

The parasternal short view is obtained at the same parasternal window, with the transducer now rotated 90° so that the marker is toward the right hip. As the transducer is tilted forward and backward, cross-sectional views are obtained at various levels of the heart (Fig. 6). The most inferior position shows the left ventricle as a doughnut-shaped structure. A mid-level view shows the left ventricle at the level of the mitral valve, which produces a "fish-mouth" appearance. The superior view shows the aortic valve with its three leaflets in a "Mercedes Benz" sign.

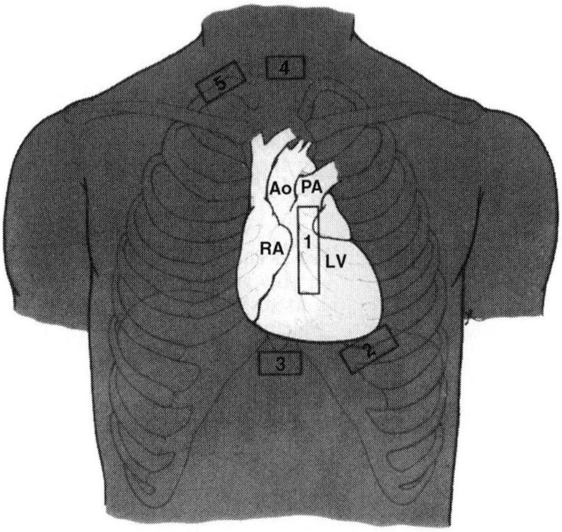

Fig. 3. Cardiac windows: 1, parasternal; 2, apical; 3, subcostal; 4, suprasternal; 5, supraclavicular. Ao, aorta; LV, left ventricle; PA, pulmonary artery; RA, right atrium. (*Adapted from* Salcedo E. Atlas of echocardiography. 2nd edition. Philadelphia: WB Saunders; 1985. p. 4; with permission.)

Apical

The final window for the emergency physician to be familiar with is the apical view. The transducer is placed on the left lateral chest wall, at the point of maximum impulse (see Fig. 3). The transducer is directed toward the patient's right shoulder, with the marker in an anterior direction.

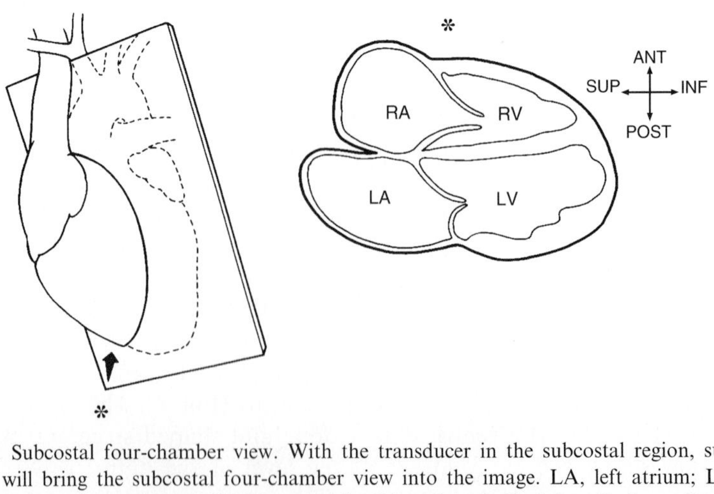

Fig. 4. Subcostal four-chamber view. With the transducer in the subcostal region, superior tilting will bring the subcostal four-chamber view into the image. LA, left atrium; LV, left ventricle; RA, right atrium; RV, right ventricle. (*From* Salcedo E. Atlas of echocardiography. 2nd edition. Philadelphia: WB Saunders; 1985. p. 32; with permission.)

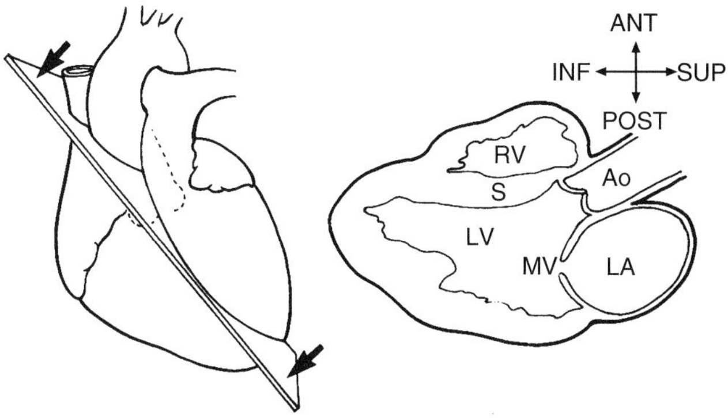

Fig. 5. Parasternal long-axis view (*arrows*). In this view, the right ventricular free wall and the right ventricular cavity (RV) are the most anterior structures. The interventricular septum (S) continues along the line of the anterior wall of the aorta (Ao) and is anterior to the left ventricular (LV) cavity. The posterior wall of the left ventricle is the most posterior structure and superiorly continues along the line of the posterior wall of the left atrium (LA). The left atrium is behind the aorta and is separated from the left ventricle by the mitral valve (MV). (*Adapted from* Salcedo E. Atlas of echocardiography. 2nd edition. Philadelphia: WB Saunders; 1985. p. 17; with permission.)

Imaging through this window also is enhanced by having the patient in a left lateral position. The apical view produces an image in which the heart appears to be "hanging upside-down," with visualization of all four chambers, the mitral and tricuspid valves and the pericardium (Fig. 7).

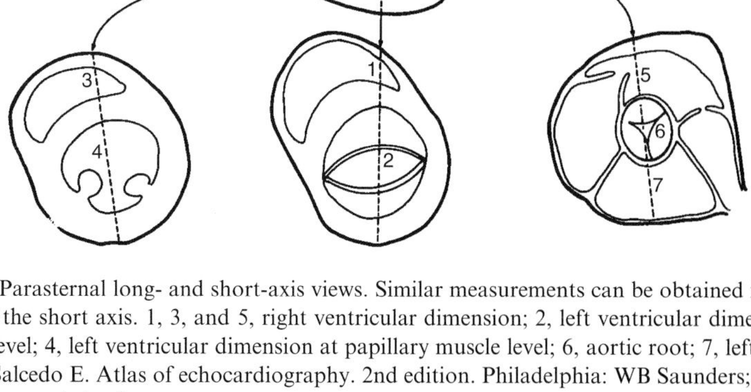

Fig. 6. Parasternal long- and short-axis views. Similar measurements can be obtained from the long or the short axis. 1, 3, and 5, right ventricular dimension; 2, left ventricular dimension at mitral level; 4, left ventricular dimension at papillary muscle level; 6, aortic root; 7, left atrium. (*From* Salcedo E. Atlas of echocardiography. 2nd edition. Philadelphia: WB Saunders; 1985. p. 48; with permission.)

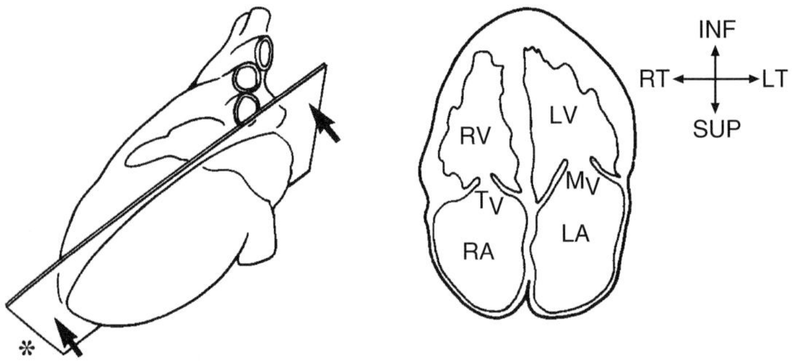

Fig. 7. Apical four-chamber view. With the transducer in the cardiac apex, the sector plane (*arrows*) is oriented parallel to the long axis of the heart. This plane encompasses both right and left ventricles (RV, LV) and both atria (RA, LA) as well as the mitral (MV) and tricuspid valves (TV). (*From* Salcedo E. Atlas of echocardiography. 2nd edition. Philadelphia: WB Saunders; 1985. p. 27; with permission.)

Pericardial effusions

Pericardial effusions have multiple causes. Some are nontraumatic (eg, malignancy, infection, chronic congestive failure, myxedema, or connective tissue diseases). Other effusions are caused by penetrating cardiac injury. Whatever the source, bedside echocardiography can be used to diagnose pericardial effusions and potential cardiac tamponade.

In normal pericardium, there is approximately 30 to 50 mL of fluid between the visceral and parietal pericardium [1]. This amount of fluid usually is not visible on ultrasound. The pericardium should appear echogenic. If there is an effusion, an anechoic space will be evident between the pericardium and the heart. With a large or rapidly developed pericardial effusion, this anechoic space surrounding the heart may be associated with diastolic collapse of the right atrium or the right ventricle [14]. A subcostal view is helpful in identifying a pericardial effusion because there is no pleural reflection between the heart and the liver. Therefore, a large effusion seen in a subcostal view is either between the pericardial or in the free abdominal space [1]. The main way to differentiate between these two locations of fluid is to understand that the pericardial fluid follows the shape of the heart. A parasternal long axis is also helpful because it allows the operator to view possible effusions in the dependent areas of the pericardium (Figs. 8 and 9).

Emergency medicine physicians can reliably perform bedside echocardiography to detect pericardial effusions [3]. Ultrasound use in the emergency department is fast, noninvasive, and easy. Depending on the image interpretation, cardiac ultrasound can direct the management of penetrating chest trauma and improve outcomes for patients with this type of injury [15]. It is especially useful in diagnosing impending cardiac tamponade when classic clinical signs are not present. Beck's triad of jugular venous distension, muffled heart sounds, and hypotension are present in less than

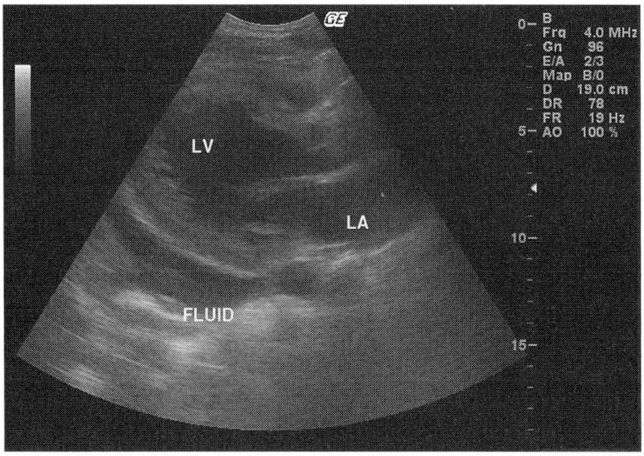

Fig. 8. Long parasternal axis view of pericardial effusion (FLUID). LA, left atrium; LV, left ventricle.

40% of patients with tamponade [16,17]. When these signs are present, it is not until late in the clinical scenario.

Even though emergency medicine physicians are fully capable of performing quality cardiac ultrasound scans, the study is operator-dependent and can be susceptible to misinterpretations. Specifically, pericardial fat can be mistaken for pericardial effusions. Epicardial fat (ie, fat over the apical portion of the heart) is commonly seen in obese patients and is routinely seen in the subcostal view. Confusing epicardial fat for pericardial effusion could result in unnecessary surgical procedures.

To prevent misinterpretations, the cardiac ultrasound be performed in more than one view. In addition, a modified subcostal view can be used to evaluate the pericardium. The probe should be angled longitudinally so that

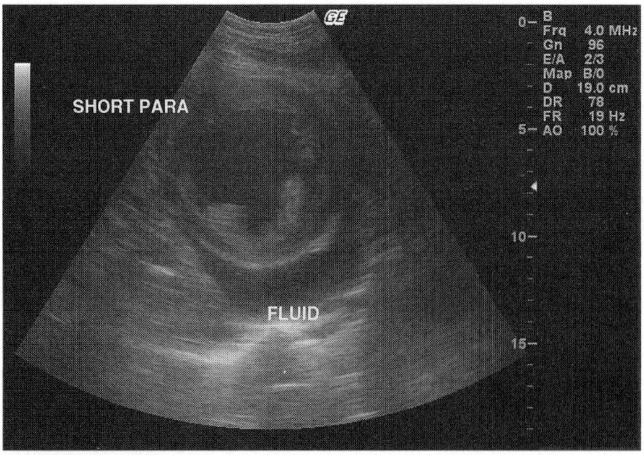

Fig. 9. Short parasternal axis view (SHORT PARA) revealing the left ventricle with surrounding effusion (FLUID).

the inferior vena cava can be seen entering the right atrium [18]. The operator will be able to view the right side of the heart adjacent to the diaphragm and any associated amount of pericardial fluid.

In addition to detecting pericardial effusion, ultrasound can be used to perform pericardiocentesis. In the emergency department, pericardiocentesis usually is a blind procedure. Risks of the procedure include pneumothorax, laceration of cardiac chambers, pneumopericardium, and liver lacerations. Ultrasound guidance may decrease the incidence of these complications. Once the pericardial effusion is visualized, the optimal needle entry site is where the fluid collection is closest to the body surface [19].

Pulseless electrical activity and near-pulseless electrical activity states

Patients in cardiac arrest present to emergency departments every day. Many emergency department physicians use the amount of "downtime" in the field or length of resuscitation before the patient's arrival to determine how long resuscitative efforts must continue. These criteria vary from physician to physician, and a great deal of time and many resources can be spent in attempts to resuscitate patients in cardiac arrest. It can be difficult to determine when to cease resuscitative efforts, especially when the monitor shows an electrical rhythm. Cardiac ultrasound can be used as a predictor in resuscitation, specifically in helping distinguish pulseless electrical activity (PEA) from near-PEA states.

Patients with PEA have an electrical rhythm but no palpable peripheral or central pulse. Patients in near-PEA states are hypotensive and have a palpable pulse, but their blood pressure cannot be obtained [20]. First, cardiac ultrasound can differentiate cardiac activity (near-PEA states) from ventricular standstill (PEA states). Second, ultrasound can identify correctable causes of PEA and allow appropriate management. Third, ultrasound-identified cardiac activity during resuscitation can be used with other factors to help predict survival outcome. Salen and colleagues [21] suggest that the combination of high levels of end tidal Co_2 and sonographic identification of cardiac activity is associated with survival from emergency department (ED) resuscitation. Patients with visualized cardiac standstill have little change in survival rates despite resuscitative efforts [22]. Therefore, cardiac ultrasound can help divide patients into risk groups, depending on whether cardiac activity is evident, and thereby help the emergency medicine physician decide if resuscitation efforts should continue.

Pulmonary embolism

Cardiac ultrasound can be used to aid in the evaluation of patients in whom pulmonary embolism is suspected. In a study of echocardiographic characteristics of pulmonary embolism, Perrier and colleagues [23] found that 75% of patients had a dilated right ventricle and 54% had abnormal septal wall movement. Often, on two-dimensional echocardiography, these patients are seen to also have a hyperkinetic left ventricle [14]. Other echocardiographic abnormalities that suggest pulmonary embolism include right ventricle hypokinesis, leftward septal deviation, and tricuspid regurgitation [24]. The detection of any of these characteristics should be combined with the clinical presentation of the patient during the diagnostic evaluation.

Estimation of central venous pressure

An evaluation of central venous pressure (CVP) is important in critically ill patients who present to the emergency department. CVP can offer information regarding a patient's hemodynamic state. It can be estimated from the observation of jugular venous distension during the physical examination; however, this information is not always readily identifiable, especially in obese patients. Bedside ultrasound offers a quick and noninvasive way to estimate CVP.

CVP can be estimated by viewing the inferior vena cava (IVC) or the internal jugular vein, both of which are easily seen on ultrasound. Normally, the inferior vena cava narrows during inspiration and distends during expiration [25]. When the CVP is elevated, the IVC will be distended throughout both the inspiration and expiratory phases of respiration. This observation indicates that a patient who is in congestive heart failure or has dyspnea or general chest pain may be overloaded with fluid. On the other hand, if the IVC is completely collapsed during inspiration, the patient may have a low CVP [26].

CVP also can be estimated by sonographically evaluating the internal jugular vein. In a patient with CVP greater than 10 cm H_2O (an elevated CVP), the internal jugular vein will appear the same size or larger than the adjacent common carotid artery in a semiupright position. In a patient with a CVP less than 0 cm H_2O (a low CVP), the internal jugular vein will appear collapsed [27]. The right internal jugular vein is the preferred vessel to scan because it is in line with the superior vena cava. However, the CVP estimation should be confirmed on the contralateral vein. Ultrasound of the internal jugular vein is a simple examination that can be performed by a sonographer of any skill level and offers a noninvasive way to estimate CVP.

Cardiac pacing

There are many indications for cardiac pacing in the emergency department (eg, asystole, polymorphic ventricular tachycardia, unstable bradycardia, type II second-degree atrioventricular block, and third-degree AV block). Cardiac pacing can be performed through a transcutaneous, transvenous, or transesophageal route; in most cases in the emergency department, the transcutaneous or the transvenous route is used. A transcutaneous approach is the preferred method of cardiac pacing in the Advanced Cardiac Life Support guidelines [28]. At times, when transcutaneous pacing is used in the ED, it is difficult to determine whether the mechanical capture was successful. Ventricular capture can occur in patients who do not have a detectable pulse or blood pressure; however, bedside ultrasound can be used to determine whether there are ventricular contractions using the subcostal view, based on associated pacer spikes on the pacemaker rhythm strip [29,30].

Transvenous pacing is performed blindly or by electrocardiographic guidance. Fluoroscopy can be used for confirming pacemaker insertion, although fluoroscopy is not always a feasible option for use in the ED. Using the subcostal view of bedside ultrasound, the operator can look for the tip of the pacemaker electrode. If the electrode touches the right ventricular apex and electrical capture is noted on the electrocardiogram, then one can conclude that the transvenous pacemaker placement was successful [31,32]. The subcostal view also is useful in this scenario because it gives a good view of all four chambers of the heart and can detect pericardial fluid, and it allows global evaluation of heart wall motion [33]. However, the caveats in using ultrasound to confirm pacemaker placement include patients who are obese and patients with chronic obstructive pulmonary disease. Both fat and air act as ultrasound barriers, making visualization of catheter tips and cardiac chambers difficult [31].

Evaluation of the patient with undifferentiated hypotension

Patients with hypotension are often seen in the emergency department. Physical examinations can be unreliable in identifying the cause of the hypotension in a timely fashion. Two-dimensional echocardiography performed at the bedside can allow the emergency medicine physician to assess global cardiac wall function. With ultrasound training, emergency medicine physicians become able to determine left ventricle function, which may provide clues as to why a patient is presenting with hypotension [34]. Based on the subjective visual interpretation of the heart, left ventricular function can be categorized as normal or as mildly, moderately, or severely dysfunctional [35]. Overall, cardiac function can provide essential information to guide management of the hypotensive patient.

Summary

The use of bedside ultrasound in the emergency department is becoming more prevalent. Specifically, two-dimensional echocardiography can provide vital information for patient management. Detecting cardiac tamponade, assessing central venous pressure, and capturing cardiac pacing are just a few of the many uses of cardiac ultrasound. Emergency physicians are capable of performing basic cardiac scans with focused training. As more ED physicians become more proficient in ultrasound skills, the uses of bedside echocardiography will continue to expand.

Acknowledgments

The authors thank Jennell S. Dickens and Linda J. Kesselring, MS, ELS, both with the Division of Emergency Medicine at the University of Maryland School of Medicine, for, respectively, typing and copyediting the manuscript.

References

[1] Rubin M. Cardiac ultrasound. Emerg Med Clin North Am 1997;15:745–62.
[2] Mayron R, Gaudio FE, Plummer D, et al. Echocardiography performed by emergency physicians: impact on diagnosis and therapy. Ann Emerg Med 1988;17(2):150–4.
[3] Mandavia DP, Hoffner RJ, Mahaney K, et al. Bedside echocardiography by emergency physicians. Ann Emerg Med 2001;38:377–82.
[4] Witting MD, Euerle BD, Butler KH. A comparison of emergency medicine ultrasound training with guidelines of the Society for Academic Emergency Medicine. Ann Emerg Med 1999;34(5):604–9.
[5] Accredation Council for Graduate Medical Education Emergency Medicine Guidelines. Available at: http://www.acgme.org/acWebsite/RRC_110/110_guidelines.asp#res. Accessed on August 1, 2005.
[6] Salcedo E. Atlas of echocardiography. 2nd edition. Philadelphia: WB Saunders; 1985. pp. 1–7.
[7] Tayal VS, Moore CL, Rose GA. Cardiac. In: Ma OJ, Mateer JR, editors. Emergency ultrasound. New York: McGraw-Hill; 2002. p. 89–127.
[8] Moore C, Promes SB. Ultrasound in pregnancy. Emerg Med Clin Am 2004;22(3):697–722.
[9] Atar S, Feldman A, Darawshe A, et al. Utility and diagnostic accuracy of hand-carried ultrasound for emergency room evaluation of chest pain. Am J Cardiol 2004;94(3):408–9.
[10] Duvall WL, Croft LB, Goldman ME. Can hand-carried ultrasound devices be extended for use by the noncardiology medical community? Echocardiography 2003;20(5):471–6.
[11] Alexander JH, Peterson ED, Chen AY, et al. Feasibility of point-of-care echocardiography by internal medicine house staff. Am Heart J 2004;147(3):476–81.
[12] Xie T, Chamoun A, McMulloch M, et al. Rapid screening of cardiac patients with a miniaturized hand-held ultrasound imager: comparison with physical examination and conventional two-dimensional echocardiography. Clin Cardiol 2004;27(4):241–5.
[13] Otto CM. Transthoracic tomographic views, normal anatomy, and flow patterns. In: Textbook of clinical echocardiography. Philadelphia: WB Saunders; 2000. p. 29–58.
[14] Heller H, Jehle D. Ultrasound in emergency medicine. Philadelphia: WB Saunders; 1995.
[15] Patel AN, Brennig C, Cotner J, et al. Successful diagnosis of penetrating cardiac injury using surgeon-performed sonography. Ann Thorac Surg 2003;76:2043–7.
[16] Thourani VH, Feliciano DV. Penetrating cardiac trauma at an urban trauma center: a 22-year perspective. Am Surg 1999;65:811–9.
[17] Whye D, Barish R, Almquist T, et al. Echocardiographic diagnosis acute pericardial effusion in penetrating chest trauma. Am J Emerg Med 1988;6:21–3.
[18] Blaivas M, DeBehnke D, Phelan MB. Potential errors in the diagnosis of pericardial effusion on trauma ultrasound for penetrating injuries. Acad Emerg Med 2000;7:1261–6.

[19] Osranek M, Bursi F, O'Leary PW, et al. Hand-carried ultrasound-guided pericardiocentesis and thoracentesis. J Am Soc Echocardiogr 2003;16:1–7.
[20] Tayal VS, Kline JA. Emergency echocardiography to detect pericardial effusion in patients in PEA and near-PEA states. Resuscitation 2003;59:315–8.
[21] Salen P, O'Connor R, Sierzenski P, et al. Can cardiac sonography and capnography be used independently and in combination to predict resuscitation outcomes? Acad Emerg Med 2001;8:610–5.
[22] Blaivas M, Fox JC. Outcome in cardiac arrest patients found to have cardiac standstill on the bedside emergency department echocardiogram. Acad Emerg Med 2001;8:616–21.
[23] Perrier A, Tamm C, Unger P, Lerch R, et al. Diagnostic accuracy of Doppler-echocardiography in unselected patients with unsuspected pulmonary embolism. Int J Cardiol 1998;65:101–9.
[24] Miniati M, Monti S, Pratali L, et al. Value of transthoracic echocardiography in the diagnosis of pulmonary embolism: results of a prospective study in unselected patients. Am J Med 12001;10:528–35.
[25] Natori H, Tamaki S, Kira S. Ultrasonographic evaluation of ventilatory effect on inferior vena caval configuration. Am Rev Respir Dis 1979;120:421–5.
[26] Randazzo MR, Snoey ER, Levitt MA, et al. Accuracy of emergency physician assessment of left ventricular ejection fraction and central venous pressure using echocardiography. Acad Emerg Med 2003;10:973–7.
[27] Lipton B. Estimation of central venous pressure by ultrasound of the internal jugular vein. Am J Emerg Med 2000;18:432–4.
[28] Emergency cardiac pacing. In: Cummins RO, editor. Advanced care life support. Dallas (TX): American Heart Association; 1997. p. 1–5.
[29] Holger JS, Lamon RP, Minnegan HJ, et al. Use of ultrasound to determine ventricular capture in transcutaneous pacing. Am J Emerg Med 2003;21:227–9.
[30] Holger JS, Minnigan HJ, Lamon RP, et al. The utility of ultrasound to determine ventricular external cardiac pacing. Am J Emerg Med 2001;19:134–6.
[31] Aguilera PA, Durham BA, Riley DA. Emergency transvenous cardiac placement using ultrasound guidance. Ann Emerg Med 2000;36:224–7.
[32] Meier B, Felner JM. Two-dimensional echocardiographic evaluation of intracardiac transvenous pacemaker leads. J Clin Ultrasound 1982;10:421–5.
[33] Macedo W, Sturmann K, Kim JM, et al. Ultrasonographic guidance of transvenous pacemaker insertion in the emergency department: a report of three cases. J Emerg Med 1999;17:491–6.
[34] Moore CL, Rose GA, Tayal VS, et al. Determination of left ventricular function by emergency physician echocardiography of hypotensive patients. Acad Emerg Med 2002;9: 186–93.
[35] McGowan JH, Cleland JGF. Reliability of reporting left ventricular systolic function by echocardiography: a systemic review of 3 methods. Am Heart J 2003;146:388–97.

ELSEVIER
SAUNDERS

Emerg Med Clin N Am
23 (2005) 1195–1217

EMERGENCY
MEDICINE
CLINICS OF
NORTH AMERICA

Cardiovascular Challenges in Toxicology

Christopher P. Holstege, MD*,
Stephen Dobmeier, BSN, CSPI

Blue Ridge Poison Center, Division of Medical Toxicology, Department of Emergency Medicine, University of Virginia, P.O. Box 800774, Charlottesville, VA 22908-0774, USA

The diagnoses and subsequent treatment of poisoned patients manifesting cardiovascular compromise challenges the most experienced emergency physician. Numerous drugs and chemicals cause cardiac and vascular disorders. Despite widely varying indications for therapeutic use, many agents share a common cardiovascular pharmacologic effect if taken in overdose. Standard advanced cardiac life support protocol care of these patients may not apply and may even result in harm if followed [1]. This chapter discusses common cardiovascular toxins and groups them into their common mechanisms of toxicity.

Epidemiology

Emergency physicians routinely evaluate and manage poisoned patients. In 2003, more than 2.3 million human exposure cases were reported to poison centers throughout the United States [1]. Of those cases, more than 500,000 (22%) were treated at health care facilities, with most of those cases evaluated in the emergency department. Cardiovascular drugs were listed as the seventh most frequently encountered human exposure in adults (40,896 cases) and the fifth leading cause of poisoning deaths. When taken in overdose, numerous other products can also produce cardiovascular toxic effects. Emergency physicians should consider the cardiac complications of specific agents at the time they are evaluating poisoned patients.

Cardiac physiology

To understand the cardiac complications of various agents, physicians must have a clear understanding of basic myocardial cell function. The

* Corresponding author.
E-mail address: ch2xf@virginia.edu (C.P. Holstege).

doi:10.1016/j.emc.2005.07.001

myocardial cell membrane in its resting state is impermeable to Na^+. The $Na^+ - K^+ -$ ATPase actively pumps three Na^+ ions out of cardiac cells while pumping in two K^+ ions to maintain a negative electric potential in the myocyte of approximately −90 mV (phase 4). Depolarization of the cardiac cell membrane is a result of the rapid opening of Na^+ channels and the subsequent massive Na^+ influx (phase 0). This Na^+ influx causes the rapid upstroke of the cardiac action potential because it is conducted through the ventricles and is directly responsible for the QRS interval of the EKG. The peak of the action potential is marked by the closure of Na^+ channels and the activation of K^+ efflux channels (phase 1). Calcium influx then occurs allowing for a plateau in the action potential (phase 2) and continued myocardial contraction. The cardiac cycle ends with closure of the Ca^{++} channels and activation of K^+ efflux channels causing the potential to again approach −90 mV (phase 3). It is this K^+ efflux from the myocardial cell that is directly responsible for the QT interval of the EKG.

General management of agents that cause cardiovascular toxicity

All patients who present to the emergency department (ED) following an overdose of agents that could result in cardiovascular toxicity should be closely monitored. The patient's airway should be patent and adequate ventilation assured. If necessary, endotracheal tube intubation should be performed. Too often physicians are lulled into a false sense of security at the time a patient's oxygen saturations are adequate on high-flow oxygen. If the patient has inadequate ventilation, the patient may be at risk for subsequent CO_2 narcosis, declining mental status, and development of a respiratory acidosis. The patient who has a poor gag reflex is at risk for the development of aspiration and prolonged hospitalization [2]. In those patients, intubation should be performed. Because laryngoscopy has been reported to induce a vagal response, administration of atropine should be considered in the bradycardic patient before intubation [3,4].

Patients who have overdosed on potential cardiovascular toxins should be placed on continuous cardiac monitoring with pulse oximetry. All patients should receive a large bore peripheral intravenous (IV) line and all symptomatic patients should have a second line placed peripheral or central. If the patient is a potential candidate for an IV pacemaker, central line placement should be placed in the right internal jugular or the left subclavian [5]. The initial treatment of hypotension consists of IV fluids. Close monitoring of the patient's pulmonary examination should be performed to assure that pulmonary edema does not develop as fluids are infused. Frequent neurologic checks should be made. In patients who experience altered mental status, the patient's glucose should be checked. Placement of a urinary catheter should be considered early in the care of symptomatic patients to monitor urinary output as an indicator of adequate renal perfusion.

Gastrointestinal decontamination should be considered only after initial supportive care has been provided and airway control has been assured. Activated charcoal (1g/kg) may be considered. Because many cardiovascular agents have sustained release preparations, multidose charcoal administration (1 g/kg first dose and 1/2 g/kg every 4 hours) should be considered along with whole bowel irrigation (Golytely at 500 mL/h for children and up to 2 L/h for adults) [6,7]. Ipecac syrup should not be administered in the ED and is contraindicated after overdose with the agents listed in this article because of the potential for rapid clinical deterioration [8]. Gastric lavage has not been shown to change outcome after overdose of these agents and can induce an unwanted vagal response [9].

Calcium channel blocker toxicity

Various calcium channel blockers (CCBs) are available by prescription. This group of agents includes derivatives from four structural classes: (1) the dihydropyridines (nicardipine, nifedipine, isradipine, amlodipine, felodipine, and nimodipine), (2) the phenylalkylamines (verapamil), (3) the benzothiazepines (diltiazem) and (4) the diarylaminopropylamine ethers (bepridil). As each agent has become available on the market over the past decade, the number of exposures has dramatically increased [1,10]. In 2003, there were 9650 CCB exposures reported to poison centers in the United States, with more than 1000 of those exposures categorized as moderate or major outcomes accounting for 57 deaths [1].

Pathophysiology

The CCBs discussed earlier inhibit the voltage sensitive L-type calcium channel within the cell membrane [11]. This channel resides in heart and vascular smooth muscle cell membranes. The inhibition of this channel prevents movement of Ca^{++} from extracellular sites through the cell membrane to intracellular sites. The inhibition of Ca^{++} influx within the conduction system results in slowing of conduction; potential first-, second-, and third-degree heart blocks; bradycardia; bundle branch blocks; and junctional and ventricular escape rhythms [12]. Decreased intracellular Ca^{++} within the myocardial cells results in decreased contractility and decreased cardiac output. Blockade of Ca^{++} influx within the vascular smooth muscle cells results in vasodilation. Decreased cardiac output coupled with vasodilation may result in profound hypotension [12].

The CCBs have also been associated with profound hyperglycemia refractory to standard doses of insulin [13]. CCB-mediated blockade of insulin release and the blockade of peripheral insulin receptors have been suggested as the possible etiology [14].

In animal models and human case series, verapamil and diltiazem have also been associated with cardiac Na^{+} channel blockade [13,15]. This blockade can result in a delay of phase 0 of depolarization, subsequent QRS prolongation, and further potential for dysrhythmias [13].

Clinical features

Hypotension is a common sign associated with toxicity from CCBs. Initially, the patient may complain of lightheadedness or dizziness, especially upon standing. Depending on the agent ingested, reflex tachycardia may not be seen. As levels of CCBs increase, the patient may develop marked hypotension, various heart blocks, bradydysrhythmias, acute mental status changes, oliguria, hyperglycemia, acidosis, syncope, asystole, and death [16,17]. Symptomatic CCB-overdose patients are prone to development of pulmonary edema, and frequent pulmonary reassessments should be made [18].

Management

A symptomatic acute CCB overdose can be one of the most challenging poisonings encountered by the emergency physician. Initial management of all CCB-toxic patients should be treated in the manner discussed in the section Entitled "General Management of Agents That Cause Cardiovascular Toxicity." Atropine may be considered in an attempt to reverse symptomatic bradycardia at doses of 1 to 2 mg IV for adults (0.02 mg/kg in children, minimum of 0.15 mg and a maximum of 1 mg); however, atropine may be ineffective at reversing the bradycardia [16,19].

In symptomatic CCB poisonings, an IV calcium infusion should be considered early in the care [20]. Before central venous access, calcium gluconate may be infused through peripheral line access. Recall that 10 mL of 10% calcium gluconate (93 mg Ca^{2+} or 4.6 mEq Ca^{2+}) provides less bioavailable calcium than 10 mL of 10% calcium chloride (272 mg Ca^{2+} or 13.6 mEq Ca^{2+}). However, calcium chloride has been reported to cause marked tissue necrosis if it extravasates while being infused through peripheral venous access [21]. After central venous access is obtained, calcium chloride may be infused. The exact infusion doses of calcium and targeted calcium levels have not been well delineated [22]. An initial dose of 10 mL of 10% or 1 g in adults (20 mg/kg or up to 1 g in children) administered IV is an appropriate starting dose. This dose may be repeated and titrated to clinical effect. Increasing the patient's ionized calcium may lead to further sedation, nausea, and vomiting.

Glucagon may be beneficial in the management of the CCB overdose [23–26]. Glucagon raises intracellular cyclic adenosine monophosphate (cAMP) concentrations that in turn open cell membrane calcium channels. A starting dose of 5 mg (50 μg/kg in children) of IV glucagon (diluted in 10 mL and infused over 1–2 minutes) should be considered, with repeat dosing administered as needed. A glucagon infusion at 5–10 mg/hr (50 μg/kg/h in children) may be considered. Glucagon at this dosage may induce emesis that could lead to aspiration in the sedate, nonintubated patient. When mixing glucagon, use normal saline and avoid using the glucagon package diluent. The package diluent contains 0.2% phenol and might hypothetically result in toxicity in high doses.

High-dose insulin drips have been advocated in CCB overdose. Experimental models suggest a superior effect of this therapy in the canine model compared with other therapies [27]. Human case reports also suggest the efficacy of these drips [13,28–30]. The optimal dose of insulin is unclear [31]. Insulin infusions can be initiated at 0.2 U/kg/h and titrated upward every hour to euglycemic effect and hemodynamic effect. Supplemental glucose may be necessary to maintain euglycemia. Serum glucose and potassium levels should be monitored closely during therapy.

Catecholamine infusions may be considered after the above therapies fail to give adequate response. Epinephrine and norepinephrine have been used in the management of CCB toxicity [32,33]. Dobutamine, a direct β_1-adrenergic agonist, may be of benefit, but adequate studies of its effect in CCB toxicity are lacking [33]. The phosphodiesterase inhibitors, amrinone and milrinone, have also been reported to be of benefit following CCB toxicity.

Recently, sodium bicarbonate infusions have been advocated in the management of CCB toxicity [13,15]. Patients with prolonged QRS (>100 ms), acidosis, or persistent hypotension despite the above methods should be considered candidates for a trial of sodium bicarbonate in doses noted in the section entitled "Sodium Channel Blocker Toxicity."

Pacemakers, intra-aortic balloon pump, extracorporeal membrane oxygenation, and cardiopulmonary bypass may all be considered in cases not responding to pharmacologic therapy [33,34]. Vasopressin has been reported to reverse hypotension following some overdoses, but a recent study does not support the use of vasopressin monotherapy in shock secondary to CCB toxicity [35]. None of the CCBs are amendable to hemodialysis or hemoperfusion because of their large size, high protein binding, or large volume of distribution.

Disposition

Asymptomatic CCB overdose patients with normal ECGs and ingestions of nonsustained release products may be observed in the ED for 4 hours [36]. If they remain asymptomatic and the ECG remains unchanged, they may be discharged to a nonmonitored setting. An asymptomatic patient acutely overdosing on a sustained release product should be admitted to a monitored bed for observation [36,37]. Any symptomatic CCB patient should be admitted to a monitored setting until complete resolution of symptoms occurs [38].

Beta-blocker toxicity

ß-adrenergic receptor antagonists are increasingly used because of their efficacy in the treatment of hypertension, ischemic heart disease, and arrhythmias. Numerous beta-blockers (BBs) are available on the market. These agents share in common the mechanism of competitive ß-adrenergic receptor antagonism. Some of these agents have equal affinity for β_1 and β_2 receptors (ie, propranolol), whereas others are selective and have greater β_1 than β_2-receptor–blocking activity (ie, metoprolol). Some agents also block other receptors, such as α-adrenergic receptors (ie, labetalol), cardiac Na^+ channels (ie, propranolol), and cardiac potassium efflux channels (ie, sotalol) [39,40].

Pathophysiology

BBs competitively inhibit the ß-adrenergic receptor. Inhibition of β_1-receptors results in a decrease in the force and rate of myocardial contraction, a decrease in AV node conduction velocity, and a decrease in renin secretion. Inhibition of β_2-receptors results in a decrease in glycogenolysis, decrease in gluconeogenesis, and decrease in relaxation of smooth muscles in blood vessels, bronchi, and the gastrointestinal tract.

Clinical features

In acute overdose (OD), BBs most pronounced effect is on the cardiovascular system [25,41]. Bradycardia, heart blocks, and hypotension are the hallmarks of significant BB toxicity [42]. Dyspnea may occur and be the result of congestive heart failure or bronchospasm. Coma, grand mal seizures, and changes in mental have been reported. Hypoglycemia may occur, especially in young children [43].

Management

The initial management of all patients presenting after an acute overdose of BBs or presenting with significant toxicity should be treated as in the manner discussed above in the "General Management of Agents That Cause Cardiovasacular Toxicity" section. Atropine may be considered in an attempt to reverse bradycardia at doses of 1–2 mg IV (0.02 mg/kg in children, minimum of 0.15 mg and a maximum of 1 mg). In previous BB intoxications, atropine has shown inconsistent effects in reversing bradycardia and hypotension [44].

Glucagon infusion should be considered in symptomatic BB-toxic patients [25,26,44]. ß-adrenergic stimulation raises intracellular cAMP concentrations that in turn regulate ion channels. When ß-adrenergic receptors are inhibited, intracellular cAMP levels decrease. Glucagon increases intracellular cAMP through nonadrenergic pathways [45]. A starting dose of 5–10 mg in adults (50 μg/kg in children) of IV glucagon (diluted in 10 mL and infused over 1–2 minutes) should be considered and can be repeated if necessary. Glucagon can be infused at 5 mg/h for adults

(50 μg/kg/h in children). For further information on glucagon therapy, see the section entitled "Calcium Channel Blocker Toxicity."

Calcium demonstrates efficacy at reversing the hypotensive effects of toxicity in animal models and human case reports [25,46–48]. Dosing of calcium should be performed at dosage noted in the CCB section.

Insulin infusions have been advocated for BB toxicity based on an animal model [49]. The exact mechanism of this therapy is unclear, but it is believed to be secondary to increased myocardial glucose use resulting from the high-dose insulin drips.

Catecholamine infusions may be considered after the therapies discussed earlier fail to give adequate response. Epinephrine and norepinephrine have been used in the management of BB toxicity. Dopamine has been used. Recall that dopamine at low concentrations (1–5 μg/kg/min) effects dopamine receptors in renal, mesenteric, and coronary beds leading to vasodilation. At somewhat higher concentrations (5–10 μg/kg/min), dopamine exerts positive ionotrophic effects by acting on $ß_1$-adrenergic receptors. It is not until dopamine is infused at high concentrations (>10 μ/kg/min), that dopamine effects $ß_1$-adrenergic receptors and leads to vasoconstriction and elevated blood pressure. Unlike the direct $ß_1$-adrenergic agonist activity of epinephrine and norepinephrine, dopamine does not have significant direct activity and instead induces norepinephrine release at the $ß_1$-adrenergic receptor. Dobutamine, a direct $ß_1$-adrenergic agonist, may be of benefit but adequate studies of its effect in BB toxicity are lacking [32]. Isoproterenol is a potent, nonselective ß-adrenergic agonist and may also be considered [46,50].

Sodium bicarbonate infusions have been advocated in the management of propranolol toxicity because of propranolol's cardiac Na^+ channel-blockading activity [8,51]. Propranolol overdoses with prolonged QRS (>100 milliseconds), acidosis, or persistent hypotension despite the above therapies should be considered candidates for a trial of sodium bicarbonate in doses noted in the section entitled "Sodium Channel Blocker Toxicity."

The phosphodiesterase inhibitors (ie, amrinone, milrinone) and aminophylline increase cAMP concentrations and, therefore, would theoretically be useful in BB toxicity. Animal models and case reports suggest improved survival with their use, but their efficacy beyond the use of glucagon is questionable [52,53]. Pacemaker insertion, balloon pump, and bypass may all be considered in cases not responding to pharmacologic therapy [54]. Extracorporeal removal has been reported with specific BBs with small volumes of distribution and low protein binding (atenolol, nadolol, and acebutolol), but removal is technically difficult if there is coexisting hypotension [55,56].

Disposition

Asymptomatic BB overdose patients who produce normal ECGs and ingestions of nonsustained release BB should be observed in the ED for at least 6 hours [8,41]. If they remain asymptomatic and the ECG remains unchanged, they may be discharged to a nonmonitored setting. Asymptomatic patients acutely overdosing on a sustained release BB or sotalol should be admitted to a monitored bed for observation. Symptomatic BB-toxic patient should be admitted to a monitored setting until complete resolution of symptoms occurs.

Sodium channel blocker toxicity

The ability of drugs to block cardiac Na^+ channels has been well described in several previous literature reports [57]. This Na^+ channel-blockading activity has been described as a membrane stabilizing effect, a local anesthetic effect, or a quinidinelike effect. Agents associated with myocardial Na^+ channel blockade are listed in Table 1.

Pathophysiology

Cardiac voltage-gated Na^+ channels reside in the cell membrane and open in response to depolarization of the cell. The Na^+ channel blockers bind to the transmembrane Na^+ channels and decrease the number available for depolarization. This binding creates a delay of Na^+ entry into the cardiac myocyte during phase 0 of depolarization. As a result, the upslope of depolarization is slowed and the QRS complex widens.

Clinical features

Myocardial Na^+ channel-blocking drugs comprise a diverse group of pharmaceutical agents (see Table 1). As a result, patients poisoned with these agents have various clinical presentations. For example, cyclic antidepressants, propoxyphene, and cocaine may result in anticholinergic, opioid, and sympathomimetic syndromes respectively. In addition, these agents may affect not only the myocardial Na^+ channels, but also other myocardial ion channels, such as the Ca^{++} influx and K^{++} efflux channels. EKG changes and rhythm disturbances not related entirely to the drug's Na^+ channel-blocking activity may result.

Sodium channel blockers result in widening of the QRS complex [58,59]. In some cases, the QRS complexes may take the pattern of recognized bundle branch blocks. In the most severe cases, the QRS prolongation becomes so profound that it is difficult to distinguish between ventricular and supraventricular rhythms [60]. Continued prolongation of the QRS may result in a sine wave pattern and eventual asystole. Sodium channel blockers may also induce a monomorphic ventricular tachycardia. Theoretically, the Na^+ channel blockers can cause slowed intraventricular conduction, unidirectional block, the development of a re-entrant circuit, and a resulting ventricular tachycardia, which can degenerate into ventricular fibrillation. Because many of the Na^+ channel-blocking agents are also anticholinergic

Table 1
Potassium and sodium channel blocking drugs and sodium-potassium-ATPase–blocking agents

K^+ efflux channel-blocking drugs	Na^+ channel-blocking drugs	$Na^+ - K^+$ ATPase-blocking agents
Antihistamines	Amantadine	Bufadienolides
astemizole	Carbamazepine	Digoxin
clarithromycin	Chloroquine	Digitoxin
diphenhydramine	Class IA antiarrhythmics	Foxglove
loratidine	disopyramide	Lily of the valley
terfenadine	quinidine	Oleander
Antipsychotics	procainamide	Red squill
chlorpromazine	Class IC antiarrhythmics	
droperidol	encainide	
haloperidol	flecainide	
mesoridazine	propafenone	
pimozide	Citalopram	
quetiapine	Cocaine	
risperidone	Cyclic antidepressants	
thioridazine	amitriptyline	
ziprasidone	amoxapine	
Arsenic trioxide	desipramine	
Bepridil	doxepin	
Chloroquine	imipramine	
Cisapride	nortriptyline	
Citalopram	maprotiline	
Clarithromycin	Diltiazem	
Class 1A antiarrhythmics	Diphenhydramine	
disopyramide	Hydroxychloroquine	
quinidine	Loxapine	
procainamide	Orphenadrine	
Class 1C antiarrhythmics	Phenothiazines	
encainide	medoridazine	
flecainide	thioridazine	
moricizine	Propranolol	
propafenone	Propoxyphene	
Class III antiarrhythmics	Quinine	
amiodarone	Verapamil	
dofetilide		
ibutilide		
sotalol		
Cyclic antidepressants		
Erythomycin		
Fluoroquinolones		
Halofantrine		
Hydroxychloroquine		
Levomethadyl		
Pentamidine		
Quinine		
Tacrolimus		
Venlafaxine		

or sympathomimetic agents, bradydysrhythmias are rare. However, the Na^+ channel-blocking agents can affect cardiac pacemaker cells. Bradycardia may occur as a result of slowed depolarization of pacemaker cells that depend upon entry of Na^+. In Na^+ channel blocker poisoning by anticholinergic and sympathomimetic drugs, the combination of a wide QRS complex and bradycardia is an ominous sign and may indicate that the Na^+ channel blockade is so profound that a tachycardia cannot be mounted in response to muscarinic antagonism or adrenergic agonism.

Management

The initial management of all patients presenting after an acute overdose of Na^+ channel-blocking agents or presenting with significant toxicity from these agents should be treated as discussed in the above section entitled "General Management of Agents That Cause Cardiovascular Toxicity." The management of Na^+ channel-blocking agents consists of administration sodium or alkalosis [61–63]. Infusion of sodium bicarbonate by intermittent bolus or by continuous infusion has been advocated. Hypertonic sodium infusion has also been shown to be effective [64]. A sodium bicarbonate infusion should be considered if any of the following criteria are met: QRS duration is greater than 100 milliseconds, persistent hypotension despite adequate hydration occurs, or dysrhythmias. Recall that a single ampule of sodium bicarbonate contains 50 mEq of Na^+ and multiple doses may be necessary to achieve clinical improvement of the patient. Sodium bicarbonate infusions can be created by mixing at least 3 ampules of sodium bicarbonate in 1 L of D5W and with the rate infused at two times maintenance. Consider adding potassium (40 mEq to a liter of D5W) to the sodium bicarbonate drip to prevent the development of hypokalemia (caused by the excretion of potassium in exchange for hydrogen ions as the kidneys attempt to correct the alkalosis). The infusion can then be adjusted to maintain a blood pH between 7.5 and 7.55. During infusions of sodium bicarbonate, close monitoring of electrolyte, pH, and fluid balance should be performed.

Hyperventilation has been shown to be effective in reversing sodium channel-blocking activity, most likely secondary to the induced respiratory alkalosis [65,66]. Lidocaine has been suggested in the treatment of ventricular dysrhythmias, though clear evidence is lacking [67]. Class IA and IC antiarrhythmics should be avoided because of their ability to block cardiac sodium channels.

Disposition

Any symptomatic patient who has ingested a potential Na^+ channel-blocking agent should be admitted and observed in a monitored setting. In the asymptomatic patient who has ingested a Na^+ channel-blocking agent, the length of observation varies. For example, a patient who has ingested amitriptyline should be observed for a minimum of 6 hours. If that patient remains asymptomatic and develops no ECG changes during that time period, they can be discharged to an unmonitored setting. Other poisonings, such as diphenhydramine, can be discharged if asymptomatic after a 4-hour postingestion observation period.

Potassium efflux blocker toxicity

Definition

Studies suggest that approximately 3% of total noncardiac prescriptions are associated with the potential for QT prolongation [68]. Potassium efflux-blocking agents competitively inhibit cellular potassium efflux during cellular repolarization; therefore, a delay in repolarization occurs corresponding with an increase in the QT interval [69]. The patient may then be at risk for polymorphic ventricular tachycardia or torsades de pointes [70]. Drugs, such as sotalol, are prescribed specifically for this mechanism [71]. Other medications possess this activity as an unwelcome side effect at therapeutic doses. Many medications, such as terfenadine and cisapride, have been removed from the United States market because of reports of torsades de pointes and sudden death in patients taking these drugs [72,73]. Other medications have rarely been reported to cause QT prolongation except when taken in massive overdose. Agents associated with QT prolongation are listed in Table 1 [68,74]. Other etiologies of prolongation of the QT interval include: (1) congenital long QT syndrome, (2) hypokalemia, (3) hypomagnesemia, (4) hypocalcemia, (5) myocardial ischemia, (6) neurological catastrophes, and (7) hypothyroidism [75].

Pathophysiology

The primary problem with K^+ channel-blocking drugs is that they prolong cardiac action potentials [76], which may lead to early afterdepolarizations (EAD), related triggered activity, and the possibility of torsades de pointes. Patients at increased risk are those with familial QT prolongation, patients who develop electrolyte abnormalities, patients on multiple agents with K^+ efflux channel-blocking activity, or patients on drugs that inhibit the metabolism of K^+ efflux channel-blocking agents resulting in the build-up to toxic levels.

Clinical features

Syncope may be associated with drug-induced QT prolongation. Palpitations, dyspnea, and sudden death may also be associated with QT prolongation. After acute overdose, the presenting signs and symptoms may not be related to the cardiac effects but to the other mechanisms of those drugs.

Management

If a patient has a prolonged QT interval caused by a potassium efflux-blocking agent, therapy should focus on immediate withdrawal of the potential cause and correction of any coexisting hypoxia or electrolyte abnormalities. The initial management of all patients presenting after an acute overdose of an agent associated with K^+ efflux blockade should be treated as discussed in the section entitled "General Management of Agents That Cause Cardiovascular Toxicity." IV magnesium sulfate is a highly effective intervention to suppress occurrence of dysrhythmias associated with QT prolongation, even though Mg^{++} does not typically result in shortening of the QT interval itself [77]. A starting dose of 2 g diluted in 10 mL D5W may be infused and titrated to effect.

In patients who experience intermittent runs of torsades not responsive to magnesium therapy, electrical overdrive pacing should be considered [78]. Pacing at rates up to 100 to 120 beats per minute is often effective at terminating torsades de pointes. In the presence of a nonperfusing rhythm, such as ventricular fibrillation, pulseless ventricular tachycardia, or torsades de pointes, unsynchronized electrical defibrillation should be performed.

Disposition

Patients with newly diagnosed prolongation of their QT interval or torsades de pointes should be admitted to a monitored setting. Symptomatic patients who have ingested these agents should also be admitted to a monitored setting.

Sodium-Potassium-ATPase—Blocker Toxicity

Cardiac glycosides (CGs) are agents that inhibit the sodium-potassium adenosine triphosphosphate ($Na^+ - K^+ -$ ATPase) pump. Digoxin is the most widely encountered CG, but numerous other similar acting agents also exist (see Table 1). Digoxin has been historically administered to treat supraventricular tachydysrhythmias and congestive heart failure, but its use has been decreasing as newer agents have been developed. Cardiac glycosides that are not prescription medications have also been associated with human toxicity, such as after ingestion of specific plants and contaminated herbal products [79–82].

Pathophysiology

The CGs inhibit active transport of Na^+ and K^+ across cell membranes by inhibiting the $Na^+ - K^+ -$ ATPase, which results in an increase in extracellular potassium and intracellular Na^+. An increased intracellular Na^+ results in a reduced transmembrane Na^+ gradient and subsequent increased activity of the $Na^+ - Ca^+$ exchanger. Intracellular calcium rises. The increased intracellular Ca^{++} augments myofibril activity in cardiac myocytes and causes a positive inotropic action. CGs also increase vagal tone that may lead to a direct antrioventricular depression and produce conduction disturbances.

Clinical features

Cardiac glycoside toxicity may result in the following dysrhythmias [83]: (1) excitant activity (atrial, junctional and ventricular premature beats and tachydysrhythmias); (2) suppressant activity (sinus bradycardia, bundle branch blocks, first-, second-, and third-degree blocks); and (3) combination of excitant and suppressant activity (atrial tachycardia with atrioventricular block, second-degree block with junctional premature beats). The most common dysrhythmia associated with toxicity induced by these agents is frequent premature ventricular beats. Bidirectional ventricular tachycardia is specific for digitalis toxicity but is rarely seen.

In addition to the cardiac manifestations, noncardiac signs and symptoms may occur in CG toxicity and vary widely depending on whether the toxicity is acute or chronic. Anorexia, nausea, vomiting, headache, fatigue, depression, dizziness, confusion, memory loss, delirium, and hallucinations have all been noted. Visual disturbances, including seeing yellow halos around objects (xanthopsia), have been reported. Not uncommonly, chronic digoxin intoxication may be misdiagnosed as a more common illness, such as influenza or gastroenteritis.

Patients suspected of having CG toxicity should have an ECG performed and a chemistry obtained. Acute toxicity most closely correlates with hyperkalemia as the $Na^+ - K^+ -$ ATPase is inhibited and extracellular K^+ rises. In chronic toxicity, hyperkalemia may not be seen because of the slow increase in K^+, allowing the kidneys to correct the imbalance. Many of those patients on chronic digoxin therapy are also on diuretics that further promote potassium excretion. Chronic toxicity associated with renal failure may result in hyperkalemia caused by the kidneys' inability to compensate.

A serum digoxin level should be obtained with therapeutic levels reported between 0.5 to 2.0 ng/mL. Serum digoxin levels should be interpreted with caution. In acute exposure, digoxin is absorbed into the plasma and then slowly redistributes into the tissues. As a result, high acute digoxin levels are not always associated with toxicity. Levels greater that 10 ng/mL at any time may be associated with significant toxicity and treatment with digoxin-specific Fab should be considered. Other CGs can cross-react with the digoxin assay, though the degree of this cross-reaction is not known. A false positive assay may result in the presence of digoxinlike immunoreactive substance seen in neonates, pregnancy, renal insufficiency, liver disease, congestive heart failure, acromegaly, and stress [84].

Management

Cardiac glycoside toxicity should always be considered in patients taking digoxin and presenting with new onset dysrhythmias, gastrointestinal complaints, or altered mental status. Meticulous attention to supportive care and a search for easily correctable conditions, such as hypoxia, hypovolemia, and electrolyte disturbances, are top priorities. Patients should always be treated as discussed in the section entitled "General Management of Agents That Cause Cardiovascular Toxicity."

In CG-poisoned patients, Fab fragments are the first-line therapy in patients who have symptomatic cardiac dysrhythmias [83,85,86]. Atropine use in animal models decreased the total percent of digoxin induced arrhythmias, delayed their onset, and changed the type of arrhythmias [87]. Cardiac pacing has been advocated for bradydysrhythmias unresponsive to atropine, but care should be exercised because the pacing wire itself may induce ventricular fibrillation. The classic antiarrhythmic of choice for ventricular dysrhythmias is phenytoin because it increases the ventricular fibrillation threshold in the myocardium and enhances conduction through the AV node. Lidocaine has been advocated for treatment of ventricular dysrhythmias caused by digitalis toxicity, although it does not affect AV nodal conduction. Few reports exist of the use of amiodarone for digoxin toxicity. Amiodarone has been reported to be effective in case reports of digoxin induced dysrhythmias [88]. Quinidine and procainamide are contraindicated in digitalis toxicity because they depress AV nodal conduction and may worsen cardiac toxicity. Electrical cardioversion of the digitalis-toxic patient must be performed with extreme caution and considered only as a last resort. A low energy setting (eg, 10–25 W/s) should be used and preparations made to treat potential ventricular fibrillation.

Supplemental potassium may be beneficial in chronic digitalis toxicity when diuretic-induced hypokalemia is a factor. It should be given cautiously because renal failure may be the cause of chronic digitalis toxicity. Potassium should not be routinely administered to the acutely poisoned patient because hyperkalemia is common. Patients who have acute CG poisoning and exhibit hyperkalemia may be treated with IV glucose, insulin, and sodium bicarbonate or continuous inhaled beta agents, such as albuterol (if no tachydysrhythmia or ectopy), although these therapies may be ineffective. The exchange resin, sodium polystyrene sulfonate, also may be considered. However, the increased serum potassium level reflects a change in potassium distribution and not an increase in total body potassium stores. The use of agents such as exchange resins may lead to total body potassium depletion and subsequent problems once the digitalis toxicity has abated. Hemodialysis may be of benefit in a CG-poisoned patient who has uncontrolled hyperkalemia. A theoretical concern exists that treating CG-induced hyperkalemia with IV calcium may enhance digitalis cardiac toxicity and should probably be avoided until further data is available.

Hypomagnesemia has been reported in a significant number of patients who are chronically CG-toxic. IV administration of magnesium has been shown to counteract ventricular irritability from digitalis toxicity [89]. The recommended dose of magnesium for malignant ventricular dysrhythmias is 2 to 4 g (10–20 mL of a 20% solution) given IV for longer than 1 minute. Magnesium should be infused more slowly in patients who are ectopic and are hemodynamically stable. Magnesium may also be helpful in treating hyperkalemia. It should be used with extreme caution in renal failure patients.

A milestone in the treatment of CG poisoning has been the development of drug-specific antibodies. Digoxin-specific Fab fragments (Digibind or DigiTab) are antibody fragments produced by enzymatic cleavage of sheep immunoglobulin (IgG) antibodies to digoxin. Fab fragments can reverse digitalis-induced dysrhythmias, conduction disturbances, myocardial depression, and hyperkalemia in severely poisoned patients. Most patients have an initial response to CG-toxic dysrhythmias within 30 minutes of Fab administration and those who respond have complete resolution by 4 hours. Animal studies and case reports have demonstrated the efficacy of Fab fragments to the CGs contained in plants. Adverse reactions to Fab administration have been few and include rare but mild hypersensitivity reactions, precipitous drops in serum potassium, and supraventricular tachydysrhythmias previously controlled by digoxin.

Fab fragment therapy is indicated for severely intoxicated patients who do not immediately respond to conventional therapies, have CG-induced dysrhythmias that threaten or result in hemodynamic compromise, and have hyperkalemia ($K^+ \geq 5.0$ mEq/L). Often, chronically poisoned patients can be managed by discontinuing digoxin and close observation. However, the threshold for treatment with Fab should be lower in chronically poisoned patients who exhibit signs of cardiac toxicity or who have any of the predisposing conditions: (a) chronic pulmonary disease, (b) hypokalemia, (c) hypothyroidism, (d) renal insufficiency, or (e) underlying cardiac disease [90]. If patients are managed conservatively, the Fab dose to be administered should be calculated (Box 1) and the Fab fragments made available at the bedside while the patient is monitored for worsening toxicity.

Although serum digoxin levels should not be the sole factor in determining the need to administer Fab, dosage calculations for Fab are based on the serum digoxin level or estimated body load of digoxin. Equimolar doses of antibody fragments are required to achieve neutralization. Forty milligrams of Fab (1 vial) binds 0.6 mg of digoxin. A severely toxic patient in whom the quantity ingested is unknown should be given 5 to 10 vials at a time and the clinical response observed. If cardiac arrest is imminent or has occurred, the dose can be given as a bolus. Otherwise, it should be infused over 30 minutes. In contrast, patients who experience chronic therapeutic overdose often have only mildly elevated digoxin levels and respond to 1 to 2 vials of Fab. The recommended dose for a given patient can be determined using the tables in the package insert or by contacting a regional poison center or toxicology consultant.

Box 1. Digoxin-specific Fab fragment dosing calculations

1) If the patient has chronic toxicity where the digoxin level is at steady state:

$$\text{Number of vials of Fab} = [(\text{serum digoxin level}) \times (\text{patient's weight in kg})]/100$$

2) If the patient has an acute overdose and the exact amount taken is known:

$$\text{Number of vials of Fab} = [(\text{amount of digoxin ingested in mg}) \times (0.80)]/40$$

3) If the amount ingested is unknown and Fab is indicated, 5–10 vials should be given.

Free digoxin levels are decreased to zero within 1 minute of Fab fragment administration, but total serum digoxin levels are markedly increased. Because most assay methods measure bound and free digoxin (total), high digoxin levels are seen after Fab fragment therapy but have no correlation with toxicity. Serum levels may be unreliable for several days after Fab treatment. The digoxin-Fab complex is excreted in the urine and in patients who undergo renal failure, elimination of the digoxin-Fab complex is prolonged, and free digoxin levels gradually increase over hours after Fab administration. Rebound CG toxicity is rare but has been reported. Hemodialysis does not enhance elimination of digoxin-Fab complex.

Disposition

All patients who receive Fab fragments require continued monitoring in an intensive care unit for at least 24 hours. For the chronically poisoned elderly patient, modifying the outpatient treatment regimen by discontinuing the use of a CG or providing a more reliable method of drug administration with close clinical follow-up may avert further toxic episodes.

Methylxanthine toxicity

The methylxanthines comprise a class of agents consisting of theophylline and caffeine. Theophylline used in treatment of lung disease has decreased over the past decade and, therefore, toxicity from this class of agents has also decreased. However, because of the potential for rapid cardiovascular compromise, emergency physicians should also be aware of these agents.

Pathophysiology

At least four mechanisms have been proposed for the pro-arrhythmic potential of methylxanthine overdoses. First, methylxanthines increase circulating catecholamines [91–94]. Second, methylxanthines inhibit phosphodiesterase [95]. Increased circulating catecholamines after methylxanthine overdose increases β_1-receptor stimulation. Stimulation of β_1-receptors increases intracellular cAMP by G-protein stimulation of adenylate cyclase. The activity of cAMP is prolonged because of its decreased metabolism because phosphodiesterase is inhibited by methylxanthines. Subsequently, β_1-receptor effects are exaggerated and tachydysrhythmias are induced. Third, methylxanthines increase myocardial intracellular calcium. Methylxanthines induce release of calcium from the sarcoplasmic reticulum and block calcium's re-uptake into the sarcoplasmic reticulum [96–98]. This resulting increase in cytosolic calcium may provoke dysrhythmias. Methylxanthines, therefore, block cardiac A2 receptors that are antiarrhythmic [99].

Hypotension is also commonly seen following overdoses of methylxanthines and is believed to be caused by two mechanisms [100]. First, methylxanthine-induced tachydysrhythmias lead to inadequate filling of the heart and subsequent decrease in cardiac output. Second, increased catecholamines stimulate β_2-receptors that increase intracellular cAMP. Augmentation of β_2-stimulation and phosphodiesterase inhibition leads to a prolonged effect of cAMP and subsequent vasodilation with resulting hypotension.

Clinical effects

Clinically, methylxanthine intoxication is associated with nausea, vomiting, tremors, mental status changes, and seizures. Reports of methylxanthine-induced cardiac dysrhythmias abound in the literature [101–105]. Hypotension can be profound and resilient to standard therapies.

Management

All methylxanthine-intoxicated patients should be managed as discussed earlier. For patients manifesting signs of excitation of the central nervous system (ie, tremors, clonus, hypereflexia), phenobarbital or benzodiazepines should be administered early before frank seizures occur.

Persistent hypotension unresponsive to IV fluids should be treated with a direct alpha-one agonist such as phenylephrine. Vasopressin has been used in a case of refractory hypotension from a caffeine overdose [106]. Two vasopressin-receptor subtypes. V1 receptors are located on vascular smooth muscle and mediate vasoconstriction. This V1-receptor activation mediates vasoconstriction by receptor-coupled activation of phopholipase C and release of calcium from intracellular stores, by way of the phosphoinositide cascade, and extracellular stores, by way of calcium channels located on the cell membrane. Vasopressin is a potent vasoconstrictor for skin, skeletal muscle, fat, pancreas, and thyroid gland. Vasopressin causes less vasoconstriction in mesenteric, coronary, and cerebral circulations probably because of a nitrous oxide (NO)-mediated vasodilating effect of vasopressin on these circulations [107]. In addition, vasopressin potentiates the contractile effects of catecholamines. V2 renal receptors, which cause the antidiuretic effects of vasopressin, are present in the renal collecting duct system and endothelial cells. Kidney V2 receptors interact with adenyl cyclase to increase intracellular cAMP and trigger the release of more water channels to appear on the cell surface with resultant increased re-absorption of water in the collecting duct [108]. The reported rate of the vasopressin infusions vary, with most infusions beginning at 0.03–0.07 units/min and are titrated to effect. Potential adverse side effects of vasopressin include organ ischemia, myocardial infarction, hypersensitivity reactions, skin necrosis, and rhabdomyolysis.

Various techniques to enhanced elimination of methylxanthines have been reported in the literature. Multidose activated charcoal has been advocated in the treatment of methylxanthine toxicity to prevent further absorption of drug and to enhance elimination by gut dialysis [109]. Hemodialysis has been shown to significantly enhance elimination following theophylline and caffeine overdose. Cases of severe methylxanthine toxicity have been treated with peritoneal dialysis, but this modality is less efficient at drug clearance than hemodialysis [110–112]. The use of charcoal hemoperfusion has been reported in theophylline poisoning. However, no clear indication exists demonstrating that charcoal hemoperfusion provides increased methylxanthine clearance over hemodialysis [113].

Summary

Multiple agents exist that can result in human cardiovascular toxicity. The management of the toxicity of each agent should follow a rationale approach. Many agents have multiple mechanisms of toxicity. The first step in the care of poisoned patients focuses on good supportive care.

References

[1] Watson WA, Litovitz TL, Klein-Schwartz W, et al. 2003 annual report of the american association of poison control centers toxic exposure surveillance system. Am J Emerg Med 2004;22(5):335–404.

[2] Isbister GK, Downes F, Sibbritt D, et al. Aspiration pneumonitis in an overdose population: frequency, predictors, and outcomes. Crit Care Med 2004;32(1):88–93.

[3] Soni N, Baines D, Pearson IY. Cardiovascular collapse and propranolol overdose. Med J Aust 1983;2(12):629–30.
[4] Cheong KF, Manivannan GK, Yau GH. Asystole following laryngoscopy and endotracheal intubation: a case report. Ann Acad Med Singapore 1996;25(2):283–5.
[5] Papasteriadis EG, Afentoglou SN, Athanasopoulos CB, et al. The use of the subclavian vein for temporary transvenous pacemaker therapy. Angiology 1983;34(7):480–3.
[6] Salhanick SD, Shannon MW. Management of calcium channel antagonist overdose. Drug Saf 2003;26(2):65–79.
[7] Position paper: whole bowel irrigation. J Toxicol Clin Toxicol 2004;42(6):843–54.
[8] Reith DM, Dawson AH, Epid D, et al. Relative toxicity of beta blockers in overdose. J Toxicol Clin Toxicol 1996;34(3):273–8.
[9] Pond SM, Lewis-Driver DJ, Williams GM, et al. Gastric emptying in acute overdose: a prospective randomised controlled trial. Med J Aust 1995;163(7):345–9.
[10] Litovitz TL, Schmitz BF, Matyunas N, et al. 1987 annual report of the american association of poison control centers national data collection system. Am J Emerg Med 1988;6(5): 479–515.
[11] DeRoos F, ed. Calcium channel blockers. In: DeRoos F, Goldfrank L, editors. Goldfrank's toxicologic emergencies. 7th edition. New York: McGraw Hill; 2002.
[12] Henrikson CA, Chandra-Strobos N. Calcium channel blocker overdose mimicking an acute myocardial infarction. Resuscitation 2003;59(3):361–4.
[13] Holstege C, Kirk M, Furbee R. Wide complex dysrhythmia in calcium channel blocker overdose responsive to sodium bicarbonate therapy [abstract]. J Toxicol Clin Toxicol 1998; 36(5):509.
[14] Kline JA, Raymond RM, Schroeder JD, et al. The diabetogenic effects of acute verapamil poisoning. Toxicol Appl Pharmacol 1997;145(2):357–62.
[15] Tanen DA, Ruha AM, Curry SC, et al. Hypertonic sodium bicarbonate is effective in the acute management of verapamil toxicity in a swine model. Ann Emerg Med 2000;36(6): 547–53.
[16] Ramoska EA, Spiller HA, Winter M, et al. A one-year evaluation of calcium channel blocker overdoses: toxicity and treatment. Ann Emerg Med 1993;22(2):196–200.
[17] Satar S, Acikalin A, Akpinar O. Unusual electrocardiographic changes with propranolol and diltiazem overdosage: a case report. Am J Ther 2003;10(4):299–302.
[18] Sami Karti S, Ulusoy H, Yandi M, et al. Non-cardiogenic pulmonary oedema in the course of verapamil intoxication. Emerg Med J 2002;19(5):458–9.
[19] Howarth DM, Dawson AH, Smith AJ, et al. Calcium channel blocking drug overdose: an Australian series. Hum Exp Toxicol 1994;13(3):161–6.
[20] Ashraf M, Chaudhary K, Nelson J, et al. Massive overdose of sustained-release verapamil: a case report and review of literature. Am J Med Sci 1995;310(6):258–63.
[21] Semple P, Booth C. Calcium chloride; a reminder. Anaesthesia 1996;51(1):93.
[22] Isbister GK. Delayed asystolic cardiac arrest after diltiazem overdose; resuscitation with high dose intravenous calcium. Emerg Med J 2002;19(4):355–7.
[23] Papadopoulos J, O'Neil MG. Utilization of a glucagon infusion in the management of a massive nifedipine overdose. J Emerg Med 2000;18(4):453–5.
[24] Snook CP, Sigvaldason K, Kristinsson J. Severe atenolol and diltiazem overdose. J Toxicol Clin Toxicol 2000;38(6):661–5.
[25] Bailey B. Glucagon in beta-blocker and calcium channel blocker overdoses: a systematic review. J Toxicol Clin Toxicol 2003;41(5):595–602.
[26] Doyon S, Roberts JR. The use of glucagon in a case of calcium channel blocker overdose. Ann Emerg Med 1993;22(7):1229–33.
[27] Kline JA, Leonova E, Raymond RM. Beneficial myocardial metabolic effects of insulin during verapamil toxicity in the anesthetized canine. Crit Care Med 1995;23(7):1251–63.
[28] Boyer EW, Shannon M. Treatment of calcium-channel-blocker intoxication with insulin infusion. N Engl J Med 2001;344(22):1721–2.

[29] Boyer EW, Duic PA, Evans A. Hyperinsulinemia/euglycemia therapy for calcium channel blocker poisoning. Pediatr Emerg Care 2002;18(1):36–7.
[30] Rasmussen L, Husted SE, Johnsen SP. Severe intoxication after an intentional overdose of amlodipine. Acta Anaesthesiol Scand 2003;47(8):1038–40.
[31] Yuan TH, Kerns WP II, Tomaszewski CA, et al. Insulin-glucose as adjunctive therapy for severe calcium channel antagonist poisoning. J Toxicol Clin Toxicol 1999;37(4):463–74.
[32] Kalman S, Berg S, Lisander B. Combined overdose with verapamil and atenolol: treatment with high doses of adrenergic agonists. Acta Anaesthesiol Scand 1998;42(3):379–82.
[33] Proano L, Chiang WK, Wang RY. Calcium channel blocker overdose. Am J Emerg Med 1995;13(4):444–50.
[34] Durward A, Guerguerian AM, Lefebvre M, et al. Massive diltiazem overdose treated with extracorporeal membrane oxygenation. Pediatr Crit Care Med 2003;4(3):372–6.
[35] Sztajnkrycer MD, Bond GR, Johnson SB, et al. Use of vasopressin in a canine model of severe verapamil poisoning: a preliminary descriptive study. Acad Emerg Med 2004;11(12): 1253–61.
[36] Belson MG, Gorman SE, Sullivan K, et al. Calcium channel blocker ingestions in children. Am J Emerg Med 2000;18(5):581–6.
[37] Tom PA, Morrow CT, Kelen GD. Delayed hypotension after overdose of sustained release verapamil. J Emerg Med 1994;12(5):621–5.
[38] Adams BD, Browne WT. Amlodipine overdose causes prolonged calcium channel blocker toxicity. Am J Emerg Med 1998;16(5):527–8.
[39] Love JN, Howell JM, Newsome JT, et al. The effect of sodium bicarbonate on propranolol-induced cardiovascular toxicity in a canine model. J Toxicol Clin Toxicol 2000;38(4):421–8.
[40] Alderfliegel F, Leeman M, Demaeyer P, et al. Sotalol poisoning associated with asystole. Intensive Care Med 1993;19(1):57–8.
[41] Love JN, Howell JM, Litovitz TL, et al. Acute beta blocker overdose: factors associated with the development of cardiovascular morbidity. J Toxicol Clin Toxicol 2000;38(3): 275–81.
[42] Love JN, Enlow B, Howell JM, et al. Electrocardiographic changes associated with beta-blocker toxicity. Ann Emerg Med 2002;40(6):603–10.
[43] Chavez H, Ozolins D, Losek JD. Hypoglycemia and propranolol in pediatric behavioral disorders. Pediatrics 1999;103(6, pt 1):1290–2.
[44] Peterson CD, Leeder JS, Sterner S. Glucagon therapy for beta-blocker overdose. Drug Intell Clin Pharm 1984;18(5):394–8.
[45] White C. A review of potential cardiovascular uses of intravenous glucagon administration. J Clin Pharmacol 1999;39(5):442–7.
[46] Love JN, Hanfling D, Howell JM. Hemodynamic effects of calcium chloride in a canine model of acute propranolol intoxication. Ann Emerg Med 1996;28(1):1–6.
[47] Pertoldi F, D'Orlando L, Mercante WP. Electromechanical dissociation 48 hours after atenolol overdose: usefulness of calcium chloride. Ann Emerg Med 1998;31(6):777–81.
[48] Brimacombe J. Use of calcium chloride for propranolol overdose. Anaesthesia 1992;47(10): 907–8.
[49] Kearns W, Schroeder D, Williams C, et al. Insulin improves survival in a canine model of acute beta-blocker toxicity. Ann Emerg Med 1997;29(6):748–57.
[50] Lewis M, Kallenbach J, Germond C, et al. Survival following massive overdose of adrenergic blocking agents (acebutolol and labetalol). Eur Heart J 1983;4(5):328–32.
[51] Shanker UR, Webb J, Kotze A. Sodium bicarbonate to treat massive beta blocker overdose. Emerg Med J 2003;20(4):393.
[52] Whitehurst VE, Vick JA, Alleva FR, et al. Reversal of propranolol blockade of adrenergic receptors and related toxicity with drugs that increase cyclic AMP. Proc Soc Exp Biol Med 1999;221(4):382–5.
[53] Kollef MH. Labetalol overdose successfully treated with amrinone and alpha-adrenergic receptor agonists. Chest 1994;105(2):626–7.

[54] Lane AS, Woodward AC, Goldman MR. Massive propranolol overdose poorly responsive to pharmacologic therapy: use of the intra-aortic balloon pump. Ann Emerg Med 1987; 16(12):1381–3.
[55] Salhanick SD, Wax PM. Treatment of atenolol overdose in a patient with renal failure using serial hemodialysis and hemoperfusion and associated echocardiographic findings. Vet Hum Toxicol 2000;42(4):224–5.
[56] Rooney M, Massey KL, Jamali F, et al. Acebutolol overdose treated with hemodialysis and extracorporeal membrane oxygenation. J Clin Pharmacol 1996;36(8):760–3.
[57] Kolecki PF, Curry SC. Poisoning by sodium channel blocking agents. Crit Care Clin 1997; 13(4):829–48.
[58] Harrigan RA, Brady WJ. ECG abnormalities in tricyclic antidepressant ingestion. Am J Emerg Med 1999;17(4):387–93.
[59] Liebelt EL, Ulrich A, Francis PD, et al. Serial electrocardiogram changes in acute tricyclic antidepressant overdoses. Crit Care Med 1997;25(10):1721–6.
[60] Brady WJ, Skiles J. Wide QRS complex tachycardia: ECG differential diagnosis. Am J Emerg Med 1999;17(4):376–81.
[61] Kerr GW, McGuffie AC, Wilkie S. Tricyclic antidepressant overdose: a review. Emerg Med J 2001;18(4):236–41.
[62] Hoffman JR, Votey SR, Bayer M, et al. Effect of hypertonic sodium bicarbonate in the treatment of moderate-to-severe cyclic antidepressant overdose. Am J Emerg Med 1993; 11(4):336–41.
[63] Bou-Abboud E, Nattel S. Relative role of alkalosis and sodium ions in reversal of class I antiarrhythmic drug-induced sodium channel blockade by sodium bicarbonate. Circulation 1996;94(8):1954–61.
[64] Hoegholm A, Clementsen P. Hypertonic sodium chloride in severe antidepressant overdosage. J Toxicol Clin Toxicol 1991;29(2):297–8.
[65] Bessen HA, Niemann JT, Haskell RJ, et al. Effect of respiratory alkalosis in tricyclic antidepressant overdose. West J Med 1983;139(3):373–6.
[66] Nousaine DA. Hyperventilation versus bicarbonate therapy for alkalinization in tricyclic antidepressant overdose. West J Med 1981;135(2):160–1.
[67] Pentel PR, Benowitz NL. Tricyclic antidepressant poisoning. Management of arrhythmias. Med Toxicol 1986;1(2):101–21.
[68] De Ponti F, Poluzzi E, Montanaro N, et al. QTc and psychotropic drugs. Lancet 2000; 356(9223):75–6.
[69] Sides GD. QT interval prolongation as a biomarker for torsades de pointes and sudden death in drug development. Dis Markers 2002;18(2):57–62.
[70] Nelson LS. Toxicologic myocardial sensitization. J Toxicol Clin Toxicol 2002;40(7): 867–79.
[71] Munro P, Graham C. Torsade de pointes. Emerg Med J 2002;19(5):485–6.
[72] Kyrmizakis DE, Chimona TS, Kanoupakis EM, et al. QT prolongation and torsades de pointes associated with concurrent use of cisapride and erythromycin. Am J Otolaryngol 2002;23(5):303–7.
[73] Horowitz BZ, Bizovi K, Moreno R. Droperidol–behind the black box warning. Acad Emerg Med 2002;9(6):615–8.
[74] De Ponti F, Poluzzi E, Montanaro N. QT-interval prolongation by non-cardiac drugs: lessons to be learned from recent experience. Eur J Clin Pharmacol 2000;56(1):1–18.
[75] Priori SG, Cantu F, Schwartz PJ. The long QT syndrome: new diagnostic and therapeutic approach in the era of molecular biology. Schweiz Med Wochenschr 1996;126(41):1727–31.
[76] Anderson ME, Al-Khatib SM, Roden DM, et al. Cardiac repolarization: current knowledge, critical gaps, and new approaches to drug development and patient management. Am Heart J 2002;144(5):769–81.
[77] Kaye P, O'Sullivan I. The role of magnesium in the emergency department. Emerg Med J 2002;19(4):288–91.

[78] Monraba R, Sala C. Percutaneous overdrive pacing in the out-of-hospital treatment of torsades de pointes. Ann Emerg Med 1999;33(3):356–7.

[79] Eddleston M, Warrell DA. Management of acute yellow oleander poisoning. QJM 1999; 92(9):483–5.

[80] Eddleston M, Rajapakse S, Rajakanthan, et al. Anti-digoxin fab fragments in cardiotoxicity induced by ingestion of yellow oleander: a randomised controlled trial. Lancet 2000;355(9208):967–72.

[81] Eddleston M, Ariaratnam CA, Sjostrom L, et al. Acute yellow oleander (Thevetia peruviana) poisoning: cardiac arrhythmias, electrolyte disturbances, and serum cardiac glycoside concentrations on presentation to hospital. Heart 2000;83(3):301–6.

[82] Tuncok Y, Kozan O, Cavdar C, et al. Urginea maritima (squill) toxicity. J Toxicol Clin Toxicol 1995;33(1):83–6.

[83] Kirk MA, Judge BS. Cardiac Glycoside Poisoning. In: Irwin RS, Rippe JM, editors. Intensive care medicine. 5th edition. Boston: Lippincott Williams & Wilkins; 2003.

[84] Avendano C, Alvarez JS, Sacristan JA, et al. Interference of digoxin-like immunoreactive substances with TDx digoxin II assay in different patients. Ther Drug Monit 1991;13(6): 523–7.

[85] Woolf AD, Wenger TL, Smith TW, et al. Results of multicenter studies of digoxin-specific antibody fragments in managing digitalis intoxication in the pediatric population. Am J Emerg Med 1991;9(2, Suppl 1):16–20.

[86] Woolf AD, Wenger T, Smith TW, et al. The use of digoxin-specific Fab fragments for severe digitalis intoxication in children. N Engl J Med 1992;326(26):1739–44.

[87] Kaplanski J, Weinhouse E, Martin O. Modification of digoxin induced arrhythmogenicity in adult rats following atropine administration. Res Commun Chem Pathol Pharmacol 1983;39(1):173–6.

[88] Maheswaran R, Bramble MG, Hardisty CA. Massive digoxin overdose: successful treatment with intravenous amiodarone. Br Med J (Clin Res Ed) 1983;287(6389):392–3.

[89] Reisdorff EJ, Clark MR, Walters BL. Acute digitalis poisoning: the role of intravenous magnesium sulfate. J Emerg Med 1986;4(6):463–9.

[90] Taboulet P, Baud FJ, Bismuth C. Clinical features and management of digitalis poisoning–rationale for immunotherapy. J Toxicol Clin Toxicol 1993;31(2):247–60.

[91] Ishida S, Ito M, Takahashi N, et al. Caffeine induces ventricular tachyarrhythmias possibly due to triggered activity in rabbits in vivo. Jpn Circ J 1996;60:157–65.

[92] Bellett S, Roman L, DeCastro O, et al. Effect of coffee ingestion on catecholamine release. Metabolism 1969;18:288–91.

[93] Benowitz N, Osterloh J, Goldschlager N, et al. Massice catecholamine release from caffeine poisoning. JAMA 1982;248:1097–8.

[94] Benowitz N. Clinical pharmacology of caffeine. Annu Rev Med 1990;41:277–88.

[95] Abott P. Caffeine: a toxicological overview. Med J Aust 1986;145:518–21.

[96] Paspa P, Vassalle M. Mechanism of caffeine-induced arrhythmias in canine cardiac Purkinje fibers. Am J Cardiol 1984;53:313–9.

[97] Boutjdir M, El-Sherif N, Gough W. Effects of caffeine and ryanodine on delayed afterdepolarizations and sustained rhythmic activity in 1-day-old myocardial infarction in the dog. Circulation 1990;81:1393–400.

[98] Hess P, Wier W. Excitation-contraction coupling in cardiac Purkinje fibers: effects of caffeine on the intracellular [Ca^{2+}] transient, membrane currents, and contraction. J Gen Physiol 1984;83:417–33.

[99] Schreieck J, Richardt G. Endogenous adenosine reduces the occurrence of ischemia-induced ventricular fibrillation in rat heart. J Mol Cell Cardiol 1999;31:123–34.

[100] Parr MJ, Anaes FC, Day AC, et al. Theophylline poisoning–a review of 64 cases. Intensive Care Med 1990;16(6):394–8.

[101] Zimmerman P, Pulliam J, Schwengels J, et al. Caffeine intoxication: a near fatality. Ann Emerg Med 1985;14:1227–9.

[102] Price K, Fligner D. Treatment of caffeine toxicity with esmolol. Ann Emerg Med 1990;19: 85–7.

[103] Chopra A, Morrison L. Resolution of caffeine-induced complex dysrhythmia with procainamide therapy. J Emerg Med 1995;13:113–7.

[104] Leson C, McGuigan M, Bryson S. Caffeine overdose in an adolescent male. Clin Toxicol 1988;26:407–15.

[105] Shannon M. Life-threatening events after theophylline overdose: a 10-year prospective analysis. Arch Intern Med 1999;159(9):989–94.

[106] Holstege CP, Hunter Y, Baer AB, et al. Massive caffeine overdose requiring vasopressin infusion and hemodialysis. J Toxicol Clin Toxicol 2003;41(7):1003–7.

[107] Aki Y, Tamaki T, Kiyomoto H, et al. Nitric oxide may participate in V2 vasopressin-receptor-mediated renal vasodilation. J Cardiovasc Pharmacol 1994;23(2):331–6.

[108] Knepper MA, Nielsen S. Kinetic model of water and urea permeability regulation by vasopressin in collecting duct. Am J Physiol 1993;265(2, pt 2):F214–24.

[109] Lim TK, Tan CC. Treatment of severe theophylline toxicity with oral activated charcoal and haemodialysis–a case report. Singapore Med J 1988;29(6):601–3.

[110] Walsh I, Wasserman GS, Mestad P, et al. Near-fatal caffeine intoxication treated with peritoneal dialysis. Pediatr Emerg Care 1987;3(4):244–9.

[111] Gitomer JJ, Khan AM, Ferris ME. Treatment of severe theophylline toxicity with hemodialysis in a preterm neonate. Pediatr Nephrol 2001;16(10):784–6.

[112] Okada S, Teramoto S, Matsuoka R. Recovery from theophylline toxicity by continuous hemodialysis with filtration. Ann Intern Med 2000;133(11):922.

[113] Higgins RM, Hearing S, Goldsmith DJ, et al. Severe theophylline poisoning: charcoal haemoperfusion or haemodialysis? Postgrad Med J 1995;71(834):224–6.

ELSEVIER
SAUNDERS

Emerg Med Clin N Am
23 (2005) 1219–1231

EMERGENCY
MEDICINE
CLINICS OF
NORTH AMERICA

Emergency Medical Service Aspects of Emergency Cardiac Care

Daniel G. Hankins, MD*, Anuradha Luke, MD

Daniel G. Hankins, MD, Department of Emergency Medicine, Mayo Clinic, 200 1st Street South West, Rochester, MN 55905, USA

Every year there are 1.25 million people who have an acute myocardial infarction (AMI) in the United States. Many of these patients die, with half of AMI deaths occurring within the first hour of symptom onset before the patient receives medical attention [1–3]. Evidence exists that early intervention with reperfusion translates into a better clinical outcome and lower mortality in these patients [4–6]. The Gruppo Italiano per la Sperimentazione della Streptochinasi nell'Infarto Miocardico (GISSI) trial demonstrated at least a 17% mortality reduction if thrombolysis was used for AMI in less than 6 hours of onset of symptoms [4]. An evaluation of pooled data from multiple trials revealed that there was an absolute reduction in mortality in those patients presenting within one hour of symptom onset of 65 lives saved per 1000 treated. Every hour thereafter resulted in a reduction of benefit of 1.6 lives per 1000 patients [7]. Potential exists for prehospital interventions to greatly influence the early access to definitive cardiac care. Issues, such as reducing the delay interval (the time from onset of symptoms to call for help), use of emergency medical services (EMS) versus private vehicle, and prehospital ECG are being investigated as factors that may speed care. Additionally, a body of literature exists that investigates the use of prehospital thrombolysis and its feasibility and success in certain populations.

Problems of access: delay interval

The time to treatment is dependent on a number of variables and time points. The patient experiencing symptoms first has to recognize the symptoms and attribute them to a heart condition. They then have to decide

* Corresponding author.
E-mail address: hankins.daniel@mayo.edu (D.G. Hankins).

doi:10.1016/j.emc.2005.07.006 **emed.theclinics.com**

to seek help. A time delay occurs from the call for assistance to arrival of assistance and, lastly, a delay occurs from arrival of help to arrival at hospital. Numerous studies have examined the time delay from onset of symptoms to call for help and found that about one third to one half of patients delay for more than 4 hours before calling for help [8,9]. The median time delay is approximately 2 hours [9,10]. Investigators have tried to identify factors that lead to increased delay in seeking help with the intention of directed intervention in these subpopulations. Meischke and colleagues [1], in a retrospective chart review of 2947 patients with AMI transported by emergency medical services (EMS), report a greater delay in seeking help in female patients, older patients, and those that had a history of angina, congestive heart failure (CHF), and diabetes. A history of prior AMI was related to a shorter delay interval in their study, which contrasted with the Worcester heart study [11] that revealed a longer time delay in patients with prior myocardial infarction. The National Registry of Myocardial Infarction 2 (NRMI2) data supported Meischke's findings while examining over 300,000 patients with AMI in the United States over a 3-year period. The investigators in this case found delay intervals were prolonged for women, older patients, nonwhite patients, and patients who had diabetes and hypertension. They also found a shorter delay interval for acutely sicker patients (ie, cardiogenic shock) and those with prior history of AMI or angioplasty [9]. The data are less clear with regards to race, education, and socioeconomic status.

Other investigators have attempted to identify factors that contribute to a delay in calling for help. Hypotheses demonstrate that this may be related to lack of knowledge, denial of symptoms, concerns of cost, self-treatment, and embarrassment about being wrong. The Rapid Early Action for Coronary Treatment (REACT) trial attempted to evaluate the community knowledge base of AMI symptoms. They evaluated 20 communities in five regions in the United States and found the greatest level of knowledge was in the non-Hispanic white population, the more educated and higher income groups, and in the older age groups [10]. Meischke and colleagues [12] in 1995 reported results of telephone interviews with patients admitted to the hospital who were experiencing suspected MI. The main reason for delay was because the patient thought the symptoms would go away, because they were not severe enough, or that they were caused by another illness [12].

Several reports exist of community-wide educational programs that have attempted to reduce this patient delay [13–15]. These programs have met with limited success in increasing the number of EMS calls and the number of emergency department (ED) visits for chest pain but have not demonstrated a change in delay times. Also, a quick drop off occurred of these benefits after the educational campaign ended. Perhaps the most compelling of these studies is the REACT trial that evaluated 10 matched pairs of communities that received an 18-month intensive public intervention to increase knowledge or did not and followed them for change in delay intervals. Delay times did not differ between the two groups although the campaign did lead to a 20% increase in the use of EMS [15].

Some subpopulations in the United States delay longer than others in seeking help for AMI symptoms. Many reasons exist for not seeking help sooner, including lack of confidence in the seriousness of the symptoms. Whatever attempts have been made to further the population's education about the need for earlier action have met with limited success. The investigators of these studies have suggested that these prior attempts have been too little, too short, and target the wrong audience. They suggest a new approach with continuous exposure to the educational message rather than abandon the public-education avenue.

Emergency medical services use

The use of EMS by patients with symptoms of AMI has been theorized to be of benefit for a number of reasons. EMS is able to treat potentially life-threatening complications, such as cardiac arrest and arrhythmias; transportation may be available to cardiac specialized hospitals and may shorten time to reperfusion therapy. In addition, they can start caring for patients immediately with important adjuvant therapy, such as oxygen and aspirin. Reports have documented between 23% and 42% of people who have AMI use EMS [8,13,16–18]. Reasons documented for lack of use of EMS includes lack of severity of symptoms, not thinking about calling 911, or the belief that self-transporting is faster [12]. In a subgroup analysis of REACT data, 89% of respondents intended to use EMS if witnessing a cardiac event; however, only 23% used the service for a personal cardiac event [16].

Further investigation of EMS-use reveals that EMS users are more likely to have a prior history of heart failure, stroke, or coronary artery disease (CAD). EMS users have also been shown to be sicker as evidenced by a higher Killip classification or by more clinical signs of heart failure [2,8]. No clear difference is documented based on ethnicity, sex, and education, [15] although one study demonstrated a slight female:male predominance [2]. Supporting the contention that patients self-select with the sicker patients choosing EMS, Becker and colleagues [19] evaluated the incidence of cardiac arrest in chest-pain patients using EMS versus self-transporting. The cardiac arrest rate in the EMS group was 5.6% versus 0.35% in the self-transporting group [19].

Hutchings and colleagues [18] evaluated the time to treatment with EMS-use versus private transport use using REACT trial data. Private transportation did demonstrate a faster arrival time to the ED of 35 versus 39 minutes for EMS users. If you consider the intervention by EMS initial care then the time to initial care was 6 minutes versus 32 minutes ($P < .001$) in the EMS versus private transporter group. Furthermore, the door to needle time in the EMS group was significantly lower (32 versus 49 minutes,

$P < .001$) and time from decision to seek care to thrombolysis was also significantly lower (75 versus 92 minutes, $P = .042$) [18]. Cabrita and colleagues [8] support these finding in their study investigating the impact of EMS on the management of AMI. Of the 140 out of 531 patients who had AMI that used EMS, the time from symptom onset to door was significantly faster (150 versus 219 minutes, $P < .001$). Delays to reperfusion were similar between two groups with no significant difference noted in symptom onset to reperfusion therapy. There were more primary angioplasty procedures (PCI) performed in the EMS group. Of note, despite the higher severity of illness in the EMS group, the hospital mortality did not differ between the two groups [8]. Canto et al also demonstrated that patients who presented by EMS had 24% greater odds of receiving PTCA or fibrinolysis. There was a 12 minute difference between door to lysis and 31 minute difference in door to PTCA. Mortality in the EMS group was higher but the patients were sicker [2]. In summary, the use of EMS may get the care to the patient sooner and perhaps speed time to definitive treatment.

The emergency medical services system response

Cardiovascular events thus comprise a large proportion of time-dependent emergencies encountered by out-of-hospital care providers. For the purpose of this discussion, emergency 911 calls and interfacility transports are considered to be part of an integrated out-of-hospital transportation system.

The EMS system, including both ground and rotor-wing, has evolved over the last 30 years. Emergency 911 cardiac calls are primarily handled by basic life support (BLS) and advanced life support (ALS) ground ambulances that transport patients to the hospital. The first contact that the EMS system has with a cardiac patient is through the call-taker for the 911 system. Pre-arrival instructions are given for bystander intervention in cardiac events. Some controversy surrounds the issue of pre-arrival instructions for cardiopulmonary resuscitation (CPR) (ie, should rescue breathing and chest compressions be instructed or just chest compressions?). For bystanders who are distraught, compressions alone may be more effective and easier to instruct over the phone [20]. This situation is currently unsettled; some systems have dispatchers instruct the bystander in doing compressions only and some instruct in the performance of traditional CPR. Once the ambulance arrives, basic interventions, such as airway management, defibrillation, oxygen, aspirin, and nitroglycerin sublingually, can be performed by advanced- and basic- level ground ambulances depending on local medical care guidelines. In most systems, first responders initiate the most time-dependent interventions involving airway breathing, circulation, and defibrillation with good success before the ambulance arrives. Police first response with defibrillators is becoming increasingly common in EMS systems [21–23]. Systems' differences may exist, however, that limit the efficacy of police defibrillation, because some systems have not found differences in survival from ventricular fibrillation with police defibrillation [24,25]. The use of defibrillators by police and other first responders needs to be integrated into the EMS system with strong medical oversight to work properly. The system needs to have continuous scrutiny to make sure that correct interventions are occurring in a timely fashion. Advanced services' paramedics may also administer more advanced pharmacologic interventions, such as morphine, diuretics, and beta- blockers, for cardiac emergencies as appropriate by local guidelines and state law.

Another therapeutic modality becoming more common in EMS systems is noninvasive ventilation. Out-of-hospital continual positive airway pressure (CPAP) and bilevel positive airway pressure (BiPAP) machines are becoming available for use in acute respiratory distress, which is often cardiac-related. The patient can then be treated for acute respiratory failure without intubation before lapsing into acute respiratory arrest [26]. A difficulty in the use of BiPAP/CPAP is finding a machine that does not use vast quantities of oxygen quickly thus using all of the oxygen in the ambulance within 5 to 10 minutes. Hospital equipment often does not translate well to being used in the out-of-hospital arena.

Circumstances exist that may warrant an air medical response to the scene of a cardiovascular emergency because of time and distance factors. Air medical services, in general, do few medical scene calls and most of those are cardiac arrests. In one series from Pennsylvania, only 30 cardiac-scene flights occurred over a 10-year period out of 8106 flights total [27]. The air medical service had little impact on the outcome of cardiac arrests. Air medical transport may make a difference in 911 ambulance calls with "intercepts" of ambulances coming into a tertiary center with a patient who has an acute coronary syndrome or stroke. This "intercept" may need to be activated if the patient deteriorates enroute or if the patient is ill enough at the time of the 911 call to compel the ambulance personnel to initiate activation of the air service through their dispatch center while the ambulance goes enroute to the hospital. This "intercept" is most useful in the context of rural volunteer services that have long transport times to the hospital because it brings tertiary care to the patient who might otherwise get basic care. More sophisticated care can be initiated so the patient's symptoms of the acute coronary syndrome can be alleviated or to treat other cardiovascular emergencies, such as stroke, pulmonary edema, or cardiac arrest. The use of air intercepts of ground ambulances in a regional EMS system requires strong medical oversight with review of these instances and cooperation among dispatch centers and ground and air services. Planning must include safety training for law enforcement and ground ambulance personnel involved in establishing a safe landing zone. Establishing prearranged landing zones for meetings between incoming ambulances and the aircraft help to improve chances for a safe intercept. The use of helicopter intercepts and scene flights are region or state dependent and not useful at all in some large urban areas [28].

Prehospital ECG

As part of the paradigm shift toward earlier and more aggressive therapy, prehospital ECGs have emerged as a tool to expedite treatment for AMI. Prehospital programs have chosen to obtain the ECG and transmit them to a base hospital for physician reading or have a computer-generated reading that is then discussed with the base hospital physician. A recent study from the Netherlands comparing the two modalities found no difference in accuracy or time delay [29]. A meta-analysis of the literature about the diagnostic performance of out-of-hospital ECG for the diagnosis of AMI demonstrated the sensitivity to be 68% and the specificity 97% [30].

Karagounis and colleagues [31] in 1990 evaluated the impact of field-transmitted ECG on time to treatment. They reported no time difference to obtain ECG for the 34 patients in the field ECG group versus the 37 patients in the nonfield ECG group. Six out of 34 patients in the field ECG group had AMI and received thrombolysis at 48 minutes after hospital arrival versus 68 minutes in 6 out of 37 patients in the nonfield ECG group. When compared with historical controls the median time to treatment was 103 minutes [31].

Kereiakes and colleagues [32], as part of the Cincinnati Heart Project, evaluated the importance of EMS transport either alone or in combination with cellular transmitted ECG. They prospectively evaluated four groups of patients with AMI who presented to ED: (1) patients self-transporting, (2) patients transported by local community ambulance, (3) patients transported by specially trained ambulances, and (4) patients transported by specially trained ambulances with ECG. In the first three groups, the median time delay from arrival to treatment was not significantly different. In the last group the time to treatment was a median of 30 minutes compared with almost 60 minutes in the other groups [32].

The findings in the NRMI-2 study of 70,763 patients contradict the findings of the prior two studies. It was an observational report of the characteristics and outcomes of patients who had a prehospital ECG. Surprisingly only 3768 (5%) had a prehospital ECG. The median time from symptom onset to ECG was notably longer in the prehospital ECG group (120 versus 108 minutes). Explanation that the investigators offer is that there may have been a selection bias to perform ECGs in the ambulance on patients with longer transport times thereby falsely elevating the delays. They do contend that prehospital ECGs have the potential for moving the diagnosis of AMI to before arrival, which may lead to earlier mobilization of hospital resources and earlier intervention with potential for better outcomes [33].

The Myocardial Infarction Triage and Intervention (MITI) project in their first phase evaluated the feasibility of performing prehospital thrombolysis. As part of this feasibility study they demonstrated that there was clear time saving with performing ECGs in the field. The door-to-treatment time in the prehospital ECG group was shorter than the in-hospital ECG group (64 versus 75 minutes) [34].

The National Heart Attack Alert Program Coordinating Committee published recommendations in a 1995 guideline regarding the staffing and equipping of EMS for treating AMI. Their recommendations included encouragement of the use of prehospital 12-lead ECG and cellular transmission to facilitate early identification of AMI and expedite time to treatment in the hospital [3].

The use of prehospital ECG has also been extended to use in BLS vehicles. A recent pilot study evaluated the change in scene times when BLS providers performed field ECGs. Scene times increased by 5 minutes. Receiving physicians agreed the 93.6% of the ECGs were appropriately performed and found them to be moderately helpful. The providers, however, did not perform ECGs on about half of the eligible patients. The suggestion by the investigators is that with increased training this statistic could be improved [35].

Although the findings are somewhat conflicted, the generally accepted principle is that prehospital ECGs if performed without a great increase in scene time may actually expedite care once the patients reach the hospital. The ideal is an ECG performed that can be transmitted to a base hospital where it can be interpreted by a physician. This process theoretically should alert the base hospital early and allow for preparation for more definitive therapy before patient arrival. If success can be consistently demonstrated at an ALS level, perhaps this can also be performed by BLS services. Areas of further study should focus on demonstrating a clinical benefit and a cost benefit analysis of performing prehospital ECGs.

Prehospital thrombolysis

As discussed earlier, a clear clinical benefit has been demonstrated by the use of reperfusion therapy in patients who have AMI. This benefit is time dependent [4–7], which has been translated to the investigation of the use of prehospital thrombolysis to expedite definitive care. Much of the information has originated in Europe where the use of prehospital thrombolysis is fairly common. The major difference in the European ambulance system is that it is staffed by physicians, whereas ambulances in the United States are staffed with paramedics and BLS providers. Potential barriers to the use of prehospital thrombolysis in the United States include complexity of administering thrombolytic drugs, concerns about adverse effects, fear of treating the wrong disorders, such as aortic dissection leading to catastrophic effects, and concerns about nonphysicians performing the therapy with its attendant legal implications.

Gibler and colleagues [36] in 1991 described a study where the investigators in two cites evaluated patients for their potential for thrombolysis by performing and transmitting prehospital ECGs. In Nashville and Cincinnati, the number of patients who have AMI found to be candidates for thrombolysis accounted for only 4.8% of 562 patients. The investigators concluded from this that there were few patients in the prehospital setting that were actual candidates for thrombolysis; it also raised concerns that the paramedics would lose skills in administration of these potentially dangerous drugs [36].

Subsequent large studies in Europe and the United States demonstrated some benefit for the use of prehospital thrombolysis. In a randomized, double-blind, placebo-controlled trial, the European Myocardial Infarction Project (EMIP) Group evaluated patients who had AMI and presented within 6 hours of symptom onset. The patients were randomized to treatment with anistreplase in the prehospital setting versus the hospital setting. Median time to treatment in the prehospital group was 130 versus 190 minutes in the hospital group. Incidences of bleeding complications, strokes, cardiovascular arrest, and shock were equal in the two groups. Overall 30-day mortality was 9.7% in the prehospital group versus 11.1% in the hospital group. This 13% difference in mortality was not statistically significant; however, it did suggest a mortality benefit to earlier treatment [31]. The MITI trial randomized 360 patients with ST-elevation myocardial infarction for less than 6 hours to treatment in the prehospital setting or the hospital setting. The time to treatment was 77 minutes versus 110 minutes in the two groups ($P < .001$). However, no difference in mortality was demonstrated. In a subgroup analysis, those treated within 70 minutes of symptom onset had a mortality benefit. Incidences of serious bleeding, stroke, and cardiac arrest occurred equally [37].

Based on these and smaller reports, the American College of Emergency Physicians (ACEP) published guidelines for the use of thrombolysis in the prehospital setting. The ACEP did not endorse routine use of prehospital thrombolysis until further research had been done. If there was going to be research into these areas, the ACEP recommended rigorous training in the correct identification of appropriate patients, recognition of contraindications, preparation and administration of thrombolytics agents, and recognition and treatment of complications. It also recommended cellular transmission of ECG data, clear online medical oversight, and informed consent of patients [38].

In 1997, the National Heart Attack Alert Program concluded that prehospital thrombolysis reduced mortality in the subgroup of patients who required long transport times [3]. Morrison and colleagues [39] performed a meta-analysis of 6 randomized control trials comparing prehospital to in-hospital thrombolysis and did reveal an approximately 60-minute time saving. Additionally, the investigators concluded that a significant short-term mortality benefit existed but could not comment on a long-term mortality benefit to prehospital thrombolysis. Their recommendations for a shorter transit time are to use ECGs to expedite definitive care but not necessarily to use thrombolytics [39]. Further confirmation of the potential benefit of prehospital thrombolysis in more rural areas can be found in the study by Pedley and colleagues [40] who demonstrated a 73-minute median time saving in rural patients who received prehospital versus in-hospital thrombolysis [40].

Over the last several years, studies have focused on the use of bolus thrombolytic drugs to increase their ease of use in the prehospital setting. The Early Retavase-Thrombolysis in Myocardial Infarction trial evaluated the use of bolus reteplase in the prehospital setting versus historical controls of in-hospital thrombolysis. The trial demonstrated a time saving of 32 minutes. The time to ST resolution was reduced among patients treated with prehospital lysis. The study was limited by comparison to historical controls [41]. Another study from the Netherlands evaluated time to treatment with the use of reteplase versus anistreplase or streptokinase in two different cities. Time saving was approximately 20 minutes (81 minutes versus 104 minutes) with the use of bolus drug. No difference in the mortality or strokes existed between the two groups, although there was a trend toward the increased use of rescue angioplasty in the reteplase group [29].

In summary, prehospital thrombolysis is possible if done in a well-trained and well-regulated environment with the use of prehospital ECG to confirm diagnosis. The treatment seems to lead to substantial time savings to definitive therapy and perhaps confer some mortality benefit, which may be of more use in settings where the time to definitive treatment is an issue, such as rural settings with prolonged transportation time.

An additional issue is the use of primary angioplasty (PCI) as the definitive therapy of choice. In a quantitative review of studies comparing PCI to thrombolytic therapy for AMI, Weaver and colleagues [42] reviewed 10 randomized trials and found a 34% reduction in 30-day mortality in the PCI group. Angioplasty was also associated with a significant reduction in death or nonfatal infarction (7.2% versus 11.9%, $P < .001$), stroke (0.7% versus 2.0%, $P = .007$) and hemorrhagic stroke (0.1% versus 1.1%, $P < .001$). The investigators concluded that PCI was superior to thrombolysis for treatment of patients who have AMI [42]. Another multicenter trial of 840 AMI patients demonstrated a 60-minute time saving of prehospital thrombolysis over PCI. Median delay from onset of symptoms to prehospital thrombolysis was 130 minutes versus 190 minutes for the PCI group; however, rescue angioplasty done immediately in 26% of prehospital group. No difference existed in mortality but a trend toward more nonfatal myocardial infarction and nonfatal stroke in the thrombolysis group. The investigators conclude that prehospital thrombolysis is as good as PCI if the patient is then transported to a hospital with 24-hour angioplasty capability because of the need for rescue angioplasty in many patients [6]. This may not be feasible in most areas of the United States because there are few institutions that have 24-hour angioplasty capability. Although if the transportation time to a center that is capable of performing PCI is short, this method appears to be preferable to prehospital thrombolysis.

Public access defibrillation

Although no one denies the usefulness of early defibrillation, one controversial area of discussion over the past several years has been the proliferation of defibrillators in public places. Many controversies surround their use. Asaeda, Clair, and Gabriel [43] found that the barriers encountered in New York City to public access defibrillation (PAD) were: (1) personnel issues: who and how to train among the myriad of possible workers in New York City; (2) liability: does the good samaritan law protect these activities? Or what if a defibrillator is not placed somewhere that it should be?; (3) cost: "everything seemed to cost money"; (4) equipment issues: which defibrillator to choose and what guidelines to use for the algorithm of the machine; (5) placement of devices: where should they be placed for maximum efficacy?; and (6) use of the device: who would use the automated external defibrillators (AEDs)? employees only? or would it truly be *public* access defibrillation? Any locale has to deal with these issues. In the zeal to get AEDs out there, not enough attention has been paid to training lay people involved, quality control, and integration with the EMS system. The impact PAD has on cardiac arrests is still unclear. A retrospective review of 3 years of paramedic calls in Pittsburgh questioned the utility of PAD. Nursing homes and dialysis centers accounted for 94% of the 27 locations that had two or more cardiac arrests during the study. Three Rivers Stadium had more than two arrests but was covered by ALS ambulance personnel who had defibrillators. The conclusion was that: "Other than nursing homes and dialysis centers, there were no identifiable high-risk locations for nonresidential out-of-hospital cardiac arrests within the City of Pittsburgh" [44]. Rational placement of AEDs with oversight by the EMS system medical director to insure integration into the system is imperative.

Interfacility transports

The other major aspect of transportation of cardiovascular patients is interfacility transfer. With the recent increased emphasis on time to PCI to save as much myocardium as possible, the method of transfer from primary care hospital to tertiary care center with availability of a heart catheterization laboratory has assumed greater importance. The mode of transportation, whether air or ground, depends on time, distance, and illness severity of the patient. Although no large studies have been completed that show a difference between ground and air transports for cardiac patients, there are two studies underway in Ohio and England [45,46]. The authors' own experience indicates that flight medical crews are more aggressive about starting new interventions in cardiac patients and in titrating existing drips to a higher level. Although we demonstrated that patients had less chest pain and tended to spend less time in the hospital, it was too small a study for statistical significance [47]. The decision to fly a patient or send a patient by ground has many complex facets and is dictated by local and logistical factors.

Summary

In conclusion, the out-of-hospital arena is in a state of flux when it comes to treating cardiovascular disease and its complications. Many new treatment modalities are being tested for utility in out-of-hospital care. The entire system from dispatch to first responders to medics and air medical crews is being scrutinized for ways to streamline and improve cardiac care. Strokes, for instance, were once considered a BLS, almost nonemergent transport and are now emergent critical care transports, perhaps best done by air [48]. Out-of-hospital care of patients with cardiovascular disease are cared for best in a system where the "right crew in the right vehicle transports the right patient" [49].

References

[1] Meischke H, Eisenberg MS, Larsen MP. Prehospital delay interval for patients who use emergency medical services: the effect of heart related medical conditions and demographic variables. Ann Emerg Med 1993;22(10):1597–601.

[2] Canto JG, Zalenski RJ, Ornato JP, et al. Use of emergency medical services in acute myocardial infarction and subsequent quality of care: observations from the national registry of myocardial infarction 2. Circulation 2002;106:3018–23.

[3] National Heart Attack Alert Program Coordinating Committee Access to Care Subcommittee. Staffing and equipping emergency medical services systems: rapid identification and treatment of acute myocardial infarction. Am J Emerg Med 1995;13:58–66.

[4] GISSI. (Gruppo Italiano per lo Studio della Streptochinasi nell'Infarcto Miocardico). Effectiveness of intravenous thrombolytic treatment in acute myocardial infarction. Lancet 1986;1:397–402.

[5] The Global Utilization of Streptokinase and t-PA for Occluded Coronary Arteries (GUSTO) Angiographic Investigators. The effects of tissue plasminogen activator, streptokinase, or both on coronary artery patency, ventricular function, and survival after acute myocardian infaction. N Engl J Med 1993;329:1615–22.

[6] Bonnefoy E, Lapostolle F, Leizorovicz A, et al. Primary angioplasty versus prehospital fibrinolysis in acute myocardial infarction: a randomized study. Lancet 2002;360:825–9.

[7] Boersma E, Maas ACP, Deckers JW, et al. Early thrombolytic treatment in acute myocardial infarction: reappraisal of the golden hour. Lancet 1996;348:771–5.

[8] Cabrita B, Bouyer-Dalloz F, L'Huillier I, et al. Beneficial effects of direct call to emergency medical services in acute myocardial infarction. Eur J Emerg Med 2004;11(1):12–8.

[9] Goldberg RJ, Gurwitz JH, Gore JM. Duration of, and temporal trends (1994–1997) in, prehospital delay in patients with acute myocardial infarction: the second national registry of myocardial infarction. Arch Intern Med 1999;159:2141–7.

[10] Goff DC, Sellers DE, McGovern PG, et al. Knowledge of heart attack symptoms in a population survey in the United States: the REACT trial. Arch Intern Med 1998;158: 2329–38.
[11] Yarzebski J, Goldberg RJ, Gore JM, et al. Temporal trends and factors associated with extent of delay to hospital arrival in patients with acute myocardial infarction: the Worcester heart attack study. Am Heart J 1994;128:255–63.
[12] Meischke H, Ho MT, Eisenberg MS, et al. Reasons patients with chest pain delay or do not call 911. Ann Emerg Med 1995;25(2):193–7.
[13] Ho MT, Eisenberg MS, Litwin PE, et al. Delay between onset of chest pain and seeking medical care: the effect of public education. Ann Emerg Med 1989;18(7):727–31.
[14] Eppler E, Eisenberg MS, Schaeffer S, et al. 911 and emergency department use for chest pain: results of a media campaign. Ann Emerg Med 1994;24(2):202–8.
[15] Luepker RV, Raczynski JM, Osganian S, et al. Effect of a community intervention on patient delay and emergency medical service use in acute coronary heart disease: the Rapid Early Action for Coronary Treatment (REACT) trial. JAMA 2000;284(1):60–7.
[16] Brown AL, Mann NC, Daya M, et al. Demographic, belief, and situational factors influencing the decision to utilize emergency medical services among chest pain patients. Circulation 2000;102:173–8.
[17] Gurwitz JH, McLaughlin TJ, Willison DJ, et al. Delayed hospital presentation in patients who have had acute myocardial infarction. Ann Intern Med 1997;126(8):593–9.
[18] Hutchings CB, Mann NC, Daya M, et al. Patients with chest pain calling 911 or self-transporting to reach definitive care: which mode is quicker? Am Heart J 2004;147(1): 35–41.
[19] Becker L, Larsen MP, Eisenberg MS. Incidence of cardiac arrest during self-transport for chest pain. Ann Emerg Med 1996;28(6):612–6.
[20] Hallstrom A, Cobb L, Johnson E, et al. Cardiopulmonary resuscitation by chest compression alone or with mouth-to-mouth ventilation. N Engl J Med 2000;342:1546–53.
[21] White RD, Hankins DG, Bugliosi TF. Seven years' experience with early defibrillation by police and paramedics in an emergency medical services system. Resuscitation 1998;39: 145–51.
[22] Mossesso VN, Davis EA, Auble TE, et al. Use of automated external defibrillators by police officers for treatment of out-of-hospital cardiac arrest. Ann Emerg Med 1998;32: 200–7.
[23] Davis EA, McCrorry J, Mossesso VN. Institition of a police automated external defibrillation program: concepts and practice. Prehosp Emerg Care 1999;3:60–5.
[24] Groh WJ, Newman MM, Beal PE, et al. Limited response to cardiac arrest by police equipped with automated external defibrillators: lack of survival benefit in suburban and rural Indiana- the police as responder automated external defibrillation evaluation (PARADE). Acad Emerg Med 2001;8:324–30.
[25] van Alem AP, Vrenken RH, de Vos R, et al. Use of automated external defibrillator by first responders in out-of-hospital cardiac arrest: prospective controlled trial. BMJ 2003;327: 1312–6.
[26] Craven RA, Singletary N, Bosken L, et al. Use of bilevel positive airway pressure in out-of-hospital patients. Acad Emerg Med 2000;7:1065–8.
[27] Jones JB, Leicht M, Dula DJ. A 10-year experience in the use of air medical transport for medical scene calls. Air Med J 1998;17:7–12.
[28] Asaeda G, Cherson A, Giordano L, et al. Utilization of air medical transport in a large urban environment: a retrospective analysis. Prehosp Emerg Care 2001;5:36–9.
[29] Lamfers EJP, Schut A, Hooghoudt THE, et al. Prehospital thrombolysis with reteplase: the Nijmegen/Rotterdam study. Am Heart J 2003;146(3):479–83.
[30] Ioannidis JPA, Salem D, Chew PW, et al. Accuracy and clinical effect of out-of-hospital electrocardiography in the diagnosis of acute cardiac ischemia: a meta-analysis. Ann Emerg Med 2001;37(5):461–70.

[31] Karagounis L, Ipsen SK, Jessop MR, et al. Impact of field-transmitted electrocardiography on time to in-hospital thrombolytic therapy in acute myocardial infarction. Am J Cardiol 1990;66:786–91.
[32] Kereiakes DJ, Gibler WB, Martin LH, et al, of Cincinnati Heart Project Study Group. Relative importance of emergency medical system transport and the prehospital electrocardiogram on reducing hospital time delay to therapy for acute myocardial infarction: a preliminary report from the Cincinnati Heart Project. Am Heart J 1992;123: 835–40.
[33] Canto JG, Rogers WJ, Facc LJB, et al. The prehospital electrocardiogram in acute myocardial infarction: is its full potential being realized? J Am Coll Cardiol 1997;29(3): 498–505.
[34] Weaver WD, Eisenberg MS, Martin JS, et al. Myocardian infarction triage and intervention project-phase I: patient characteristics and feasibility of prehospital initiation of thrombolytic therapy. J Am Coll Cardiol 1990;15(5):925–31.
[35] Provo TA, Frascone RJ. 12-lead electrocardiograms during basic life support care. Prehosp Emerg Care 2004;8:212–6.
[36] Gibler WB, Kereiakes DJ, Dean EN, et al. Prehospital diagnosis and treatment of acute myocardial infarction: a North-South perspective. Am Heart J 1991;121:1–11.
[37] Weaver WD, Cerqueira M, Hallstrom AP, et al. Prehospital-initiated vs hospital-initiated thrombolytic therapy: The Myocardial Infarction Triage and Intervention Trial. JAMA 1993;270:1211–6.
[38] Benson NH, Maningas PA, Krohmer JR, et al. Guidelines for the prehospital use of thrombolytic agents. Ann Emerg Med 1994;23(5):1047–8.
[39] Morrison LJ, Verbeek PR, McDonald AC, et al. Mortality and prehospital thrombolysis for acute myocardial infarction: a meta-analysis. JAMA 2000;283(20):2686–92.
[40] Pedley DK, Bisset K, Connolly EM, et al. Prospective observational cohort study of time saved by prehosptial thrombolysis for ST elevation myocardial infarction delivered by paramedics. BMJ 2003;327(7405):22–6.
[41] Morrow DA, Antman EM, Sayah A, et al. Evaluation of the time saved by prehospital initiation of reteplase for ST-elevation myocardial infarction: results of the Early Retavase-Thrombolysis in Myocardial Infarction (ER-TIMI) 19 trial. J Am Coll Cardiol 2002;40(1): 71–7.
[42] Weaver WD, Simes RJ, Betriu A, et al. Comparison of primary coronary angioplasy and intravenous thrombolytic therapy for acute myocardial infarction: a quantitative review. JAMA 1997;278(23):2093–8.
[43] Asaeda G, Clair JJ, Gabriel E. Public-access defibrillation—New York City's experience. Prehosp Emerg Care 2002;6:489–91.
[44] Frank RL, Rausch MA, Menegazzi JJ, et al. The locations of non-residential out-of-hospital cardiac arrests in the City of Pittsburgh over a three-year period: implications for automated external defibrillator placement. Prehosp Emerg Care 2001;5:247–51.
[45] Jaynes CL, Blevins G, Weman HA. Evaluating interfacility ground and air transport of the critical cardiac patient. Air Med J 2002;21:37–41.
[46] Oberg KC, Kociszewski C, Dubovsky J, et al. Cardiac patient air medical transport in the northeast region of the United States. Prehosp Emerg Care 1998;2:297–303.
[47] Berns KS, Hankins DG, Zietlow SP. Comparison of air and ground transport of cardiac patients. Air Med J 2001;20:1–4.
[48] Thomas SH, Kociszewski C, Schwamm LH, et al. The evolving role of helicopter emergency services in the transfer of stroke patients to specialized centers. Prehosp Emerg Care 2002;6: 210–4.
[49] Clawson JJ, Dernocoeur K. Principles of emergency medical dispatch. 2nd edition. Salt Lake City (UT): National Academy of Emergency Medical Dispatch; 1998.

ELSEVIER
SAUNDERS

Emerg Med Clin N Am
23 (2005) 1233–1249

EMERGENCY
MEDICINE
CLINICS OF
NORTH AMERICA

Cardiovascular Emergencies in the Pediatric Patient

William A. Woods, MD[a,*],
Michael A. McCulloch, MD[b]

[a]*Departments of Emergency Medicine and Pediatrics, University of Virginia Health System, PO Box 800699, Charlottesville, VA 22908, USA*
[b]*Department of Pediatrics, University of Virginia Health System, PO Box 800386, Charlottesville, VA 22908, USA*

Children with heart disease may present to the emergency department (ED) in many stages of life. They can present with undiagnosed congenital heart disease with their disease undiagnosed, after a temporizing procedure has been performed or after definitive repair. The practicing emergency physician needs to be prepared to make the diagnosis of congenital heart disease and to recognize complications common after a surgical correction of heart disease. Children can also present at any stage of life with syncope or chest pain; therefore, emergency physicians must also be comfortable with the most common types of heart disease associated with these symptoms.

The purpose of this article is to describe the physiology and presentation of undiagnosed congenital heart disease, to describe the complications that can occur after a staged or definitive repair, and to discuss acquired heart disease in children.

Evaluation of the child who has suspected congenital heart disease

The first step in recognizing a previously undiagnosed congenital heart disease is being familiar with the common presentations. In general, patients with significant congenital heart disease present with signs and symptoms of congestive heart failure (CHF), cyanosis, or shock. Infants manifest CHF as feeding difficulty, tachypnea, fussiness, or agitation. Physical examination

* Corresponding author.
E-mail address: waw9h@virginia.edu (W.A. Woods).

doi:10.1016/j.emc.2005.07.003

may reveal a murmur, tachypnea, diaphoresis, feeding intolerance, or hepatomegaly. In this setting, any murmur, especially if present in diastole, must be addressed. If a murmer is benign, it is imperative the emergency physician seek reassurance from the primary physician or a consultant.

Central cyanosis refers to excessive dissociated hemoglobin and is classically visible in the lips and mucous membranes [1]. Data suggest that 3 to 5 g/dL of dissociated hemoglobin are necessary before central cyanosis becomes visible [2–4]. Peripheral cyanosis, by comparison, is a manifestation of poor peripheral perfusion. In this situation, a decreased flow of oxygenated blood to the periphery exists with an increased oxygen extraction at the end organs. Often the lips and mucous membranes are spared. Thus, peripheral cyanosis can occur without hypoxia. Affected children can present with central and peripheral cyanosis. This combination can be seen when children with hypoplastic left heart syndrome (HLHS) or critical coarctation of the aorta present in shock.

The second step in identifying congenital heart disease is classifying the lesion. Significant congenital heart disease can be broken down into two groups: mixing and obstructive lesions. Mixing lesions can result in a left-to-right shunt (oxygenated blood mixes with deoxygenated blood and exits the heart into the pulmonary system) as in atrial or ventricular septal defects. These patients can present with pulmonary edema, heart failure, inadequate peripheral perfusion, and peripheral cyanosis. Mixing lesions can also result in a right-to-left shunt (deoxygenated blood mixes with oxygenated blood and exits the heart into the systemic circulation) as in a teenager with pulmonary hypertension as a result of an undiagnosed atrial septal defect. Right-to-left lesions may present with central cyanosis and progress to peripheral cyanosis, as seen in children having hypercyanotic episodes ("Tet spells").

Symptomatic obstructive lesions can be a result of intracardiac obstruction (eg, valvular atresia or stenosis) or extracardiac obstruction caused by atrectic vasculature (eg, pulmonary atresia). Obstructive lesions may present after closure of the ductus arteriosis, as in coarctation of the aorta. These patients often demonstrate peripheral cyanosis signs and symptoms of CHF or shock. Severe CHF may result in hypoxia with secondary central cyanosis.

Obstructive lesions that present in the ED are typically caused by closure of the ductus arteriosis. Other forms of obstruction lesions are usually identified in the nursery. Ductal dependent lesions typically become symptomatic within the first two weeks of life; however, reports of children up to 6 weeks old presenting with HLHS or coarcation are not uncommon.

This classification scheme is not perfect. For example, the child who develops HLHS may return home from the nursery with a mixing lesion balanced to keep them asymptomatic. When the ductus arteriosis closes the infant develops an obstruction to peripheral flow. This obstruction results in peripheral cyanosis, yielding an infant in shock. Although not perfect, thinking of congenital heart disease in these terms help the treating emergency physician manage the patient until able to reach definitive care. No matter how complicated the congenital heart disease lesion, stabilizing treatment depends only on considering mixing and considering obstruction to flow; therefore, further attempts at classifying the lesions are unnecessary. Further description of cardiac lesions are not presented here. The reader is referred to standard texts [5,6] if interested and is urged to consider this classification system to deal with the lesions not listed in the standard texts, the proverbial "scrambled heart."

One lesion poorly suited for this categorization is transposition of the great vessels. Children with this condition have a mixing lesion until the ductus closes, typically within the first 3 days of life. After closure, children suddenly develop severe central cyanosis due to significantly decreased mixing between the pulmonary and systemic circulations.

The third step in identifying children with undiagnosed congenital heart disease is the diagnostic evaluation in the emergency department. The initial diagnostic evaluation is the attempt at classification done by the history and physical examination. Further workup should be done to verify this suspicion. Blood pressures in all four extremities can identify an obstructive ductal dependent lesion presenting after closure of the ductus arteriosis. Blood pressures higher in the arms than the legs suggest a lesion becoming symptomatic with closure of the ductus arteriosis. Recording oxygen saturations in pre- and postductal extremities also assists in identifying a ductal dependent lesion. If blood pressures are adequate and comparable in all four extremities but oxygen saturations are lower in the legs, then right to left shunting is occurring at the ductus arteriosus after the takeoff of the head and neck vessels. The child, thus, has an open ductus arteriosis with a right to left shunt.

Chest radiography can identify a particularly abnormal heart size or shape. Radiography can also assist with determining the degree of pulmonary blood flow. A child who has a ventricular septal defect with mixing left-to-right may have pulmonary edema present on chest radiograph. Conversely, a child who has developed a ventricular septal defect and pulmonary atresia may have central cyanosis from right-to-left mixing across the defect, and that child may have a paucity of pulmonary vascularity on chest radiograph.

Similar to adults with shortness of breath, in children it may be difficult to determine if hypoxia is caused by a pulmonary or cardiac problem. The hyperoxygenation test may assist the physician in making this distinction. Arterial oxygenation should be greater than 150 mm Hg if a child is allowed to breath 100% oxygen for 10 minutes and there is a respiratory cause for the hypoxia. Values less than 100 mm Hg suggest congenital heart disease with a mixing lesion as the cause for the hypoxia [4].

No diagnostic evaluation of the child who has suspected congenital heart disease is complete without the consideration of alternative diagnoses, such as dehydration, sepsis, intracranial hemorrhage, pneumonia, and hypoglycemia.

The final step when identifying children who have undiagnosed congenital heart disease is to initiate ED therapy. The aggressiveness of the initial therapy is determined by the classification of the lesion, the tempo of presentation, and the severity of the child's clinical condition. Mixing lesions typically present with gradual onset of symptoms, unless an associated obstructive ductal dependent lesion also exists. Left-to-right mixing lesions may worsen from supplemental oxygenation if pulmonary edema is present. The pulmonary vasculature differs from the systemic vasculature in that oxygen is a vasodilator; therefore, supplemental oxygen may cause a decrease in pulmonary artery pressure with a resultant increase in pulmonary edema and worsening central cyanosis. Alternatively, positive pressure ventilation may improve the shunt fraction. The increase in pulmonary artery pressure with positive pressure ventilation may decrease pulmonary blood flow (which is already excessive) and reduce central cyanosis (improve oxygenation).

Right-to-left lesions may improve with oxygenation. Again, oxygen decreases pulmonary vascular resistance, lessening the right-to-left shunt and improving oxygenation. Supplemental oxygen has a minimal effect on arterial oxygenation unless the shunt fraction alters because the inadequate flow of blood through the pulmonary vasculature enters the left atrium 100% saturated with oxygen. Conversely, positive pressure ventilation may increase pulmonary vascular resistance, worsening the shunt fraction and worsening arterial oxygenation. Intravenous (IV) fluid administration may be beneficial in these children and should be considered.

In the case of a hypercyanotic episode, or "tet spell," a child with the tetralogy of Fallot has an acute worsening of the right-to-left shunt after an increase in the intracardiac obstruction or decrease in systemic vascular resistance. In this case, placing the child in the knee chest position or compressing the abdominal aorta [7] increases systemic vascular resistance and may acutely decrease the right-to-left shunt.

Acute obstructive lesions presenting in the ED typically do so after closure of the ductus arteriosis. Infusion of prostaglandins may open the ductus, relieving the obstruction, and allowing the child to stabilize until they are able to reach definitive care. Complications of prostaglandin infusion include apnea, a mild decrease in systemic vascular resistance and nonpathologic hyperthermia [8,9]. Although unstudied, conventional teaching is that the risk for apnea increases with higher infusion rates. Initial infusion rate is controversial. Some clinicians prefer to start at a higher dose (0.10–0.20 μg/kg/min) and decrease the dose after the ductus reopens. Other investigators prefer to start at a lower dose (0.05 μg/kg/min) and increase the dose every 15 to 20 minutes until an effect is achieved. Although there is concern that starting prostaglandins in a child who has sepsis and not congenital heart disease, may worsen resuscitation and outcome as a result of the decrease in systemic vascular resistance, no data support or refute this concern. Careful administration of a bolus of IV fluids may be beneficial in these children.

Corrected congenital heart disease

ED care of the child who has corrected congenital heart disease has received little attention in the emergency medicine literature; however, care of these children also can follow simple principles, allowing the emergency physician a starting place until consultation can be obtained.

Once a child is diagnosed with congenital heart disease, they may be discharged home with medical management until they grow large enough, which decreases their surgical mortality risk. They may also undergo a temporizing or initial surgical repair. Finally, children undergo definitive repair. They may present to the ED with a wide variation in original anatomy in various stages of surgical repair. Fortunately for the emergency physician, a few principles apply to these repairs.

One common problem across all surgical repairs is stenosis at the extracardiac surgical anastomosis. In this situation, the child resorts to presurgical physiology because whatever repair performed to encourage flow has become stenotic, resisting additional flow. Consider, for example, a child who has had a repair of coarctation of the aorta. If stenosis develops at the anastomosis, the child presents with symptoms of an obstructive lesion. Peripheral cyanosis in the lower extremities with decreased pulses results. Another example is the child who had a Blalock-Taussig shunt placed after diagnosis with tricuspid valve atresia with an associated hypoplastic right ventricle and pulmonary artery stenosis. Blood exits the right atrium directly into the left atrium. A Blalock-Taussig shunt is typically a gortex graft from the right subclavian artery to the right pulmonary artery. This shunt is a temporizing procedure, which creates a left-to-right shunt, allowing adequate mixing until the child grows. If stenosis develops at the anastomosis, the child may develop lessening pulmonary blood flow (which may be visible with comparison chest radiographs) with an increase in central cyanosis. The result is the child's preoperative physiology.

Another common complication in postsurgical patients is arrhythmias. Practically all patients that have undergone surgery for congenital heart disease are at increased risk for sudden death from a presumed ventricular arrhythmia. Those procedures that do not increase the risk for sudden death are an atrial septal defect repair and patent ductus arteriosis ligation. Box 1 provides a list of common procedures associated with an increased risk for sudden death. No child who has undergone these procedures should be discharged from the ED after presentation with syncope or palpitations unless thoroughly discussed with the child's cardiologist.

Box 1. Corrected congenital heart disease lesions associated with sudden death

High Risk
Tetralogy of Fallot
Aortic stenosis
Transposition of the great arteries
Coarctation of the aorta
Atrioventricular septal defect
Pulmonary stenosis
Anomalies that undergo the Fontan procedure

Low Risk
Ventricular septal defect

Because of the increased atrial pressures present before and sometimes after surgery, many of these patients are also at increased risk for atrial arrhythmias. Arrhythmias can also arise from the cardiac chamber manipulated during surgery. For example, a suture in the ventricular septal defect repair can be a focus of ventricular arrhythmia.

The final group of complications includes those specific to a particular surgical repair. The Fontan repair is the procedure with the longest list of serious complications. The Fontan (Fig. 1) is typically performed in the case of single ventricle physiology. The most effective ventricle becomes the systemic ventricle, whereas the superior and inferior vena cava drain directly into the right pulmonary artery. Box 2 contains a list of the most common complications of a Fontan procedure presenting after discharge from the hospital. Thromboembolism can occur in the pulmonary or systemic circulation. Thrombotic complications occurred in 25% of patients within 4 years after surgery in one study [10]. Twenty-five percent of these thrombi were in the systemic arterial circulation, whereas 75% were in the pulmonary circulation [10]. Many of the complications arise from the persistent increased central venous pressure that develops to drive pulmonary blood flow [11,12]. If a fenestrated Fontan is performed, a "pop-off valve" exists between the inferior vena cava and the right atrium. Because of the fenestration, it is possible for these children to develop cyanosis with a significant right to left shunt across the fenestration.

The Blalock-Taussig shunt is a temporizing procedure whereby the right subclavian artery is anastomosed to the right main pulmonary artery. In addition to the risks for stenosis at the anastomosis, these shunts may thrombos when a child is dehydrated. Additionally, the ipsilateral vertebral artery may have been intentionally ligated to prevent a basilar steal phenomenon. The long-term risks of this ligation are unknown.

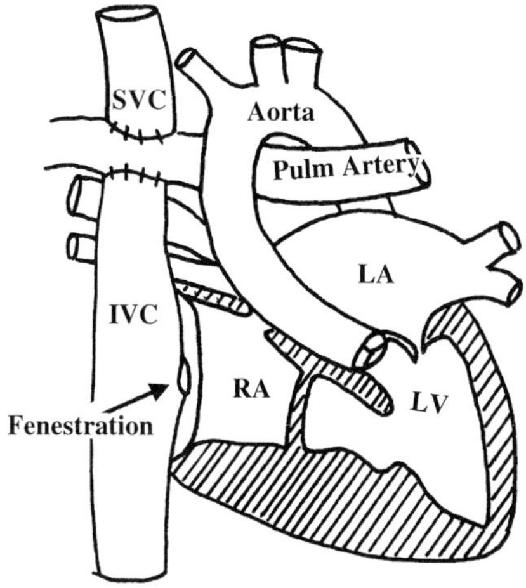

Fig. 1. Fenestrated Fontan in repair of tricuspic atresia with resultant hypoplastic right ventricle. Inferior vena cava and superior vena cava drain into right pulmonary artery. Fenestration into the right atrium from the inferior vena cava.

Surgical repair of coarctation of the aorta carries another set of postoperative risks. One recent series details the complications of 383 patients available for follow-up of 580 patients who had repair. Aneurysmal dilation at the sight of the coarctation occurred in 2% of patients. Two patients had massive hemoptysis from an aortobronchial fistula. Intracardiac stenosis requiring surgery occurred in three patients, and one patient had a rupture of a sinus of Valsalva aneurysm [13].

Heart transplantation

Children presenting to the ED after orthotopic heart transplantation have complications that differ from other children who have corrected

Box 2. Complications that may occur after a Fontan procedure

Thromboembolism
Thrombosis
Increased central venous pressure
Ascites
Pulmonary effusion
Pericardial effusion
Protein-losing enteropathy
Atrial arrhythmia
Sudden death

congenital heart disease and require separate attention. These children may present to the ED with an invasive infection, acute/chronic rejection or with posttransplant lymphoproliferative disorder.

Infectious complications in transplant recipients may be caused by viral, bacterial, protozoan, or fungal infections. Most bacterial infections occur within the first month after transplant. Viral infections predominate over the following month. Throughout the life of the transplant recipient, an increasing risk for protozoan or fungal infections exists [14].

In a review of 74 outpatient febrile episodes in 22 pediatric heart transplant patients, 22 of 74 (30%) were considered serious and required inpatient therapy [15]. Three episodes were pneumonia, two were caused by cytomegalovirus (CMV) infections, and two were caused by streptococcic infection. One child in the series died.

No data are available to reassure the emergency physician that clinical presentation or acute laboratory evaluation can exclude the presence of bacterial illness in the transplanted patient who has an acute illness. In a small series, pneumococcal bacteremia occurred in 9 of 80 patients (11%) at 3 to 48 months posttransplant [16]. Of those 9 children, 3 had pneumonia, 2 presented with otitis media, and 1 child had petechiae and purpura. Most of these children, but not all, had a temperature higher than 101°F at presentation.

Pneumocystis carinii pneumonia (PCP) can present with symptom durations from 1 to 2 days to 2 weeks [17]. In this small series, all 10 patients had tachypnea and room air oxygen saturations less than 95%.

CMV is a recognized cause of morbidity in the transplant recipient [18]. CMV infections can present as a mononucleosis-type syndrome, an interstitial pneumonitis, a hepatitis, or as a gastrointestinal disease. The symptoms are typically nonspecific and include headache, myalgias, abdominal pain, and diarrhea. CMV-mononucleosis differs from Epstein-Barr Virus (EBV) mononucleosis because it does not include pharyngitis, tonsillitis, or splenomegaly.

Acute rejection has been defined as the clinical decision to intensify immunosuppression in association with histopathology or dysfunction [19]. The distinction between acute and chronic rejection does not refer to the time of onset after transplantation. Acute rejection is a more fulminant process than chronic rejection. Children may be asymptomatic or present in cardiogenic shock. Common symptoms include fever, myalgias and vomiting. Chest pain may occur, but is uncommon. The electrocardiogram may show a decreased R wave amplitude and an increased QRS duration; however, these findings are not sensitive. Laboratory findings are not helpful. There is no data to suggest that cardiac enzymes are reliably elevated with acute rejection. Elevated hepatic transaminases, although nonspecific for acute rejection, always suggest an invasive complication in the transplant recipient.

Chronic rejection differs microscopically from acute rejection. The clinical manifestation of chronic rejection is accelerated atherosclerosis.

Symptoms are caused by ischemia or infarction and usually include decreased exercise tolerance or malaise. Patients may also present after syncope or sudden death. As with acute rejection, no specific laboratory, or ECG findings exist to secure this diagnosis.

Posttransplant lymphoproliferative disorder (PTLD) is typically a B-cell lymphoma associated with transplant patients [20,21]. The cause is most likely a result of EBV. Presenting symptoms include fever, malaise, a mononucleosis-type syndrome, palpable lymphadenopathy, or mass effect from tumor location. The most common location of the masses are (in descending order): abdomen, thorax, head and neck, and brain [21]. Abdominal PTLD may present with abdominal pain, hepatomegaly, splenomegaly, an abdominal mass, gastrointestinal bleeding, anemia, intussusception, diarrhea, or a protein-wasting enteropathy [21].

In caring for the transplant recipient with an acute illness, the emergency physician should perform several steps. A careful history allows the treating physician to identify a clinical syndrome consistent with a self-limited or more aggressive illness. Noncompliance with the immunosuppressive regimen and PCP prophylaxis increases the risk for acute rejection [22] or acute PCP infection [17]. After a careful physical examination, a chest radiograph and ECG should be obtained in all children who experience an unclear symptom complex. A comparison ECG is necessary because changes including right bundle branch block, left atrial enlargement, and right ventricular hypertrophy are not associated with clinical deterioration [23]. Laboratory studies should include a complete blood count with differential, serum electrolytes, hepatic transaminases, and blood cultures.

The admission recommendations are unclear for children who develop an obvious etiology for their symptoms. The emergency physician should consider admission for any child who experiences a significant fever or fever history. Children with vomiting without a history clearly suggestive of acute viral gastroenteritis are also a concern. Dehydration should be treated more aggressively in transplant recipients because of the nephrotoxicity of their immunosuppressive regimens.

Infective endocarditis

Infective endocarditis refers to a condition in which an organism infects the valves, endocardium, or other cardiac structures. The term acute bacterial endocarditis refers to a fulminant illness whereby death can occur within weeks. Subacute bacterial endocarditis refers to an indolent course evolving over months. The most common bacterial causes of infective endocarditis are *Staphylococcus aureus*, *Streptococcus pyogenes* and *Streptococcus viridans*. The most common symptoms in patients who have infective endocarditis are fever, malaise, chest and abdominal symptoms, and arthralgias. Physical findings may include embolic events, a changing or new murmur, splenomegaly, and petechiae. The classically described findings of

Roth spots, Osler's nodes, Janeway lesions, and splinter hemorrhages are uncommon. The most common laboratory abnormalities in patients who have infective endocarditis are elevated erythrocyte sedimentation rate (ESR), anemia, hematuria, and positive blood cultures.

Children who have congenital heart disease are at an increased risk for bacterial endocarditis. Surgical manipulations of the aortic valve or aorta are the highest risk anomalies. Surgically corrected septal defects or right-sided lesions are at a low risk. The cause of the initial bacteremia leading to endocarditis is frequently unknown. In the most comprehensive series available, a precipitating event could be identified in only 87 of 214 cases of endocarditis in patients who had congenital heart disease [24]. Of these 87, 42 cases were associated with dental procedures and 10 were associated with skin infections. Interestingly, patients received appropriate endocarditis prophylaxis in one half of the cases occurring after dental procedure [24].

The extensive series by Li and Somerville [24] does not list any cases of bacterial endocarditis occurring after traumatic injury. Current recommendations do not suggest endocarditis prophylaxis for cases of traumatic injury [25,26]. Investigators state that prophylaxis is not indicated for urethral catheterization without infection or for endotracheal intubation [25,26]; however, one investigator recommends prophylaxis for urethral catheterization in the face of a urinary tract infection [26].

Endocarditis prophylaxis is indicated for all patients with congenital heart disease. Prophylaxis is not indicated for patients at least 6 months from a surgically repaired ventricular septal defect or patent ductus arteriosis without residual defect. Patients with an isolated atrial septal defect do not require prophylaxis before repair or 6 months after complete repair [25,26]. Box 3 details the current dosing regimen recommended by the American Heart Association for infective endocarditis prophylaxis.

Arrhythmias or congestive heart failure in children

Not all cardiac causes of acute illness in children are a result of congenital heart disease. Children may present to the ED with syncope, palpitations, chest pain, or shortness of breath. The following section describes the most common pathologic cardiac conditions that may result in ED presentation. Before starting though, it is necessary to have an understanding of the normal age-related progression of the pediatric ECG.

Normal changes in the pediatric ECG

The pediatric ECG is an evolving process, changing on a nearly weekly basis as pulmonary vascular resistance (PVR) decreases, left ventricular (LV) mass increases relative to right ventricular mass (RV), and various other changes occur in the developing cardiovascular system. Though the basic premises are unchanged, physicians must be familiar with these age-

Box 3. Endocarditis prophylaxis recommendations

Dental, oral, respiratory tract, or esophageal procedures
Give 1 hour before procedure:
Amoxicillin (50 mg/kg with a maximum of 2.0 g) by mouth.
No follow-up dose recommended.

Genitourinary or gastrointestinal procedures in high risk patients
Give within 30 minutes of starting procedure:
Ampicillin (50 mg/kg with a maximum of 2.0 g) and
Gentamicin (1.5 mg/kg not to exceed 120 mg) IV.
Give 6 hours after the procedure:
Ampicillin or amoxicillin (25 mg/kg with a maximum of 1.0 g).

For more information see: Committee on Rheumatic Fever, Endocarditis, and Kawasaki Disease. Prevention of bacterial endocarditis: recommendations by the American Heart Association. JAMA 1997;277:1794–1801; Circulation 1997;96:358–66; JADA 1997;128:1142–50.

related variations associated with pediatric ECG to correctly interpret its data. This discussion focuses on this and anatomic variations specific to the pediatric population from birth to 2 months of age to help physicians accurately detect anomalies during this critical period.

Most of the age-related variations demonstrated in the pediatric ECG are because of the changes in the ratio of LV to RV mass. As PVR continues to decrease relative to systemic vascular resistance (SVR), RV dominance rapidly wanes from an LV/RV ratio of 0.8 to 1.5 by 1 month of age. Concurrent with these changes is a gradual decrease in the severity of the right QRS axis deviation. The precordial R/S ratios also change, increasing and decreasing in the left and right precordial leads, respectively. As a point of reference, the newborn ECG may demonstrate a complete reversal of the adult R/S progression, but by 1 month of age, the R/S ratio is typically greater than 1 in V6 and between 1–6 months of age, the R/S ratio in V2 also approaches 1. During this last age range, it is not uncommon to erroneously suspect bilateral ventricular hypertrophy based on the large precordial QRS deflections.

T waves are typically dynamic during the first week of life. At birth the T waves are upright in V1 and V6 with the vector anterior and to the left. Within a few days the vector changes rightward leaving flattened or inverted T waves laterally. By the end of the first week of life, the T wave axis changes posterior and leftward, producing inverted T waves in lead V1 and upright T waves in lead V6. The inverted T wave in V1 may not turn upright until late adolescence.

Supraventricular tachycardia

Pediatric arrhythmias in the first 2 months are rare but can become hemodynamically significant. The most commonly experienced arrhythmia in this age group is supraventricular tachycardia (SVT), generally producing narrow complex heart rates greater than 240 beats per minute. At these rates, P waves (if present) are often buried in the preceding T waves making it difficult to differentiate an atrial from a nodal focus. SVT is not, however, always associated with a heart rate greater than 240. An inappropriately elevated heart rate in an otherwise calm or sleeping infant is SVT until proven otherwise. Any infant found to have an initial episode of SVT should be thoroughly evaluated by a pediatric cardiologist to rule out problems, such as SVT-induced CHF, anatomic anomalies (ie, Ebstein's anomaly), or a reentrant/aberrant pathway as with Wolff-Parkinson-White (WPW) syndrome. The prognosis for infants with SVT is excellent with 60% to 90% of patients experiencing complete remission of symptoms by 6 to 12 months of age.

Wolff-Parkinson-White syndrome

WPW syndrome is associated with ventricular pre-excitation by way of an accessory pathway between the atria and ventricles. These accessory pathways do not demonstrate the obligatory pause as seen in the atrioventricular node. As a result, ventricular pre-excitation is responsible for the short PR interval and delta waves frequently detected on ECG.

WPW typically occurs spontaneously; however, familial clusters have been described. Pre-excitation can be intermittent, making true prevalence in the population difficult to define. WPW frequently coincides with congenital cardiac abnormalities, including Ebstein's anomaly, hypertrophic cardiomyopathy, and atrial septal defects.

The WPW syndrome refers to a patient with symptoms of tachyarrhythmias in the face of ECG evidence of pre-excitation. Three ECG features are described: (1) short PR interval (<0.12 seconds), (2) a prolonged QRS duration (>0.12 seconds), and (3) a delta wave or a slow gradual upslope leading into the QRS complex. The degree of pre-excitation detected on the ECG depends on the relative conduction times between the atrioventricular node and the accessory pathway. Measures to slow conduction through the atrioventricular node may make an accessory pathway more prominent. Described methods include Valsalva or vagal maneuvers and adenosine therapy.

Not all patients with ECG evidence of pre-excitation are symptomatic. Most of those with symptoms are limited to chest discomfort, dizziness, syncope, or shortness of breath [27]. The most common arrhythmias in this population are atrial fibrillation and orthodromic reciprocating tachycardia. Orthodromic reciprocating tachycardia is a type of paroxysmal supraventricular tachycardia that allows antegrade conduction down the atrioventricular node and retrograde conduction in the accessory pathway. Episodes of the less common antidromic tachycardia place the patient at higher risk for ventricular fibrillation [28].

Although atrial fibrillation is common in patients who have WPW, its occurrence in the presence of rapid conduction across an accessory pathway may predispose a patient to ventricular fibrillation [29,30]. Medications that slow conduction across the atrioventricular node should not be used in patients who develop atrial fibrillation and WPW syndrome. Agents, such as digoxin, calcium channel blockers, beta-blockers, and adenosine, may increase the risk for ventricular fibrillation. Procainamide or amiodarone are drugs of choice for rate control in this situation.

Anomalous coronary artery

Anomalous origin of a coronary artery, although a rare form of congenital heart disease, can cause myocardial ischemia in the infant or syncope in the young adult. Many types of congenital coronary artery abnormalities are described [31]; however, the two most common variations that cause symptoms are discussed here.

The left main coronary artery may arise from the pulmonary artery. This rare lesion occurs in 1 of 300,000 children [32]. Infants with this anomaly present after infarction or with angina. Children with angina may be diagnosed with colic due to inconsolable crying, especially after feeding. In Mahle's series [33], the most common finding in the 11 children identified were cardiomegaly on chest radiography and ischemia on ECG [32]. The classic ECG finding are deep Q waves in leads I and aVL with poor R-wave progression across the precordium [31].

If the left coronary artery originates from within the right coronary sinus or from the right coronary artery, syncope and sudden death may occur in adolescence. Syncope and sudden death are most common if the left coronary artery courses between the pulmonary artery and aorta. Left coronary artery blood flow may be asymptomatic until, classically, flow is impaired by external compression from the aorta and pulmonary artery leading to ischemia, arrhythmia, or sudden death. This occurs during exertion when cardiac output increases causing a mild dilation in diameter of the aortic and pulmonary artery roots. Detection of this lesion requires diagnosis of acute ischemia or clinical suspicion confirmed by echocardiography or catheterization.

Kawasaki Disease

Kawasaki Disease (KD), formerly described as mucocutaneous lymph node syndrome, was originally defined by Kawasaki in a series of 50 cases in 1967 [34]. KD is an acute febrile syndrome of childhood of uncertain etiology that is also the leading cause of acquired heart disease and myocardial infarction (MI) in children in the United States. Eighty percent of all cases occur in children less than 5 years old. KD is rare in infants less than 4 months old and in adults.

Diagnostic criteria for KD include fever of at least 5 days, and four of the following five findings: (1) nonpurulent bilateral bulbar conjunctivitis, (2) polymorphous exanthema, (3) cervical lymphadenopathy, (4) involvement of the extremities, and (5) changes in the lips and oral cavity (injected pharynx or lips, fissured lips or strawberry tongue). The polymorphous rash is typically truncal without vesicles. Lymph nodes must be at least 1.5 cm in diameter. Extremity involvement includes edema and erythema of the hands and feet followed by periungual desquamation. Other findings in children who have Kawasaki Disease may include extreme irritability, arthritis, gallbladder hydrops, mild hepatitis, uveitis, urethritis, aseptic meningitis, or myocarditis. Laboratory abnormalities may include thrombocytosis (usually in the second and third weeks of illness), elevated sedimentation rate, sterile pyuria, and proteinuria. At its peak, the platelet count may exceed 1,000,000. ECG changes that may be detected during the acute phase include PR prolongation, corrected QT prolongation, and T-wave flattening.

Children may have symptoms of myocarditis or pericarditis during the acute phase; this is typically self-limited. Aneurysms of the coronary arteries may develop during the second and third weeks of illness. Those with aneurysms may suffer acute MI. While occurring in less than 3% of patients, MI typically occurs within 1 year of onset of symptoms and frequently within 3 months of onset of symptoms. MIs may be silent, or the child may present with abdominal pain, vomiting, or crying.

Treatment in the acute phase of Kawasaki Disease in the ED is supportive. Intravenous fluids are typically required because the children have had poor oral intake with increased insensible losses. Aspirin therapy and intravenous gamma-globulin have been shown to decrease complication rates; however, these therapies would not typically be started without appropriate consultation.

Myocarditis

Myocarditis refers to an inflammatory disease of the myocardium that is not caused by acute ischemia. Myocarditis, then, is a clinico-pathologic diagnosis, which does not refer to a specific etiology. While most myocarditis in the United States is viral, the cause can be bacterial, rickettsial, protozoal, parasitic, fungal, autoimmune or pharmacologic [35,36]. Coxsackie B virus, an enterovirus, and adenovirus are the most common viral causes of myocarditis. While newborns are particularly susceptible to coxsackie B myocarditis, all ages are at risk. Presenting symptoms include fever, poor appetite, irritability, sudden death, diaphoresis, pallor, and congestive heart failure. Older children may not present until dilated cardiomyopathy is already present. Older patients are more likely to present with a gradual onset of congestive heart failure, or atrial or ventricular arrhythmias.

The electrocardiogram may demonstrate sinus tachycardia, low-voltage QRS complexes, and inverted or low-voltage T waves. Wide Q waves and ST-segment changes may also be apparent. The chest radiograph typically shows a dilated heart and pulmonary edema. Treatment is supportive until the child can be transferred to a center whereby aggressive diagnostic evaluation and therapy can be performed.

Hypertrophic cardiomyopathy

Hypertrophic cardiomyopathy, in this section, refers to the idiopathic condition sometimes referred to as idiopathic hypertrophic subaortic stenosis or familial hypertrophic subaortic stenosis. Hypertrophic cardiomyopathy can also be a descriptive diagnosis that includes cardiac conditions secondary to obstructive congenital heart disease (aortic stenosis) or an inborn error of metabolism (glycogen storage disease).

The left ventricular hypertrophy in hypertrophic cardiomyopathy is variably asymmetric and, at the cellular level, myocardial cells are organized in a bizarre fashion. Commonly, this condition is a result of mutations in the cardiac myosin heavy-chain gene. A familial component commonly exists to this disorder.

Clinical manifestations are typically caused by obstruction of flow or arrhythmias. The disorganized contraction of the hypertrophic section of ventricle results in subaortic outflow obstruction during systole. The increased ventricular pressure required to overcome this obstruction results in increased myocardial-wall stress and oxygen demand. Arrhythmias may result from this ischemia or may result from the arrhythmogenic foci of the bizarrely arranged myocardial fibers.

Physical examination of the child who has developed hypertrophic cardiomyopathy may reveal a systolic murmur exacerbated by a Valsalva maneuver or by standing. The murmur is best detected at the left lower sternal boarder or at the apex. A prominent left ventricular lift may exist on palpation. ECG frequently reveals left ventricular hypertrophy and ST-segment and T-wave changes. Chest radiograph is typically normal. Treatment at presentation is limited to supportive therapy for the patient's clinical condition. Consultation is necessary even in children who experience only mild symptoms.

Summary

Although the myriad of congenital heart lesions and their surgical repairs can seem overwhelming, ED evaluation and care of children who experience these conditions requires the practitioner to understand a few principles. A solid understanding of the physiology of cyanosis helps the clinician determine the appropriate diagnostic studies and interpret the results. Remembering common patterns of postsurgical complications allows the physician to initiate treatment in the child who has surgically corrected congenital heart disease, even if the family cannot relate the surgical history to the physician. Finally, reviewing the common pathologic cardiac causes of CHF and syncope should allow the physician to appropriately exclude a pathologic cause of syncope or palpitations in a child.

References

[1] Lees MH. Cyanosis of the newborn infant. J Pediatr 1970;77:484–98.
[2] Goss GA, Hayes JA, Burdon JG. Deoxyhaemoglobin concentratins in the detection of central cyanosis. Thorax 1988;43:212–3.
[3] Martin L, Khalil H. How much reduced hemoglobin is necessary to generate central cyanosis. Chest 1990;97:182–5.
[4] Yabek SM. Neonatal cyanosis: reappraisal of the response to 100% oxygen breathing. Am J Dis Child 1984;138:880–4.
[5] Garson A, Bricker JT, Fisher DJ, et al, editors. The science and practice of pediatric cardiology. 2nd edition. Baltimore (MD): Williams & Wilkins; 1998.
[6] Allen HD, Gutgesell HP, Clark EB, et al, editors. Moss and Adams' heart disease in infants, children, and adolescents: including the fetus and young adult. 6th edition. Baltimore (MD): Lippincott, Williams & Wilkins; 2001.
[7] Baele PL, Rennottee MTE, Veyckemans FA. External compression of the abdominal aortareversing tetralogy of Fallot cyanotic crisis. Anesthesiology 1991;75:146–9.
[8] Saxena A, Shara M, Kothari SS, et al. Prostaglandin E1 in infants with congenital heart disease: Indian experience. Indian Pediatr 1998;35:1063–9.
[9] Lewis AB, Free MD, Heymann MA, et al. Side effects of therapy with prostaglandin E1 in infants with critical congenital heart disease. Circulation 1981;64:893–8.
[10] Jahangiri M, Ross DB, Redington AN, et al. Thromboembolism after the Fontan procedure and its modifications. Ann Thorac Surg 1994;58:1409–14.
[11] Somerville J. The complex lesions: problems in the adult survivors. Schweiz Med Wochenschr 1993;123:2060–4.
[12] Kaulitz R, Luhmer I, Bergmann F, et al. Sequelae after modified Fontan operation: postoperative haemodynamic data and organ function. Heart 1997;78:154–9.
[13] Manganas C, Iliopoulos J, Chard RB, et al. Reoperation and coarctation of the aorta in children. Ann Thorac Surg 2001;72:1222–4.
[14] Schowengerdt KO, Naftel DC, Seib PM, et al. Infection after pediatric heart transplantation: results of a multi-institutional study. J Heart Lung Transplant 1997;16:1207–16.
[15] Crandall WV, Norlin C, Bullock EA, et al. Etiology and outcome of outpatient fevers in pediatric heart transplant patients. Clin Pediatr (Phila) 1996;35:437–42.
[16] Stovall SH, Ainley KA, Mason EO, et al. Invasive pneumococcal infections in pediatric cardiac transplant patients. Pediatr Infect Dis J 2001;20:946–50.
[17] Janner D, Bork J, Baum M, et al. Pneumocystis carinii pneumonia in infants after heart transplantation. J Heart Lung Transplant 1996;15:758–63.
[18] Green M, Wald ER, Fricker FJ, et al. Infections in pediatric orthotopic heart transplant recipients. Pediatr Infect Dis J 1989;8:87–93.
[19] Boucek RJ, Boucek MM. Pediatric heart transplantation. Curr Opin Pediatr 2002;14:611–9.
[20] Holmes RD, Sokol RJ. Epstein-Barr virus and post-transplant lymphoproliferative disease. Pediatr Transplant 2002;6:456–64.

[21] Pickhardt PJ, Siegel MJ, Hayashi RJ, et al. Posttransplantation lymphoproliferative disorder in children: clinical, histopathologic, and imaging features. Radiology 2000;217: 16–25.

[22] Chartrand C, Servando ES, Chartrand S. Risk factors for acute rejections after pediatric heart transplantation. Transplant Proc 2001;33:1732–4.

[23] Shreve MR, Crosson JE, Eusebio EJ, et al. Electrocardiographic changes during long-term follow-up of pediatric heart transplant recipients. Am J Cardiol 1993;71:1253–6.

[24] Li W, Somerville J. Infective endocarditis in the grown-up congenital heart (GUCH) population. Eur Heart J 1998;19:166–73.

[25] Dajani AS, Taubert KA, Wilson W, et al. Prevention of bacterial endocarditis: recommendations by the American Heart Association. JAMA 1997;277:1794–801.

[26] Durack DT. Prevention of infective endocarditis. N Engl J Med 1995;332:38–44.

[27] Munger TM, Packer DL, Hammill SC, et al. A population study of the natural history of Wolff-Parkinson-White syndrome in Olmsted County, Minnesota, 1953–1989. Circulation 1993;87:866–73.

[28] Al-Khatib SM, Pritchett ELC. Clinical features of Wolff-Parkinson-White syndrome. Am Heart J 1999;138:403–13.

[29] Prystowsky EN, Fananapazir L, Packer DL, et al. Wolff-Parkinson-White syndrome and sudden cardiac death. Cardiology 1987;74(Suppl 2):67–71.

[30] Dreifus LS, Haiat R, Watanabe Y, et al. Ventricular fibrillation: a possible mechanism of sudden death in patients with Wolff-Parkinson-White syndrome. Circulation 1971;43: 520–7.

[31] Herlong JR. Congenital coronary artery anomalies. In: Garson A, Bricker JT, Fisher DJ, et al, editors. The science and practice of pediatric cardiology. 2nd edition. Baltimore (MD): Williams & Wilkins; 1998. p. 1647–66.

[32] Keith JD. Anomalous origin of the left coronary artery from the pulmonary artery. Br Heart J 1959;21:149–61.

[33] Mahle WT. A dangerous case of colic: anomalous left coronary artery presenting with paroxysms of irritability. Ped Em Care 1998;14:24–7.

[34] Kawasaki T, Kousaki F. Febrile oculo-oro-cutaneo-acrodesquamatous syndrome with or without acuter nonsuppurative cervical lymphadenitis in infancy and children: clinical observations of 50 cases. Jpn J Allergol 1967;16:178.

[35] Friedman RA, Schowengerdt KO, Towbin JA. Myocarditis. In: Garson A, Bricker JT, Fisher DJ, et al, editors. The science and practice of pediatric cardiology. 2nd edition. Baltimore (MD): Williams & Wilkins; 1998. p. 1777–94.

[36] Towbin JA. Myocarditis. In: Allen HD, Gutgesell HP, Clark EB, et al, editors. Moss and Adams' heart disease in infants, children, and adolescents: including the fetus and young adult. 6th edition. Baltimore (MD): Lippincott, Williams & Wilkins; 2001. p. 1197–215.

EMERGENCY MEDICINE CLINICS OF NORTH AMERICA

ELSEVIER SAUNDERS

Emerg Med Clin N Am 23 (2005) 1251–1271

Cumulative Index 2005

Note: Page numbers of article titles are in **boldface** type.

A

0733-8627/05/$ - see front matter
doi:10.1016/S0733-8627(05)00097-0

D

E

N

O

Q

R

S

T

United States Postal Service

Statement of Ownership, Management, and Circulation

1. Publication Title	2. Publication Number	3. Filing Date
Emergency Medicine Clinics of North America	0 7 3 3 - 8 6 2 7	9/15/05
4. Issue Frequency	5. Number of Issues Published Annually	6. Annual Subscription Price
Feb, May, Aug, Nov	4	$170.00

7. Complete Mailing Address of Known Office of Publication (*Not printer*) (*Street, city, county, state, and ZIP+4*)

Elsevier Inc.
6277 Sea Harbor Drive
Orlando, FL 32887-4800

Contact Person: Gwen C. Campbell
Telephone: 215-239-3685

8. Complete Mailing Address of Headquarters or General Business Office of Publisher (*Not printer*)

Elsevier Inc., 360 Park Avenue South, New York, NY 10010-1710

9. Full Names and Complete Mailing Addresses of Publisher, Editor, and Managing Editor (*Do not leave blank*)

Publisher (*Name and complete mailing address*)

Tim Griswold, Elsevier Inc., 1600 John F. Kennedy Blvd., Suite 1800, Philadelphia, PA 19103-2899

Editor (*Name and complete mailing address*)

Karen Sorensen, Elsevier Inc., 1600 John F. Kennedy Blvd., Suite 1800, Philadelphia, PA 19103-2899

Managing Editor (*Name and complete mailing address*)

Heather Cullen, Elsevier Inc., 1600 John F. Kennedy Blvd., Suite 1800, Philadelphia, PA 19103-2899

10. Owner (*Do not leave blank. If the publication is owned by a corporation, give the name and address of the corporation immediately followed by the names and addresses of all stockholders owning or holding 1 percent or more of the total amount of stock. If not owned by a corporation, give the names and addresses of the individual owners. If owned by a partnership or other unincorporated firm, give its name and address as well as those of each individual owner. If the publication is published by a nonprofit organization, give its name and address.*)

Full Name	Complete Mailing Address
Wholly owned subsidiary of	4520 East-West Highway
Reed/Elsevier Inc., US Holdings	Bethesda, MD 20814

11. Known Bondholders, Mortgagees, and Other Security Holders Owning or Holding 1 Percent or More of Total Amount of Bonds, Mortgages, or Other Securities. If none, check box → ☐ None

Full Name	Complete Mailing Address
N/A	

12. Tax Status (*For completion by nonprofit organizations authorized to mail at nonprofit rates*) (*Check one*)
The purpose, function, and nonprofit status of this organization and the exempt status for federal income tax purposes:
☐ Has Not Changed During Preceding 12 Months
☐ Has Changed During Preceding 12 Months (*Publisher must submit explanation of change with this statement*)

(*See Instructions on Reverse*)

PS Form **3526**, October 1999

13. Publication Title: Emergency Medicine Clinics of North America

14. Issue Date for Circulation Data Below: August 2005

15. Extent and Nature of Circulation		Average No. Copies Each Issue During Preceding 12 Months	No. Copies of Single Issue Published Nearest to Filing Date
a. Total Number of Copies (*Net press run*)		3225	3000
b. Paid and/or Requested Circulation	(1) Paid/Requested Outside-County Mail Subscriptions Stated on Form 3541. (*Include advertiser's proof and exchange copies*)	2034	1952
	(2) Paid In-County Subscriptions Stated on Form 3541 (*Include advertiser's proof and exchange copies*)		
	(3) Sales Through Dealers and Carriers, Street Vendors, Counter Sales, and Other Non-USPS Paid Distribution	365	386
	(4) Other Classes Mailed Through the USPS		
c. Total Paid and/or Requested Circulation [*Sum of 15b. (1), (2), (3), and (4)*] →		2399	2338
d. Free Distribution by Mail (*Samples, compliment-ary, and other free*)	(1) Outside-County as Stated on Form 3541	120	103
	(2) In-County as Stated on Form 3541		
	(3) Other Classes Mailed Through the USPS		
e. Free Distribution Outside the Mail (*Carriers or other means*)			
f. Total Free Distribution (*Sum of 15d. and 15e.*) →		102	103
g. Total Distribution (*Sum of 15c. and 15f.*) →		2501	2441
h. Copies not Distributed		724	559
i. Total (*Sum of 15g. and h.*) →		3225	3000
j. Percent Paid and/or Requested Circulation (*15c. divided by 15g. times 100*)		96%	96%

16. Publication of Statement of Ownership
☐ Publication required. Will be printed in the **November 2005** issue of this publication. ☐ Publication not required

17. Signature and Title of Editor, Publisher, Business Manager, or Owner

Jean Fanucci – Executive Director of Subscription Services — Date: 9/15/05

I certify that all information furnished on this form is true and complete. I understand that anyone who furnishes false or misleading information on this form or who omits material or information requested on the form may be subject to criminal sanctions (including fines and imprisonment) and/or civil sanctions (including civil penalties).

Instructions to Publishers

1. Complete and file one copy of this form with your postmaster annually on or before October 1. Keep a copy of the completed form for your records.
2. In cases where the stockholder or security holder is a trustee, include in items 10 and 11 the name of the person or corporation for whom the trustee is acting. Also include the names and addresses of individuals who are stockholders who own or hold 1 percent or more of the total amount of bonds, mortgages, or other securities of the publishing corporation. In item 11, if none, check the box. Use blank sheets if more space is required.
3. Be sure to furnish all circulation information called for in item 15. Free circulation must be shown in items 15d, e, and f.
4. Item 15h., Copies not Distributed, must include (1) newsstand copies originally stated on Form 3541, and returned to the publisher, (2) estimated returns from news agents, and (3), copies for office use, leftovers, spoiled, and all other copies not distributed.
5. If the publication had Periodicals authorization as a general or requester publication, this Statement of Ownership , Management, and Circulation must be published; it must be printed in any issue in October or, if the publication is not published during October, the first issue printed after October.
6. In item 16, indicate the date of the issue in which this Statement of Ownership will be published.
7. Item 17 must be signed.

Failure to file or publish a statement of ownership may lead to suspension of Periodicals authorization.

PS Form **3526**, October 1999 (*Reverse*)

Changing Your Address?

Make sure your subscription changes too! When you notify us of your new address, you can help make our job easier by including an exact copy of your Clinics label number with your old address (see illustration below.) This number identifies you to our computer system and will speed the processing of your address change. Please be sure this label number accompanies your old address and your corrected address—you can send an old Clinics label with your number on it or just copy it exactly and send it to the address listed below.

We appreciate your help in our attempt to give you continuous coverage. Thank you.

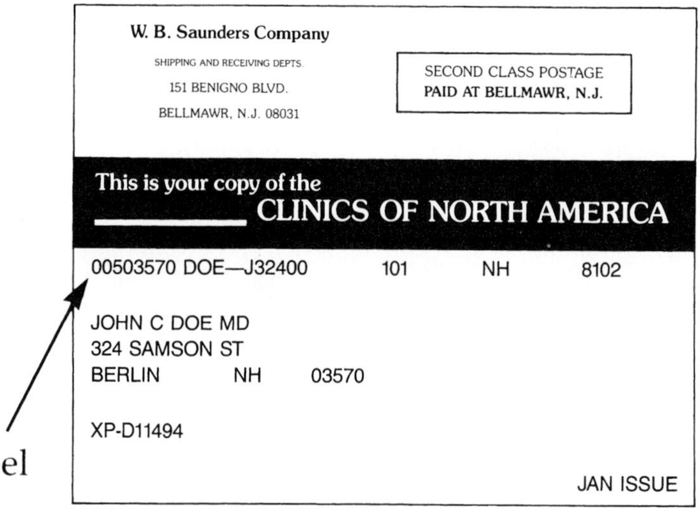

Your Clinics Label Number

Copy it exactly or send your label along with your address to:
W.B. Saunders Company, Customer Service
Orlando, FL 32887-4800
Call Toll Free 1-800-654-2452

Please allow four to six weeks for delivery of new subscriptions and for processing address changes.